D0077159

## DATE DUE

**Unless Recalled Earlier**

| | | |
|---|---|---|
| FEB 13 1993 | | |
| MAR - 8 1993 | | |
| MAR 29 1993 | | |
| MAY - 3 1993 | | |
| | | |
| | | |
| | | |
| | | |
| | | |
| | | |
| | | |
| | | |
| | | |
| | | |
| | | |

DEMCO 38-297

# RESEARCH UTILIZATION IN THE SOCIAL SERVICES: INNOVATIONS FOR PRACTICE AND ADMINISTRATION

Anthony J. Grasso, DSW
Irwin Epstein, PhD
Editors

## SOME ADVANCE REVIEWS

"It is hard to imagine a more skillful blending of discourse and examples for a difficult subject matter — the utilization of research in social work. A monumental achievement by renowned scholars. There is nothing on the subject that equals this book's comprehensiveness. Explores a range of questions about research utilization which go well beyond the basic issues. A model of scholarly acumen. Exhaustively researched. The definitive text on this topic. Should be required reading for all graduate social work students."

**Richard M. Grinnell, Jr., PhD**
Professor and Associate Dean
Faculty of Social Work
The University of Calgary
Alberta, Canada;
Editor, *Social Work Research and Evaluation*

"A compendium of excellent [chapters] authored by outstanding social work educators. The topics covered are central to research in the profession. Overall, I found the [chapters] well-written and up-to-date. I consider this volume to be an important and useful addition to the social work research literature."

**Srinika D. Jayaratne, PhD**
Professor, School of Social Work
University of Michigan, Ann Arbor

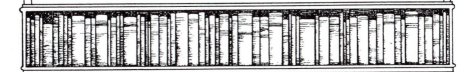

**NOTES FOR PROFESSIONAL LIBRARIANS
AND LIBRARY USERS**

This is an original book title published by The Haworth Press, Inc. Unless otherwise noted in specific chapters with attribution, materials in this book have not been previously published elsewhere in any format or language.

**CONSERVATION AND PRESERVATION NOTES**

The paper used in this publication meets the minimum requirements of American National Standard for Information Sciences — Permanence of Paper for Printed Material, ANSI Z39.48-1984.

# Research Utilization in the Social Services
## *Innovations for Practice and Administration*

## *HAWORTH* Social Administration
Simon Slavin, EdD, ACSW, Senior Editor

# Research Utilization in the Social Services
## *Innovations for Practice and Administration*

Anthony J. Grasso, DSW
Irwin Epstein, PhD
Editors

RECEIVED

NOV 1 3 1992

MSU - LIBRARY

The Haworth Press
New York • London • Norwood (Australia)

HV
91
.R47
1992

© 1992 by The Haworth Press, Inc. All rights reserved. No part of this work may be reproduced or utilized in any form or by any means, electronic or mechanical, including photocopying, microfilm and recording, or by any information storage and retrieval system, without permission in writing from the publisher. Printed in the United States of America.

The Haworth Press, Inc., 10 Alice Street, Binghamton, NY 13904-1580

**Library of Congress Cataloging-in-Publication Data**

Research utilization in the social services : innovations for practice and administration / Anthony J. Grasso, Irwin Epstein, editors.
    p.  cm.
  Includes bibliographical references and index.
  ISBN 1-56024-070-9 (alk. paper). — ISBN 1-56024-071-7 (pbk. alk. paper)
    1. Social service — United States — Technological innovations — Congresses. 2. Social service administration — United States — Technological innovations — Congresses. 3. Social service — Research — United States — Congresses. I. Grasso, Anthony J. II. Epstein, Irwin.
HV91.R47 1991
361′ .0068 — dc20
                                                91-8447
                                              CIP

# CONTENTS

# ABOUT THE EDITORS

**Anthony J. Grasso, DSW,** is Assistant Professor in the School of Social Work, University of Nevada at Las Vegas. He was formerly Director of Boysville Institute. The author of several articles on research and information utilization in social work, he is the designer of the Boysville Management Information System and several other agency-based research and information systems.

**Irwin Epstein, PhD,** is Professor of Social Work Research at Hunter College School of Social Work. A former Fulbright Scholar at the University of Wales, he has taught social work research methods and their clinical and program applications at Howard University, the University of Michigan, and the University of Warwick, in addition to Hunter College. From 1987 to 1988, he served as the first occupant of the Institute Chair at Boysville of Michigan for which he received the Hugh Whiffle Award from the Michigan Association of Childcare Agencies. He is the author of several books and articles on research and information utilization in social work.

Together Drs. Epstein and Grasso planned and co-convened the Conference on Research Utilization and have written several articles on agency-based research utilization. They have co-conducted computerization and program evaluation workshops in the United States and Canada. In addition, they serve as research utilization, management information, and evaluation consultants to several social agencies across the country.

# CONTRIBUTORS

**Martin Bloom, PhD,** is a Professor at the School of Social Work, Virginia Commonwealth University.

**Betty J. Blythe, PhD,** is an Associate Professor at the School of Social Work, University of Pittsburgh.

**Scott Briar, PhD,** is Director of the School of Social Work, Florida International University.

**Leon W. Chestang, PhD,** is Dean of the School of Social Work, Wayne State University.

**David Fanshel, PhD,** is a Professor at the Columbia University School of Social Work.

**Stephen J. Finch, PhD,** is an Associate Professor in the Department of Applied Mathematics and Statistics, State University of New York at Stony Brook.

**Anne E. Fortune, PhD,** is an Associate Professor at the School of Social Welfare, Nelson A. Rockefeller College of Public Affairs and Policy, State University of New York at Albany.

**John F. Grundy, PhD,** is a Senior Programmer and Analyst at the Columbia University School of Social Work.

**Yeheskel Hasenfeld, PhD,** is a Professor at the School of Social Welfare, University of California at Los Angeles.

**Shirley Jenkins, PhD,** is a Professor at the Columbia University School of Social Work.

**Stuart A. Kirk, PhD,** is a Professor at the Columbia University School of Social Work.

**Harold Lewis, DSW,** is Dean of the School of Social Work, Hunter College.

**Paul A. Marsters** is a Statistician with the Sterling-Winters Research Institute in Rensselaer, New York.

**Hamilton I. McCubbin, PhD,** is Dean and Professor at the School of Family Resources and Consumer Sciences, University of Wisconsin at Madison.

**Marilyn A. McCubbin, PhD,** is a Professor of Nursing, University of Wisconsin at Madison.

**Terry Mizrahi, DSW,** is a Professor at the Hunter College School of Social Work.

**David P. Moxley, PhD,** is an Assistant Professor at the School of Social Work, Wayne State University.

**Elizabeth Mutschler, PhD,** is a Professor at the School of Social Work, University of Michigan.

**Rino Patti, DSW,** is Dean at the School of Social Work, University of Southern California.

**Cindy E. Penka** is a doctoral student at the School of Social Welfare, Nelson A. Rockefeller College of Public Affairs and Policy, State University of New York at Albany.

**Melvyn C. Raider, PhD,** is an Associate Professor at the School of Social Work, Wayne State University.

**Helen Rehr, DSW,** is a Professor of Community Medicine Emerita at the Mount Sinai School of Medicine, City University of New York.

**William J. Reid, DSW,** is a Professor at the School of Social Welfare, Nelson A. Rockefeller College of Public Affairs and Policy, State University of New York at Albany.

**Sheldon D. Rose, PhD,** is a Professor at the University of Wisconsin at Madison.

**Aaron Rosenblatt, PhD,** is a Professor at the School of Social Welfare, Nelson A. Rockefeller College of Public Affairs and Policy, State University of New York at Albany.

**Jack Rothman, PhD,** is a Professor at the Center for Child and Family Policy Studies, UCLA School of Social Welfare.

**Allen Rubin, PhD,** is a Professor at the School of Social Work, University of Texas at Austin.

**John R. Schuerman, PhD,** is a Professor at The Chapin Hall Center for Children, University of Chicago and the Juvenile Protective Association of Chicago.

**Edwin J. Thomas, PhD,** is a Professor at the School of Social Work, University of Michigan.

**Tony Tripodi, PhD,** is a Professor at the School of Social Work, University of Pittsburgh.

**Harold Weissman, DSW,** is a Professor at the School of Social Work, Hunter College.

**James K. Whittaker, PhD,** is a Professor of Social Work and Director of the Social Welfare PhD Program, University of Washington. He is also a member of the National Research Advisory Committee, Boysville of Michigan.

# Foreword

Conferences sometimes constitute significant and highly visible historical milestones for a profession. Indeed, over the years many landmark developments in social work have emerged at major conferences. Perhaps the most profound of these was Dr. Abraham Flexner's keynote speech at the 1915 Conference of Charities and Corrections. Asking "Is social work a profession?" Flexner responded in the negative. Some observers regard his conference presentation as the single most important event in the growth of social work education and in the subsequent professionalization of social work.

Barely four years after Flexner's conference presentation, the Association of Training Schools for Professional Social Work emerged as the primary organization charged with promoting and strengthening social work education. The formation of this body is widely regarded as a direct outcome of Flexner's speech. The Association evolved in mission, purpose, and name until 1952 when it became the Council on Social Work Education. This organization serves today as the central body which promotes, guides, and formally accredits social work education throughout the United States. Its annual program meetings constitute a major venue for intellectual exchange within the social work profession. In their own right, they serve as a gauge of the various intellectual, educational, and practice developments within the profession. A similar function also has been served by the annual conferences sponsored by the National Association of Social Workers and the now-defunct National Conference on Social Welfare.

In like fashion, the Boysville Conference on the Future of Research and Information in Social Work constitutes another significant milestone in the progress of the social work profession, yet it is a milestone of a somewhat different order. This agency initiated conference, and the chapters in this volume, are bound to direct the profession's attention toward the next challenging frontier in its illustrious history, namely, the dissemination and application—as well as the generation—of research-based information for social work education and practice. This is an immediate and inexorable frontier that looms large for the profession. To our good fortune, however, the scope, magnitude, and key features of this rapidly emerging frontier are identified in large part by the chapters that appear in this volume. Doctors Anthony E. Grasso and Irwin Epstein have performed a major service for the social work profession by organizing the Boysville Conference and capturing its substance in the following pages.

A noteworthy historical link exists between the Boysville Conference and the Conference of Charities and Corrections. In 1915, Flexner proclaimed six criteria as essential for professional status. Social work was deemed to be particularly deficient with regard to one of these: the possession of systematically communicable methods based upon a body of scientific knowledge. The communicability and utilization of scientific information are the concerns which constitute the essential subjects of inquiry both for the Boysville Conference and the Conference of Charities and Corrections, as well as the present volume.

The primary objective of Flexner's presentation was to dissuade social workers from agitating for public recognition as an established profession. Ironically, however, its effect was to promulgate criteria that provided operational objectives for social work's subsequent drive toward public acceptance as a profession. Flexner's speech resulted in the elaboration of criteria that have served until today as standards for judging the extent of progress made by social work in its long and arduous journey toward professionalization.

From 1915 to the present, nearly every debate about social work's status as a profession has concentrated upon the extent to which it possesses a significant body of knowledge that is derived from scientific research, amenable to widespread dissemination, and applicable by practitioners in ways that are both effective and efficient. In the intervening years, however, unimaginable advances have been made in conceptualization, measurement, and computing and audiovisual technologies. All of these have import for information processing and information utilization in a vibrant and contemporary profession.

Today, the quintessential question no longer is whether social work is a profession. Rather, the more timely, fundamental, and complex question is, "How effective is social work and how can it become even more effective?" The contributors to this volume suggest a variety of ways to address, if not always answer, this formidable question. Yet they all proceed from the common assumption that social work's strength as a helping profession can be enhanced significantly through the skillful and efficient application of relevant information. Accordingly, the quality and quantity of the profession's research and information utilization activities must be regarded as a central concern.

During the past 15 years, scientific research and the dissemination and utilization of research-based information have been the focus of several special conferences. In 1976 the Social Work Training Branch of the National Institute of Mental Health funded a conference on Research Utilization in Social Work in conjunction with the Council on Social Work Education's Project on Research Utilization in Social Work. Two years later the National Institute of Mental Health and the National Association of Social Workers spearheaded a landmark national conference that focused expressly on the future of social work research. This conference brought together nearly 300 social workers who demonstrated that the profession had finally accumulated a critical mass of highly trained researchers with both the capability and the commitment to significantly advance its scientific knowledge base.

The high hopes with which these conferences were launched did not keep pace with other developments in the social work profession, however. On the one hand, doctoral programs proliferated substantially since 1978. Nearly 50 schools of social work now offer doctoral training, but fewer than 300 persons per year graduate from doctoral programs in social work and only a fraction of these pursue research careers. At the same time, the number of social work practitioners and, therefore, the demand for practice knowledge has grown dramatically.

Accredited graduate programs in social work increased from 53 in 1952 to 97 in 1987. In 1952, about 50 undergraduate social work programs were affiliated with the Council on Social Work Education, whereas in 1989 there were 362. Correspondingly, the membership of the National Association of Social Workers rose from 20,000 persons in 1955 to 127,000 in 1989. At least 70,000 additional social work graduates have not become members of the Association. Hence, it is estimated that there are more than 200,000 professional social workers in the United States. In view of these data, no other profession may experience a greater disparity than social work between its numbers of practitioners and researchers. Accordingly, the profession must attend diligently not only to the development of a scientific knowledge base but, even more, to the efficient dissemination and utilization of the full range of information that can be put to use by practitioners.

The Boysville Conference and the contents of this volume mark the end of an inordinately long hiatus in the profession's quest to promote and realize the full potential of scientific inquiry. During this period some observers have seriously doubted the profession's ability to generate, disseminate, and apply information that is based on scientific research. A major indicator of these concerns, as well as an attempt to address them, can be found in the creation two years ago of a Task Force on Research in Social Work. Established in 1988 under the auspices of the National Institute of Mental Health, this group was formed at the joint initiative of Dr. Lewis B. Judd, the Institute's Director, and the leading organizations in social work education and practice, namely, the Council on Social Work Education, the National Association of Deans and Directors of Schools of Social Work, the Group for the Advancement of Doctoral Education, and the National Association of Social Workers. The mission of the Task Force is to examine the role of research in all aspects of social work education and practice. It is expected to issue a final report in 1991.

It is important to note that the Boysville Conference was launched under the aegis of a nationally recognized social work agency and that it was co-hosted by a major school of social work. It brought together many of the nation's most experienced and highly respected leaders in social work research and information utilization. At the same time, it involved relative newcomers to the field who will inevitably become the leaders of tomorrow. Both the

Conference and this work represent the timely culmination of efforts to proceed beyond the current plateau in social work history and to advance the profession toward a higher level of development wherein social work practice is predicated upon decision making which follows from the skillful use of research-based information.

The chapters here clearly reveal the progress that has been made by social workers in recent years. They bear witness to the immense promise and the great potential of research-based information for social work practice. Likewise, they highlight the problems and the pitfalls that await the profession as it seeks to strengthen its knowledge base. The central themes of the book are the central issues of the profession: changing models of research information; research information utilization in micro-level social work practice and macro-level social work practice; and agency-based research and information utilization. The myriad of ideas that appear on the following pages are both an accurate reflection and a welcome portent of the direction of social work practice and education.

*Ronald A. Feldman*
*New York, New York*

# Introduction

Anthony J. Grasso
Irwin Epstein

In October 1976, The Social Work Training Branch of the National Institute of Mental Health funded a Conference on Research Utilization in Social Work as part of the Council on Social Work Education's Project on Research Utilization in Social Work. The conference was attended by the leading social work researchers and research instructors in the United States. Its broad purposes were:

> to spotlight research utilization, stimulate social work researchers to stimulate social work educators to rethink the teaching of research, and begin identifying ways to improve the utilization of research. (Rubin, 1979)

Participants in the conference achieved consensus on four principal themes:

1. There is a need to formulate empirically based practice models for social work in which research occupies an integral, essential role.
2. Social work research should be directed to finding solutions for the problems encountered by practitioners, with special emphasis on *developmental* research.
3. Social work students should be prepared for active participation in the research process, not only to be passive consumers of research.
4. The development of a new breed of practitioner-scientist should be cultivated and encouraged (Briar, 1979).

Over a decade has passed since the conference was held. During that period, significant advances have been made in research pedagogy, computer technology, applied research model development and testing, and the application of research to practice. Moreover, with the advent of agency-based, practice-research models (Blythe and Briar, 1985), "integrated" information systems (Mutschler and Hasenfeld, 1986), and quality assurance monitoring strategies (Nuehring and Pascone, 1986), the issue of research utilization has been brought much closer to the locus of practice. No longer is the site of research consumption and application confined to the classroom, the library, or the practitioner's study. Increasingly, the agency is the locus at which the compatibility or incompatibility of research and practice is confronted.

Such an agency is Boysville of Michigan, a private child and family treatment organization serving hundreds of troubled adolescents and their families throughout Michigan and in northern Ohio. Under the aegis of the Boysville Institute, this agency has been piloting a unique effort to integrate research and social work practice at all levels of the organization. This effort relies heavily on state-of-the-art computer technology and on original software development (Grasso and Epstein, 1989), as well as on a research-based organizational philosophy and decision-making design (Grasso and Epstein, 1987).

In addition to its investment in this innovative administrative design and its implementation, Boysville is unique in that it is engaged in studying empirically its own research utilization (Grasso, Epstein, and Tripodi, 1988). Finally, Boysville is attempting to create a research-based learning environment for Boysville staff at all levels as well as for social work students who have their fieldwork placements at the agency. By "learning environment" is meant an atmosphere in which systematically collected and computer-analyzed information is used to promote professional growth as well as agency effectiveness and efficiency. Consequently, Boysville exemplifies an agency's efforts to implement all of the themes articulated by the original Conference on Research Utilization in Social Work.

For these reasons, on May 1–2, 1989, the Boysville Institute sponsored and Wayne State University School of Social Work housed a second research utilization conference, roughly a decade later. Entitled the Conference on the Future of Research and Information in Social Work, it differed from the original in a number of fundamental ways.

First, the conference benefited from the past decade's professional, pedagogical, and programmatic experiences of a number of former conference participants. Thus, several of the most active contributors to the research-utilization literature were invited to attend and give papers on how their research perspectives have changed through their own research-utilization efforts over the previous ten years or so.

Second, the conference addressed the issue of agency-based research and information utilization. Although this topic was ignored in the earlier conference, great strides have been made in this area over the last decade. These advances were reflected in a special session and set of papers presented at the conference.

Third, the conference concerned itself with the place of computerization in social work education and practice at every organizational level. This theme was not addressed in the original conference since very little of this type of research utilization was taking place at the time.

## CONFERENCE OBJECTIVE

The objectives of the 1989 Conference on Research and Information Utilization in Social Work were to:

1. Describe new models of research and information utilization that have evolved over the past decade and make projections for future developments.
2. Describe micro-social work innovations in research and information utilization that have developed in the past ten years and make projections for future developments.
3. Describe macro-social work innovations in research and information utilization that have developed in the past ten years and make projections for future developments.
4. Describe new approaches to research and computer pedagogy that have emerged in the last decade and make projections for future developments.
5. Describe innovative models of agency-based research and in-

formation utilization, to consider the ethical implications of these innovations and to make projections with regard to future developments.

## CONFERENCE ORGANIZATION

The conference lasted two days. It was by invitation only and involved the presentation and discussion of original papers on pre-specified topics by acknowledged experts on the development and implementation of new models of research and information utilization and on research education in social work. Papers were distributed prior to the conference so that presenters were only required to do a 15-minute presentation on panels grouped by topic areas. A panel leader was responsible for leading the discussion over the next hour on the issues raised in each topic area. Additionally, leaders were responsible for writing the introduction to each of the sections of this book. This book contains the papers presented at this historic conference.

We feel that this book will be of value to those responsible for teaching and training a new generation the information based, enquiry-driven social work practitioners. The research models and innovations presented offer tools for those who would innovate, not just for the sake of innovation, but for the betterment of the field.

## REFERENCES

1. Briar, S. Introduction. *Sourcebook on Research Utilization*. A. Rubin and A. Rosenblatt, eds., Council on Social Work Education, New York. 1979: 132-140.

2. Blythe, B. and Briar, S. Developing Empirically Based Models of Practice. *Social Work*, Vol. 30 (6), 1985: 483-488.

3. Grasso, A. and Epstein, I. Management by Measurement: Organizational Dilemmas and Opportunities, *Administration in Social Work*, Vol. II (3) 1987: 89-100.

4. Grasso, A. and Epstein, I. The Boysville Experience: Integrating Practice Decision-making, Program Evaluation, and Management Information. *Computers in Human Services*, Vol. 4 (1&2), 1989: 85-95.

5. Grasso, A., Epstein, I., and Tripodi, T. Agency Based Research Utilization in a Residential Child Care Setting, *Administration in Social Work* Vol. 12 (4), 1988: 61-80.

6. Mutschler, E. and Hasenfeld, Y. Integrated Information Systems for Social Work Practice. *Social Work*, Vol. 31 (5), September-October, 1986: 345-349.

7. Nuehring, E. and Pascone, A. Single-Subject Evaluation: A Tool for Quality Assurance. *Social Work*, Vol. 31 (5), September-October, 1986: 359-365.

8. Rubin, A. Preface. *Sourcebook on Research Utilization*. A. Rubin and A. Rosenblatt, eds., Council on Social Work Education, New York. 1979: 132-140.

# INTRODUCTION TO SECTION I

## Changing Models of Practice
## in Research Utilization

### Irwin Epstein

The publication of this volume is taking place roughly a decade after the publication of *Sourcebook on Research Utilization* by the Council of Social Work Education in 1979. That volume was based on the papers presented at the historic first Conference on Research Utilization held in New Orleans in 1977. Three of the four authors of the chapters in the first section of this book presented papers at that conference. The fourth was in England at the time and could not attend. All four, however, were pioneering work on the problems and possibilities of research utilization in social work practice. Several other contributors to this volume presented papers and were in attendance at that conference, and all of us are beneficiaries of the ideas, interests, and opportunities that the conference instigated.

The subtitle of this work refers to "practice." Each of the authors of the first set of chapters have been actively engaged in the practice of research utilization in social work for over two decades. In fact, they are our most astute and prolific conceptualizers, theorizers, practitioners, evaluators, and disseminators of research utilization. As such, they are ideally suited to engage in a reflective review of how their own approaches to research utilization have evolved over the past decade and what they anticipate in the next ten years. No one in social work today is better equipped for this "back to the future" reflection than Tony Tripodi, Scott Briar, Jack Rothman, and Edwin Thomas.

First, Tony Tripodi introduces the concept of "Differential Research Utilization" as an approach to the integration of research and social work practice at various stages of micro and macro practice. To do so, he distinguishes between substantive and methodological knowledge and suggests that these forms of knowledge are most likely to be utilized when they are directly tied to practice decisions.

In the second chapter, "Integration of Practice and Research: Past, Present, and Future," Scott Briar reflects on the "Practitioner Scientist" model which he introduced in 1978 and which the University of Washington School of Social Work has been educating its students to perform for the past decade. He describes the ways in which this micro practice model has been criticized by social work researchers and the successes and failures of the educational effort to disseminate this model through former students. Finally, he considers future implications for the promotion of practice research utilization through social work education.

In "Creating Tools for Intervention: The Convergence of Research Methodologies," Jack Rothman introduces the "umbrella" concept of "Intervention Design and Development" in an effort to encompass both Thomas' D&D approach and his own "Social Research and Development (R&D)" model. Working predominantly at the macro level of practice, Rothman emphasizes the importance of an institutional base for legitimating and promoting research-based practice and the need for multidisciplinary efforts, multiple information sources, and multisite tests of practice research innovations.

Finally, Thomas describes a decade of change in his "Design and Development Model (D&D)." In so doing, he introduces the "developmental practice" model which effectively links D&D and research utilization. This linkage is intended to promote the development, evaluation, and dissemination of social work practice innovation at every level of practice.

Although their research utilization approaches differ in important ways, common to the work of each of these four scholars and practitioners is their unwavering commitment to the promotion of research utilization in social work practice.

# Differential Research Utilization in Macro and Micro Social Work Practice: An Evolving Perspective

Tony Tripodi

## INTRODUCTION

Differential research utilization comprises a series of interrelated strategies for the attainment of research integration in macro and micro social work practice. Defining research integration as the extent to which substantive and/or methodological knowledge from research is used in practice (Tripodi, 1988), differential research utilization involves the following:

1. Macro and micro practice activities are specified by developmental stages of practice; and within these stages, key decisions that must be made for the conduct of practice are delineated (Blythe and Tripodi, in press; Epstein and Tripodi, 1977; Tripodi, 1974, 1983; Tripodi and Epstein, 1980).
2. Research knowledge is divided into substantive and methodological knowledge, which is further divided into usage categories, i.e., activities regarded as important for the application of research in practice (Epstein and Tripodi, 1978; Tripodi, 1974, 1988; Tripodi and Epstein, 1978).
3. The basic strategy for applying substantive research knowledge is the assessment of research studies (Tripodi, Fellin, Meyer, 1969); while fundamental to the integration of methodological research knowledge are differential evaluation (Tripodi, Fellin and Epstein, 1971) and the incorporation of research into practice by specifying decisions within stages of program development and practice (Tripodi, 1974, 1983).
4. Research integration is achieved when substantive and/or

methodological knowledge is used as information for making decisions in practice (Tripodi and Epstein, 1978; Tripodi, 1983, 1988).

Hence, differential research utilization involves a set of procedures for integrating practice in research. It is based on the notion that macro practice, micro practice, and research are not monolithic (Briar, 1979, 1980; Fanshel, 1980; Tripodi, 1988). Within each of those areas there are different approaches founded on different assumptions and theories (Meyer, 1984; Epstein, 1985; Cohen, Sargent and Sechreist, 1986). Macro practice is broadly conceived as comprising community organization, administration, planning, and policy development and implementation (Epstein and Tripodi, 1978); micro practice is concerned with social work interventions designed to help and influence individuals, couples, groups, and families (Tripodi and Epstein, 1978); and research contains qualitative and quantitative approaches ranging from the case study to social experimentation (Tripodi, 1974, 1983, 1988).

Differential research utilization is a process that differentiates practice into key decisions within stages of development, such as in initiating programs and in forming conclusions about the nature and extent of client problems; and it then links research knowledge with those decisions. Both substantive and methodological research knowledge are regarded as information sources for practice.

The concept of differential research utilization has been evolving over 20 years from the late 1960s to the present. It is used at this conference on research utilization to represent an evolving set of strategies for research utilization with which my colleagues and I have been involved. The purpose of this chapter, therefore, is to present the primary ingredients of this perspective on research utilization, to trace its conceptual development, and to present pertinent research investigations. First, substantive knowledge will be defined, and categories of activities related to its usage will be explicated. This will be followed by the conceptual development of the assessment of research and related research activities. Second, methodological knowledge will also be defined and specified into usage categories. Then the conceptual development of differential evaluation and of incorporating research into practice with relevant research investigations will be discussed. Finally, there will be presented suggestions for future research to foster the further development of the differential utilization of substantive and methodological research knowledge.

## SUBSTANTIVE RESEARCH KNOWLEDGE

Substantive research knowledge is synonymous with the results of findings of social research (Thomas, 1967). Such knowledge can be provided in the form of levels that include increasing amounts of information (Greenwood, 1960; Tripodi, 1974, 1983): (1) hypothetical-developmental knowledge, which includes the conceptualization of phenomena as well as the articulation and specification of concepts, variables, and hypotheses; (2) qualitative and quantitative-descriptive knowledge, including historical and contextual descriptions in addition to simple facts regarding observed, empirical regularities; (3) correlational or associational knowledge about the empirical relationships of sets of two or more variables; and (4) cause-effect knowledge in the sense of causal inferences between specified sets of independent and dependent variables.

It has long been recognized by the social work profession that a desirable skill for social workers is the critical consumption of substantive knowledge from research (Tripodi, Fellin, and Meyer, 1969). This skill is central to using substantive research knowledge in terms of research assessment, qualitative reviews, and quantitative reviews (Tripodi, 1988). These categories comprise a continuum that is based on the following dimensions: skills of the user, time to complete the user task, and amounts of information about substantive research knowledge.

### Usage Categories

*Research Assessment*

Research assessment refers to the assessment of one research study, which involves judgments about the internal validity and generalizability of substantive knowledge, as well as its relevance and applicability to macro and micro social work practice (Tripodi, Fellin, and Meyer, 1969; Epstein and Tripodi, 1977; Tripodi and

Epstein, 1980). This activity can be performed by educators, students, researchers, and practitioners. Although it has been observed that not all social workers read research articles or conduct research (Rosenblatt, 1968; Kirk, Osmalov, and Fischer, 1976), it is correspondingly important to place that observation in perspective, noting that neither do all psychologists (Morrow-Bradley and Elliott, 1986), physical scientists, or engineers (Brittain, 1970). Many of the social work efforts in conceptualizing and conducting research on factors that influence the extent of substantive knowledge utilization are traceable to the behavioral sciences (Festinger and Katz, 1953) and to the Center for Research on the Utilization of Scientific Knowledge, University of Michigan (Havelock, 1971).

## Qualitative Reviews

A qualitative review involves the assessment of a series of research studies, typically subsumed under a specific domain. Each study is assessed, then all the studies are compared and contrasted to search for similarities and differences with respect to emergent themes. Such reviews are subject to the biases of the reviewer as manifest in criteria for selecting studies, acceptable degrees of internal validity and generalizability, and inferences about the studies themselves. Nevertheless, when conducted by reviewers experienced in the phenomenon being addressed and discussed in that context, these reviews can provide adequate summaries of the "state of the art" in that particular domain. This process also is employed in the analysis stage of developmental research (Thomas, 1984). Examples of these reviews are contained in doctoral dissertations and in social work journals (e.g., Tripodi and Miller, 1966; Reid and Hanrahan, 1982).

## Quantitative Reviews

Quantitative reviews, when properly conducted, include assessment of individual research studies and qualitative judgments about their similarities and differences, as well as criteria of inclusion and data synthesis techniques. Data synthesis is the use of quantitative procedures for systematically comparing research studies (Pillemer and Light, 1980; Nurius, 1984). These procedures can be relatively simple, for example, as in the use of proportions to describe research trends over time (Tripodi, 1984), or they can be more complex as in the use of effect sizes or standard scores for meta-analyses. Hogarty (1988) clearly points out the necessity for reading the individual studies prior to subjecting them to meta-analysis in his review of literature about the effectiveness of social work with the chronically mentally ill. Although there is some effort to employ meta-analysis in social work (e.g., Videka-Sherman, 1984, 1988), there continues to be a dearth of research studies that compare the relative advantages and disadvantages of various data synthesis techniques for reviewing the social work research literature.

## Assessment of Research

The conceptual development of research assessment can best be described by referring to five time periods: initial conception, 1965-1970; simplification, 1971-1975; relationship to practice decisions, 1976-1980; problem of generalizability, 1981-1985; and synthesis, 1986-present. Major conceptual developments and related research for these time periods are shown in Figure 1, where one can refer to original writings as well as sources of influence in greater detail.

Basic notions about the assessment of research were stimulated by the need of research instructors to present guidelines to social work students for evaluating and using research and by the observation that there did not appear to be sufficient differentiation in evaluating different levels of substantive research knowledge. Involved in the initial conception of the assessment of research are three major processes: classification, evaluation, and utilization (Tripodi, Fellin, and Meyer, 1969). First, a research study is categorized into its major type as a function of research purpose and the research procedures employed: experimental, quantitative, descriptive and exploratory studies (Weinberger and Tripodi, 1969). Second, a series of evaluation questions within each phase of the research process, from problem formulation to research design and data collection to data analysis and conclusions, are presented for each type of research, and those questions are employed as guidelines for evaluating the soundness of the research knowledge. Third, a set of

FIGURE 1. Major Influences on the Conceptual Development of Differential Research Utilization, 1965-1989

|  | 1965-1970 | 1971-1975 |
|---|---|---|
| Books* | Tripodi, Fellin, Meyer (1969)[1,2,3] | Tripodi, Fellin and Epstein (1971)[2,4,5] Tripodi, (1974)[1,2,3,4,5] |
| Conceptual articles, chapters, editorials | Tripodi & Miller (1967)[2] Miller & Tripodi (1966)[2] Tripodi, Epstein & MacMurray (1970)[2,4,5] | |
| Research Articles | Weinberger & Tripodi (1969)[1,3] | Stuart & Tripodi (1973)[2,5] |
| Other Major Sources | Hage & Aiken (1970)[4] Suchman (1967)[4] Rosenblatt (1968)[1,3] Festiger & Katz (1953)[1,2] Greenwood (1957, 1960)[1,3] Finestone (1959)[1,3] French (1952)[2,4] Goldstein (1962, 1963)[2,5] Thomas (1967)[1,2] | Brittain (1970)[1] Havelock (1971)[1] Briar & Miller (1971)[2,5] Carter (1972)[2,5] Gottman & Leiblum (1974)[2,5] |

*Revised Editions are not included
Legend: 1 = substantive knowledge; 2 = methodological knowledge; 3 = assessment of research; 4 = differential evaluation; 5 = incorporating research in practice stages

| 1976-1980 | 1981-1985 | 1986-1989 |
|---|---|---|
| Epstein and Tripodi (1977)[1,2,3,4,5] Tripodi and Epstein (1980)[1,2,3,4,5] | Tripodi (1983)[1,2,3,4,5] | Blythe and Tripodi (1989)[2,5] |
| Epstein, Tripodi & Fellin (1977)[2,4,5] Tripodi & Epstein (1975)[2,5] Epstein & Tripodi (1978)[2,4,5] Tripodi & Harrington (1979)[2,4,5] | Tripodi (1981)[1,2,3] Tripodi (1982)[1,2,3] Bielowski & Epstein (1984)[2,4,5] | Tripodi (1988)[1,2,3,4,5] Wedaneja, Nurius & Tripodi (1988)[2,5] Epstein & Grasso (1987)[2,5] |
| Stuart, Jayaratne & Tripodi (1976)[2,5] | Tripodi (1984)[1,3] Nurius & Tripodi (1985)[1,2,3] | Nurius, Wedenoja, Tripodi (1987)[1,2,5] Jayaratne, Talsma, Tripodi (1988)[2,5] Grasso, Epstein & Tripodi (1988)[2,5] |
| Fanshel (1980)[2] Kirk, Osmalov, Fischer (1976)[1,3] Briar (1979, 1980)[2,5] Hersen & Barlow (1976)[2,5] Thomas (1978)[2,5] Rothman (1978, 1980)[1,2,5] Rubin & Rosenblatt (1979) [1,2] Mullen (1978)[1,2,5] Jayaratne & Levy (1979)[2,5] Mutschler (1979)[2,5] | Reid & Hanrahan (1982)[1] Glass, McGaw & Smith (1981)[1,2] Shapiro & Shapiro (1982)[1,2] Bloom & Fischer (1982)[2,5] Vidaka-Sherman (1984)[2,5] Thomas (1984)[2,5] | Cohen, Sargent & Sechrest (1986)[1] Hogarty (1988)[1] Videka-Sherman (1988)[1] Morrow, Bradley & Elliott (1986)[1] Briar & Blythe (1985)[2,5] McMahon (1987)[2,5] |

guidelines are offered for applying the knowledge to social work practice, very broadly conceived (Tripodi, Fellin, and Meyer, 1969).

The chief problem with that conception was that it is too cumbersome for many students to use. Moreover, it was in the early 1970s that much concern was raised about conflicts between practice and research, barriers to utilization, and the extent to which social workers actually read research studies (Rosenblatt, 1968; Brittain, 1970; Havelock, 1971). Therefore the concept of assessment was simplified (Tripodi, 1974). Instead of categorizing by research type and relating evaluation questions to each type, the task of assessment was simplified to discern knowledge-seeking objectives of the research, and then to determine whether those objectives were attained. This was done by applying evidentiary criteria: concept translatability, hypothesis researchability, measurement accuracy, empirical generality, and internal control. These criteria were employed differentially and in combination for evaluating the achievement of knowledge objectives. Moreover, criteria for using the results of social research were reduced to these questions: "Is the knowledge relevant?" "Is the knowledge accessible?" "Are the potential users receptive to the knowledge?" "Are the value systems of the potential users consonant with the knowledge?" "Do the potential users have the capability for implementing the knowledge?" (Tripodi, 1974, p. 106).

Although that system for assessing research knowledge was simpler, it too did not provide a direct link to social work practice. The responsibility for doing so was put on the practitioner. In the late 1970s there was an increased emphasis on making the concept of assessment more relevant to social work by writing more specifically about its applications to practice decisions. Therefore, assessment principles were discussed in relation to the effectiveness and efficiency of programs selected in the planning stages of administrative practice and program development (Epstein and Tripodi, 1977) and to the choice of interventions designed to solve problems in social work practice with individuals (Tripodi and Epstein, 1980). Simultaneously, attention was given to the application of methodological knowledge to practice. Mullen (1978) developed a model for formulating practice prescriptions based on research findings, and Rothman (1978) discussed procedures for converting substantive knowledge to practice principles.

In the early 1980s two developments took place. One was the notion that a logic of research design could be specified so that designs for evaluative research could be integrated in both micro and macro practice. Research designs were articulated with respect to micro or macro units of analysis, desired levels of knowledge, and the necessary evidence for such knowledge (Tripodi, 1983). The second development was a conception of criteria and procedures for inferring generalizability, an area frequently neglected in research methodology. Qualitative judgmental procedures were suggested for conceptual generality; sampling procedures, for representativeness; replication procedures, for consistency of results; and experimental procedures for external validity control (Tripodi, 1983, pp. 89-97). In these developments the problem of generalizing substantive knowledge from research to practice was emphasized. This, in turn, led to research about generalizability in the research and practice literature (Nurius and Tripodi, 1985; Nurius, Wedenoja and Tripodi, 1987).

The present time (Tripodi, 1988) is one of synthesis, reorganization, and further development. Not only is the concept of assessment shifting in emphasis, but it is also being merged with ideas about differential evaluation and the incorporation of research knowledge in social work practice.

## *Research*

Weinberger and Tripodi (1969) devised a system for classifying research studies in social work journals, and demonstrated that a high degree of interrater reliability could be achieved. It was also shown that a typology of research can be useful for depicting trends reflected in the literature. For example, from the period 1956-60 to 1961-65 there was less emphasis on discussions about research and more attention devoted to reports of empirical research. Also, there was an increase in the percentage of studies devoted to testing hypotheses.

The content analysis of research in social work journals was extended to include the time periods 1966-70, 1971-75, and 1976-80 (Tripodi, 1984). There continued to be an increase in hypothesis-testing, but studies describing population characteristics were also in ascendance. Notably, studies concerned with seeking relationships among variables declined. In addition, time-series analysis was reported as useful for studying changes in the percentage of research articles over time.

Research on generalizations was pursued in two distinct studies. First, a classification system was devised to differentiate the degree to which generalizations in research were based on evidence accumulated by qualitative and/or quantitative procedures, such as qualitative judgment in comparing the results of studies, use of sampling procedures, and statistical testing (Nurius and Tripodi, 1985). It was found that the use of systematic procedures for inferring generalizability varied by the type of research. Quantitative-descriptive studies were more likely to employ quantitative procedures than either experimental or exploratory studies. In general, there was a low use of generalization procedures; when used, both quantitative and qualitative procedures were employed, and qualitative procedures were observed to be used slightly more often than quantitative procedures in research studies reported in two major social work research journals over a five-year span.

The second study on generalization was an analysis of practice prescriptions as reflected in the journal *Social Casework* (Nurius, Wedenoja, and Tripodi, 1987). Practice prescriptions, i.e., conclusions about what behaviors social workers should exhibit in interpersonal practice, were specified, and a typology of types of evidence used to justify those conclusions was constructed and shown to be reliable. It was observed that 35% of the 360 reviewed articles contained practice prescriptions. The primary source of justification for generalizations about practice was experience (59%), followed by the use of idiosyncratic theories, assumptions, and concepts (51%). While 35% of the generalizations included reference to the literature, it is believed that very few generalizations were based on substantive research knowledge.

## *METHODOLOGICAL RESEARCH KNOWLEDGE*

Methodological research knowledge comprises the concepts, strategies, and observational methods of social research, especially those that can be incorporated in social work for processing information pertinent to macro or micro practice decisions (Tripodi, 1974, 1988; Epstein and Tripodi, 1978; Tripodi and Epstein, 1980; Siegel, 1988; and Siegel and Reamer, 1988). This conception was initially stimulated by Goldstein (1962, 1963) who believed that interpersonal social work practice could be made more scientific by incorporating research standards and procedures for data gathering and analysis. Thomas (1967) suggested that behavioral science research methods could be employed for problems and issues relevant to social work, and that perspective was also adopted in *The Assessment of Social Research* (Tripodi, Fellin, and Meyer, 1969). For example, in an evaluation of community leadership (Bonjean, 1963), it was indicated that the methods for determining community leadership could also be used by community organizers. Uses of research concepts and methods are fundamental to the notion of research-based macro practice that is concerned with planning, monitoring, and evaluation (Epstein and Tripodi, 1977, 1978) and to the collection and analysis of information in micro practice as it progresses from assessment to termination and follow-up (Tripodi and Epstein, 1980; Blythe and Tripodi, in press).

The usage categories that follow form a continuum, based as with categories for substantive knowledge, on the knowledge and skills of the user and on the time needed to complete the activity. These categories in increasing order of difficulty are "applying research concepts," "assessing available instruments," "developing instruments," and "employing strategies for processing research information in practice" (Tripodi, 1988).

## Usage Categories

### Applying Research Concepts

Applying research concepts refers to the use of research standards and principles for analyzing information produced in practice. Goldstein (1963) advocated that practice information should be appraised for its reliability and validity, and questions should also be raised about the accuracy and reliability of classification systems. Current concerns in intervention research about procedural reliability, i.e., consistency in the delivery of practice procedures (Billingsley, White, and Munson, 1980), and shifts in the deployment of interventions (McMahon, 1987), are cases in point. Biased sampling, populations, and representative sampling are examples of other concepts that can be helpful in making valid assessments of community, organizational, and individual needs.

## Assessing Available Instruments

Assessing available instruments involves the review and use of instruments that can be employed for collecting data in practice. An evaluation of instruments is necessary prior to their effective use, and this includes an application of the concepts of reliability and validity (Tripodi and Epstein, 1980). Instruments have been available in articles, books, and monographs for many years (Tripodi, 1974); however, their use has been facilitated by the increased involvement of social workers in developing and locating them. For example, Levitt and Reid (1981) located rapid assessment instruments that can be administered easily; Hudson (1982) developed a package of measuring instruments covering such topics as marital satisfaction and self-esteem; and Corcoran and Fischer (1987) compiled a range of instruments that can be used in micro practice.

## Developing Instruments

Principles for constructing instruments such as questionnaires, interview schedules, and observational forms can be applied in social work practice. For example, questionnaires for assessing client satisfaction, community needs, and utilization of social services can be developed for macro practice, and forms and rating scales can be tailored to specific clients, groups, and families (Epstein and Tripodi, 1977; Tripodi and Epstein, 1980). Gottman and Lieblum (1974) show how self-anchored rating scales can be developed for psychotherapy and behavioral practice; Mutschler (1979) reports that social workers can be trained to adapt goal attainment scaling in work with families (Kinesuk and Sherman, 1968); and Bloom and Fischer (1982) provide principles for developing instruments for evaluating interpersonal practice effectiveness.

## Employing Strategies for Processing Research Information

Strategies for processing research information include: (1) methodologies identified with techniques, such as the survey, single-case design, experimentation, and the case study (Festinger and Katz, 1953; Hersen and Barlow, 1976), and (2) approaches that provide perspectives and ways to combine specific methodological techniques, e.g., empirically based micro practice (Briar, 1979; Jayaratne and Levy, 1979; Bloom and Fischer, 1982; Siegel, 1984), research-based macro practice (Epstein and Tripodi, 1977, 1978), program evaluation (French, 1952; Tripodi, Fellin, and Epstein, 1971; Tripodi, 1983), qualitative methodology (Epstein, 1985; Tripodi, in press), and computerized information systems (Mutschler and Hasenfeld, 1986; Epstein and Grasso, 1987; and McCullough, Farrell, and Longabaugh, 1986).

Needs-resources surveys are employed in community organization, planning, and administrative practice. Approaches to program evaluation and methodologies for evaluating micro practice effectiveness are employed by practitioners, and it is expected that these will be used increasingly since the Council on Social Work Education has mandated that social work students should be taught to evaluate their practice.

## *Differential Evaluation*

Differential evaluation can be described in a fashion similar to that of the assessment of research. Five time periods depict the major shifts in differential evaluation: initial conception, 1965-1970; modification and specification, 1971-1975; relationship to macro practice decisions, 1976-1980; merging of macro and micro practice evaluations, 1981-1985; and synthesis and integration, 1986-present. Major writings and influences on the development of this concept are observable in Figure 1.

Stimulated by Suchman's *Evaluative Research* (1967) and by consultation on management and evaluation of social programs in the war on poverty, the idea of differential evaluation was devised as a response to these observations (Tripodi, Epstein, and MacMurray, 1970). Many programs were in different stages of development and could not be evaluated in the same way; evaluators from different disciplines tended to employ the methodologies in which they were trained, irrespective of their program relevance, and social program administrators appeared to need information to help them choose consultants to conduct program evaluations.

The basic idea of differential evaluation is that different evaluation techniques are appropriate for different stages of program development: program initiation, which focuses on the planning and initial development of a program; program delivery, which is concerned with providing relevant services to appropriate clientele; and program implementation, which refers to that stage in which a program is fully operative. This conception was modified and expanded in *Social Program Evaluation* (Tripodi, Fellin, and Epstein, 1971). Differential evaluation was regarded as "a process of asking different evaluation questions of program efforts, effectiveness, and efficiency for each program stage of development, and then choosing those evaluation techniques which are most appropriate to the evaluation objectives" (Tripodi, Fellin, and Epstein, 1971, p. 12). The name for the program delivery stage was changed to "program contact" to emphasize administrative concerns with solving problems and barriers to achieving contact with designated target populations. Evaluation techniques of monitoring, research, and cost analyses were also described, as well as their utility for evaluating programs differentially.

Evaluation questions geared to efforts, effectiveness, and efficiency provided a framework for program evaluation. However, their applicability to the planning of program evaluations required more skills than were initially assumed. Moreover, the consideration of a wide range of evaluation techniques required much more knowledge than the typical administrator or evaluator possessed. Therefore, it was believed that more details about research techniques should be provided to administrators. To this end, administrative practice was conceptualized as involving stages of development analogous to program development: program planning, monitoring program contact, and evaluation of the implemented program (Epstein and Tripodi, 1977, 1978). Within each of these administrative functions, it was shown that research techniques could be employed to provide information relevant to administrative decisions. For example, principles of sampling and of questionnaire construction were used to develop needs surveys for program planning (Epstein and Tripodi, 1977). It was re-emphasized that differential evaluation is a management technique that can be employed in formative program evaluations, a perspective that was also applied to community development (Epstein, Tripodi, and Fellin, 1977).

Three innovations occurred that served to expand differential evaluation to embrace micro as well as macro practice. First, it was suggested that single-subject designs were applicable to program evaluation in the form of time-series designs that include either aggregated units from single subjects or organizational units of analysis (Tripodi and Harrington, 1979). Interrupted time-series designs could be employed simultaneously for evaluations of effectiveness for individuals and for programs, providing that programmatic and individual objectives are similar. Second, the concepts of initiation, contact, and implementation can be applied to distinguish developmental stages in micro practice that are analogous to assessment of client problems and formulation of treatment plans, implementation of treatment plans, and termination and follow-up (Tripodi, 1983, pp. 21-24). Third, a logic of evaluative research design was developed that links designs to criteria for attaining levels of knowledge for evaluating either single-case interventions or social programs (Tripodi, 1983).

Differential evaluation is now viewed as a strategy for conducting evaluations that can be used by administrators and direct service practitioners. Its purpose is to provide information that is relevant to decisions that are made at appropriate stages of development (Tripodi, 1983, 1988). Perhaps its most important idea for differential research utilization is in its specification of development stages and location of practice decisions to which information on program or practice effectiveness can be applied.

### Incorporating Research into Practice

Incorporating research into practice is a strategy that involves the following ideas: (1) research concepts, principles, and methods are tools that can produce substantive information while practice is in process; (2) micro and macro social work practice require information to be effective and efficient; (3) decisions can be specified within developmental stages of practice; and (4) information generated by research tools can provide inputs for making practice decisions. These ideas were stimulated by Goldstein (1962, 1963) who regarded social work practice and social work research as problem solving models that progressed from the identification of a problem to its solution in the form of information or direct action with clientele, and by the notions of information feedback and stages of development contained within the strategy of differential evaluation.

The evolution of these ideas can be described in the following time periods: initial conception, 1971-1975; specification and application, 1976-1980; expansion, 1981-1985; and shifting perspective, 1986-present. Basic writings are referenced in Figure 1.

In the early 1970s a strategy for research incorporation was suggested which included the specification of a practice problem-solving model into tasks and functions; a determination of the correspondence of those tasks and functions with a problem-solving model of research, e.g., practice assessment as analogous to research problem formulation; the location of research procedures employed in the research analog to practice; and a consideration of the appropriateness of those research methods for practice (Tripodi, 1974). This strategy required a great deal of knowledge about practice and research, was cumbersome, and placed too much of a burden for research utilization on practitioners. It was not pursued further.

Another strategy required more specification of research methods for the purpose of facilitating their use by practitioners (Tripodi and Epstein, 1978; Epstein and Tripodi, 1978). Social work practice is divided into fields such as administration, community organization, and interpersonal practice. Then, a problem-solving model is used to locate decisions pertinent to practice. Finally, research tools applicable to those decisions are described and illustrated. This strategy was delineated further and applied to administration and clinical social work in *Research Techniques for Program Planning, Monitoring and Evaluation* (Epstein and Tripodi, 1977) and in *Research Techniques for Clinical Social Workers* (Tripodi and Epstein, 1980).

Conceptually, the notions of differential evaluation and incorporating methodological knowledge in practice overlap. This became evident as the idea of developmental stages from differential evaluation and from problem-solving models in research and practice merged when they were applied to both macro and micro practice in *Evaluative Research for Social Workers* (Tripodi, 1983). It was indicated that evaluative information could be used to inform either micro or macro practice at various stages of development, and the logic for applying research concepts and designs was regarded as similar, but with different units of analysis for practice and program effectiveness. This is illustrated further by Epstein and Grasso (1987) who show how differential evaluation and management information from Boysville's computerized system can be integrated in practice.

The concept of incorporating research into practice shifted from the articulation of research principles to apply in practice to a greater emphasis on the foundation of practice principles that contain research concepts. Hence, guidelines for constructing and evaluating practice prescriptions were developed, which include the notions of specification of a prescription, description of appropriate populations and situations to which it is applicable, justification for generalizing the prescription, limitations of its generalizability, and suggestions for conceptually generalizing the prescription to other populations (Wedenoja, Nurius, and Tripodi, 1988).

To deal with the problem of lack of research integration due to perceived inapplicability of measurement for nonbehavioral areas of interpersonal practice (Meyer, 1984), *Measurement in Direct Social Work Practice* (Blythe and Tripodi, in press) was developed to integrate research from a perspective of interpersonal practice. Measurement is discussed with respect to a typology of practice variables, and it is further articulated in chapters devoted to decisions within practice phases. Types of practice variables are considered in reference to assessment devices, such as DSM-III and eco maps; and research concepts are embedded in principles for assessing and prioritizing client problems, forming intervention hypotheses, and proceduralizing and evaluating interventions. Furthermore, measurement is discussed in regard to practice goals of maintenance and prevention, as well as change; and data analytic and graphic procedures are presented for using research information for evaluating progress in the context of practice.

## Research

Several research investigations in the 1970s indicated that researchers and practitioners could collaborate in developing treatment procedures and research protocols to monitor and evaluate treatment effectiveness in work with predelinquents, their families and schools. Those studies demonstrated that students could be trained to employ research protocols for the implementation and evaluation of treatment (Tripodi, 1974, pp. 182-185). As examples, two investigations followed the model of research, development, training, and evaluation in which research-based practice principles were modified, adapted, and developed; research protocols were devised; practitioners were trained to carry out specified treatments and use research protocols; and treatment effectiveness was evaluated. One study was an experimental evaluation of three time-constrained behavioral treatments for predelinquents and their families (Stuart and Tripodi, 1973). The results of treatment for 15, 45, or 90 days were studied in randomized pre-test/post-test comparison designs. The 15 day treatment was evaluated as most effective on a variety of measures related to desirable behaviors in school and at home. A second investigation analyzed the effectiveness of behavioral contracting (Stuart, Jayaratne, and Tripodi, 1976). Researchers and practitioners collaborated in devising therapeutic interventions and research protocols which were employed in training students to use the interventions with junior high school teachers, predelinquents, and their families. A randomized experimental design comparing behavioral treatment with a group discussion group serving as a placebo control showed the treatment group to be more successful on measures of community adjustment.

Of significance to the merging of practice and program evaluation is a research investigation in which there was a comparison of data synthesis procedures for aggregating the results of behavioral interventions in single-case studies (Jayaratne, Tripodi, and Talsma, 1988). Behavioral interventions were used in a family service agency to deal with individual, marital, and child management problems. Most notably, it was demonstrated that results from single-case interventions could be combined for use in program evaluation. Aggregation by proportions of success resulted in different conclusions than aggregations by effect sizes, as employed in meta-analyses of time-series data. It was concluded that an analysis of proportions was simpler to calculate and interpret, and contained fewer assumptions than the use of effect sizes.

A most encouraging development for the incorporation of methodological research is the work currently being done at Boysville. One investigation concentrated on the impact of the Boysville Management Information System on staff attitudes toward research, perceptions of factors that facilitate utilization, and self-reported research utilization that bears on practice decision-making (Grasso, Epstein, and Tripodi, 1988). Of interest here are the staff's reports of research utilization: 61% reported they used research information frequently or occasionally for assessing individual client change; 60% for planning client treatment; 55% in discussion with team members; 48% with students; and 45% with supervisors. These results on the uses of methodological research knowledge are remarkable when contrasted with those studies reporting on the extent to which practitioners use substantive research knowledge. Apparently, research utilization is facilitated when methodological research knowledge is incorporated to produce information that is accessible through computerization and relevant to practice decisions, and when staff are trained to use that knowledge.

## *FUTURE CONSIDERATIONS*

The concept of differential research utilization should be applied and evaluated in the teaching of research utilization skills to students and practitioners. Basic notions of differentiation with respect to assessment and to evaluation, as well as those pertaining to stages of program and practice development, will be modified and refined as social work practice changes its emphases in response to shifting priorities and changing social problems. Although the terms micro and macro practice were used here, attention needs to be paid to meso practice as a construct that can be employed for the integration of micro and macro practice issues and concerns. When new strategies are developed for processing information, substantive and methodological research knowledge may be relatively more accessible at the time when important practice decisions must be made.

Conceptual developments also should be in response to future research that might affect key ingredients of the process of differential research utilization. Suggestions for further research related to uses of substantive and methodological research knowledge follow.

### Substantive Research Knowledge

1. There should be investigations of the reliability of assessments of research with respect to levels of knowledge attainment.
2. Qualitative reviews of research in given domains should be compared with quantitative reviews for their accuracy, efficiency, and utility.
3. Different procedures for data synthesis for quantitatively reviewing research should be compared with respect to their accuracy, efficiency, and utility.
4. Qualitative and quantitative research reviews by experienced investigators should be compared with those of inexperienced investigators in given domains of inquiry.
5. Much more attention should be devoted to the analysis of the generalizability of research results.
6. Studies on utilization of substantive knowledge should continue to be conducted in the context of social agencies to determine the extent of usage by administrators, supervisors, and line workers in actual practice. Studies of practice simulations are less likely to provide meaningful information than field studies of practice since they are less immediate and relevant to practice decisions.

### Methodological Research Knowledge

1. There should be continued methodological development of ways to combine the results of single-case evaluations for use in program evaluation.
2. One problem in the evaluation of practice is that before-after studies are not always possible. If shown to be valid, the use of retrospective procedures would facilitate practice evaluation. Therefore, there should be comparisons of measurements or dependent variables before and after treatment with retrospective procedures. These studies should focus on behaviors, attitudes, and knowledge to determine when, if at all, retrospective procedures can produce results similar to those obtained by before and after measurement.
3. The utilization of methodological research knowledge by social workers in various stages of micro and macro practice should be studied.

4. Research should be conducted on the impact of research generating systems in practice, e.g., computerized information systems of variables reflecting client progress.
5. More research should focus on the relative efficiency of interventions for achieving practice goals of maintenance and prevention.
6. There should be continued development of research instruments and forms that can be adapted for purposes of assessment, monitoring, and evaluation in macro and micro social work practice.

## REFERENCES

Bielawski, B. and Epstein, I. (1984). Assessing program stabilization: an extension of the "differential evaluation" model. *Administration in Social Work*, 8, 13-23.

Billingsley, F., White, O.R. and Munson, R. (1980). Procedural reliability: a rationale and an example. *Behavioral Assessment*, 2, 229-241.

Bloom, M. and Fischer, J. (1982). *Evaluating practice: a guide for helping professionals*. New York, NY: Sage.

Blythe, B. and Tripodi, T. (in press). *Measurement in direct social work practice*. Beverly Hills, CA: Sage.

Bonjean, C.M. (1963). Community leadership: a case study and conceptual refinement. *American Journal of Sociology*, 68, 672-681.

Briar, S. (1980). Toward the integration of practice and research. In D. Fanshel (Ed.), *Future of social work research*, 31-37. Washington, DC: National Association of Social Workers.

Briar, S. (1979). Incorporating research into education for clinical practice in social work: toward a clinical science in social work. In A. Rubin and A. Rosenblatt (Eds.), *Sourcebook on research utilization*, 132-140. New York, NY: Council on Social Work Education.

Briar, S. and Blythe, B. (1985). Agency support for the outcomes of social work services. *Administration in Social Work*, 9, 25-36.

Briar S. and Miller, H. (1971). *Problems and issues in social casework*. New York, NY: Columbia University Press.

Brittain, J.M. (1970). *Information and its users*. New York, NY: Wiley Interscience.

Carter, R. (1972). Designs and data patterns in intensive experimentation. *Course monographs: research in interpersonal influence*. Ann Arbor, MI: University of Michigan School of Social Work.

Cohen, L.H., Sargent, M.M. and Sechreist, L.B. (1986). Use of psychotherapy research by professional psychologists. *American Psychologist*, 41, 198-206.

Corcoran, K. and Fischer, J. (1987). *Measures for clinical practice*. New York, NY: The Free Press.

Epstein, I. (1985). Quantitative and qualitative methods. In R.M. Grinnell, Jr. (Ed.), *Social work research and evaluation* (2nd ed.), 263-274. Itasca, IL: F.E. Peacock.

Epstein, I. and Grasso, A.J. (1987). Integrating management information and program evaluation: the Boysville experience. In C.V. Morton, M.L. Balasone, and S.R. Guendelman (Eds.), *Preventing low birth weight and infant mortality*, 141-152. Berkeley, CA: Proceedings of the 1986 Public Health Social Work Institute, University of California, Berkeley.

Epstein, I. and Tripodi, T. (1978). Incorporating research into macro social work practice and education. *Administration in Social Work*, 2, 295-305.

Epstein, I. and Tripodi, T. (1977). *Research techniques for program planning, monitoring and evaluation*. New York, NY: Columbia University Press.

Epstein, I., Tripodi, T. and Fellin, P. (1977). Community development programs and their evaluation. In T. Tripodi, P. Fellin, I. Epstein and R. Lind (Eds.). *Social workers at work*, (2nd ed). Itasca, IL: F. E. Peacock.

Fanshel, D. (1980), (Ed.). *Future of social work research*. Washington, DC: National Association of Social Workers.

Festinger, L. and Katz, D. (1953) (Eds.). *Research methods in the behavioral sciences*. New York, NY: The Dryden Press.

Finestone, S. (1959). The critical review of a research monograph: a teaching unit in a social work research course. In *Selected papers in methods of teaching research in the social work curriculum*, 33-37. New York, NY: Council on Social Work Education.

French, D.G. (1952). *An approach to measuring results in social work*. New York, NY: Columbia University Press.

Glass, G.V., McGaw, B. and Smith, M.L. (1981). *Meta-analysis in social research*. Beverly Hills, CA: Sage.

Goldstein, H.K. (1963). *Research standards and methods for social workers*. New Orleans, LA: Hauser Press.

Goldstein, H.K. (1962). Making practice more scientific through knowledge of research. *Social Work*, 7, 108-112.

Gottman, J.M. and Leiblum, S.R. (1974). *How to do psychotherapy and how to evaluate it: a manual for beginners*. New York, NY: Holt, Rinehart and Winston.

Grasso, A.J., Epstein, I. and Tripodi, T. (1988). Agency-based research utilization in a residential child care setting. *Administration in Social Work*, 12, 61-80.

Greenwood, E. (1960). Lectures in research methodology for social welfare students. *University of California syllabus series no. 388*, Berkeley, CA: University of California.

Greenwood, E. (1960). Social work research: a decade of reappraisal. *Social Service Review*, 311-320.

Hage, J. and Aiken, M. (1970). *Social change in complex organizations*. New York, NY: Random House.

Havelock, R.G. (1971). *Planning for innovation through dissemination and utilization of knowledge*. Ann Arbor, MI: Center for Research on Utilization of Scientific Knowledge, University of Michigan.

Herson, M. and Barlow, D.H. (1976). *Single-case experimental designs: strategies for studying behavior change*. New York, NY: Pergamon Press.

Hogarty, G.E. (1988). The meta-analysis of social work practice effects with the chronic mentally ill: a critique and reappraisal of the literature. Pittsburgh, PA: Western Psychiatric Institute, The University of Pittsburgh.

Hudson, W. (1982). *The clinical measurement package: a field manual*. Homewood, IL: Dorsey Press.

Jayaratne, S. and Levy, R. (1979). *Empirical clinical practice*. New York, NY: Columbia University Press.

Jayaratne, S., Tripodi, T. and Talsma, E. (1988). Comparative analysis and aggregation of single-case data. *Journal of Applied Behavioral Science*, 24, 119-128.

Kinesuk, T.J. and Sherman, R.E. (1968). Goal-attainment scaling: a general method for evaluating comprehensive community mental health programs. *Community Mental Health Journal*, 4, 443-453.

Kirk, S.A., Osmalov, M.J. and Fischer, J. (1976). Social worker's involvement in research. *Social Work*, 2, 121-124.

Levitt, J.L. and Reid, W.J. (1981). Rapid-assessment instruments for practice. In F.W. Seidl (Ed.). *Special issue on assessment. Social Work Research and Abstracts*, 17,13-20.

McCullough, L., Farrell, A.D. and Longabaugh, R. (1986). The development of a microcomputer-based mental health information system: a potential tool for bridging the scientist-practitioner gap. *American Psychologist*, 41, 207-214.

McMahon, P.M. (1987). Shifts in intervention procedures: a problem in evaluating human service interventions. *Social Work Research and Abstracts*, 23,13-16.

Meyer, C.H. (1984) (Editorial Page). Integrating research and practice. *Social Work*, 29, 323.

Miller, H. and Tripodi, T. (1967). Information accrual and clinical judgment. *Social Work*, 12, 63-69.

Morrow-Bradley, C.M. and Elliott, R. (1986). Utilization of psychotherapy research by practicing psychotherapists. *American Psychologist*, 41, 188-197.

Mullen, E.J. (1978). The construction of personal models for effective practice: a method for utilizing research findings to guide social interventions. *Journal of Social Service Research*, 2, 45-64.

Mutschler, E. (1979). Using single-case evaluation procedures in a family and children's service agency: integration of practice and research. *Journal of Social Service Research*, 3, 115-134.

Mutschler, E. and Hasenfeld, Y. (1986). Integrated information systems for social work practice. *Social Work*, 31, 345-349.

Nurius, P.S. (1984). Utility of data synthesis for social work. *Social Work Research and Abstracts*, 20, 23-32.

Nurius P. and Tripodi, T. (1985). The use of generalization procedures in empirical social work. *Social Service Review*, 59, 239-257.

Nurius, P., Wedenoja, M. and Tripodi, T. (1987). Prescriptions, proscriptions and generalization in social work direct practice literature. *Social Casework*, 68, 589-596.

Pillemer, D.B. and Light, R.J. (1980). Synthesizing outcomes: how to use research evidence for many studies. *Harvard Educational Review*, 2, 176-195.

Reid, W.J. and Hanrahan, P. (1982). Recent evaluations of social work: grounds for optimism. *Social Work*, 27, 328-340.

Rosenblatt, A. (1968). The practitioner's use and evaluation of research. *Social Work*, 13, 53-59.

Rothman, J. (1980). *Social R and D: research and development in the human sciences*. Englewood Cliffs, NJ: Prentice-Hall.

Rothman, J. (1978). Conversion and design in the research utilization process. *Journal of Social Service Research*, 2, 117-131.

Rubin, A. and Rosenblatt, A. (Eds.), (1979). *Sourcebook on research utilization*. New York, NY: Council on Social Work Education.

Siegel, D.H. (1988). Integrating data-gathering techniques and practice activities. In R.M. Grinnell, Jr. (Ed.). *Social Work Research and Evaluation* (3rd ed.), 465-482, Itasca, IL: F.E. Peacock.

Siegel, D.H. (1984). Defining empirically based practice. *Social Work*, 29, 325-331.

Siegel, D.H. and Reamer, F.G. (1988). Integrating research findings, concepts, and logic into practice. In R. M. Grinnell, Jr. (Ed.), *Social Work Research and Evaluation*, (3rd ed.), 483-502, Itasca, IL: F. E. Peacock.

Shapiro, D.A. and Shapiro, D. (1982). Meta-analysis of comparative therapy outcome studies: a replication and refinement. *Psychological Bulletin*, 92, 581-604.

Stuart, R.B. and Tripodi, T. (1973). Experimental evaluation of three time-constrained behavioral treatments for predelinquents and delinquents. In R.D. Rubin, J. P. Brady and J.D. Henderson (Eds.). *Advances in Behavior Therapy*, Vol. 4, New York, NY: Academic Press.

Stuart, R.B., Jayaratne, S. and Tripodi, T. (1976). Changing adolescent deviant behavior through reprogramming the behavior of parents and teachers: an experimental evaluation. *Canadian Journal of Behavioral Science*, 8, 132-144.

Suchman, E.A. (1967). *Evaluative research*. New York, NY: Russell Sage Foundation.

Thomas, E.J. (1984). *Designing interventions for the helping professions*. Beverly Hills, CA: Sage.

Thomas, E.J. (1978). Generating innovation in social work: the paradigm of developmental research. *Journal of Social Service Research*, 2, 95-115.

Thomas, E.J. (1967). *Behavioral science for social workers*. New York, NY: The Free Press.

Tripodi, T. (in press). Qualitative research methodologies. In J.G. McCullagh and P. Allen-Meares (Eds.). *Conducting research in the schools: a handbook for social workers*. Des Moines, IA: Iowa Department of Education.

Tripodi, T. (1988). A typology of research knowledge for relating research to social work practice. Paper presented at the 90th Anniversary of Columbia University School of Social Work. New York, NY: Columbia University.

Tripodi, T. (1984). Trends in research publication: a study of social work journals from 1956 to 1980. *Social Work*, 29, 353-359.

Tripodi, T. (1983). *Evaluative research for social workers*. Englewood Cliffs, NJ: Prentice-Hall.

Tripodi, T. (1982) (Editorial Page). Use of data synthesis in social work. *Social Work Research and Abstracts*, 18, 2.

Tripodi, T. (1981) (Editorial Page). Research utilization. *Social Work Research and Abstracts*, 4, 2.

Tripodi, T. (1974). *Uses and abuses of social research in social work*. New York, NY: Columbia University Press.

Tripodi, T. and Epstein, I. (1980). *Research techniques for clinical social workers*. New York, NY: Columbia University Press.

Tripodi, T. and Epstein, I. (1978). Incorporating knowledge of research methodology into social work practice. *Journal of Social Service Research*, 2, 65-78.

Tripodi, T. Epstein, I. and MacMurray, C. (1970). Dilemmas in evaluation: implications for administrators of social action programs. *American Journal of Orthopsychiatry*, 40, 850-857.

Tripodi, T., Fellin, P. and Epstein, I. (1971). *Social program evaluation*. Itasca, IL: F.E. Peacock.

Tripodi, T., Fellin, P. and Meyer, H.J. (1969). *The assessment of social research*. Itasca, IL: F.E. Peacock.

Tripodi, T. and Harrington, J. (1979). Use of time-series designs for formative program evaluation. *Journal of Social Service Research*, 3, 67-78.

Tripodi, T. and Miller, H. (1966). The clinical judgment process: a review of the literature. *Social Work*, 11, 63-69.

Videka-Sherman, L. (1984). Progress report to NASW Board of Directors, Harriett, M. Bartlett Practice Effectiveness Project. New York, NY: National Association of Social Workers.

Videka-Sherman, I. (1988). Meta-analysis of research on social work practice in mental health. *Social Work*, 33, 325-338.

Wedenoja, M., Nurius, P. and Tripodi, T. (1988). Enhancing mindfulness in practice prescriptive thinking. *Social Casework*, 69, 427-433.

Weinberger, R. and Tripodi, T. (1969). Trends in types of research reported in selected social work journals, 1956-65. *Social Service Review*, 43, 438-447.

# Integration of Practice and Research:
# Past, Present, and Future

## Scott Briar

The conference a decade ago on research utilization in social work and the subsequent monograph issued from it (Briar, Weissman, and Rubin, 1981) established a useful baseline for the status of research utilization in the profession at that time. This conference offers a rare and welcome opportunity to assess what progress has been made in the last decade and the direction that research utilization by social workers may take in the future.

One of the concepts discussed in the 1977 conference was that of the practitioner-scientist, defined at that time as follows:

> This concept means not only that the same person can both practice and conduct research, but also that he or she can engage in practice and research simultaneously as a set of integrated activities. This concept makes possible an empirically based model of practice. (Briar, 1980, p. 35)

The practitioner-scientist idea was controversial then; by 1989 the controversy had lessened, but persists.

Some practitioners and practice educators argue that introduction of research techniques and objectives into the practice situation distorts and contaminates the practice process in undesirable ways. On the other hand, some researchers contend that research conducted in the practice situation by practitioners will necessarily be flawed because of the differing objectives and contexts required for the two sets of activities (Thomas, 1978).

The classic example of this issue is that of withholding treatment from persons in a control group: Is that not unethical? A case in point is a recent decision to terminate an experiment investigating the effectiveness of a drug widely used in treating mild arrythmia because early results indicated strong negative effects on patients in the experimental group compared to the control cases. In this example it was the control patients who benefited more than those receiving the treatment. It is becoming clear that this is a false issue which serves to inhibit the introduction of a scientific perspective and commitment into social work practice. To see this most clearly, one needs only to observe and listen to sensitive, clinically astute students and practitioners who are integrating research techniques in their practice and are finding these additions useful in helping their clients.

Such criticisms are somewhat surprising in view of the frequent references in the literature of social work, throughout much of its history, to the basic similarities between the scientific method and the study-diagnosis-treatment model used in social work practice. In fact, this analogy often has been invoked to support the claim that social work is a scientific profession. For more than 70 years, social work has proclaimed that it is a scientific profession without examining, until recently, what being a scientific profession means, specifically, in social work practice. One of the benefits of the recent focus on research utilization in practice is that it has forced an examination of scientific practice.

The practitioner-scientist concept also has been criticized under the erroneous assumption that the research of practitioner scientists would rely on only one set of research designs; single-system designs. It is true that the emergence of single-system methodologies has made it possible for practitioners to conduct research on the effectiveness of their practices, but that does not preclude the use of other designs which are indispensable for certain research problems and questions. Related criticisms have come from some researchers and research educators who do not accept single-system designs as legitimate research designs. It is curious that some of the same researchers who have criticized the research validity of single-system designs at the same time have urged increased use of some demonstrably less rigorous qualitative methods.

## THE PRACTITIONER-SCIENTIST: TEN YEARS LATER

Beyond the continuing controversies of the past decade, there have been several important developments related to the practitioner-scientist concept. One of the appropriate questions raised about this concept is its feasibility. If practitioners learn how to use research tools for the evaluation of their practice, will they actually use them? And even if practitioners are motivated to use these research tools, will it be feasible for practitioners to use them in view of the constraints and obstacles they encounter in their practice settings?

Some of the early studies bearing on these questions were not encouraging (Kolevzon, 1975; Morelock et al., 1981; Siegel, 1982; Welch and Granwold, 1980). Students who received instruction in research tools and methods to evaluate their own practices subsequently engaged in practice evaluation activities to no greater extent than did students in comparison groups. However, most of these studies were based on small samples of students exposed to fairly time-limited and circumscribed instruction in research methods for practice evaluation.

In 1983, Blythe reported what still is the largest and most ambitious study of practice evaluation by social work practitioners (Blythe, 1983). Blythe surveyed 341 MSW graduates (representing six consecutive cohorts, from 1977 to 1982) who had been enrolled in a practice/research integration sequence, called educational units (EU), at the University of Washington. These EUs combined into one educational sequence four required courses—two research courses and two direct practice courses—plus the practicum in the second and third quarters of the first year. The research instruction included single-system as well as other research designs.

Blythe found that about 40% of the graduate respondents used one or more research designs in their practice during the previous year, and the designs ranged from surveys and single-group pretest-posttest studies to elaborate single-system designs. Is 40% an indicator of success or failure? Although the Blythe study did not use a comparison group, the 40% figure is nearly double comparable utilization figures reported in the studies cited earlier. Ultimately, the question about success may depend on whether one sees the cup as half empty or half full. As one of the faculty involved in establishing the EUs, I said at the outset that they should be considered a success if one student in ten used research designs and techniques in his or her practice following graduation. By that criterion, 40% is impressive. That aside, it does seem highly unlikely that the rate of utilization of research designs would have occurred in the absence of some special educational efforts.

Blythe's study went beyond molar questions about use of research designs. Her questionnaire also asked the practitioners to indicate the extent to which they performed, in their work with clients, each of 13 techniques involved in the evaluation of practice. Responses to these items indicated that, on the average, the practitioners used these techniques somewhere between "sometimes" and "quite often." A similar study by Gingerich (1982) also asked practitioners why they used research evaluation techniques in their practice. The reasons given by a majority of the practitioners who used these techniques were that these techniques facilitated intervention tasks, provided evidence of progress for the client, and yielded evidence of improvement for the practitioner. In other words, when practitioners do apply evaluation techniques in their practice they do so primarily because they find them useful, not because of some categorical imperative.

It is important to note that the work of Blythe and Gingerich expands the concept of research utilization by practitioners to include the utilization of research tools and techniques, not just the application of the *findings* of research studies which previously had been the primary focus of the literature on research utilization in social work. The use of research techniques (e.g., specification of objectives and interventions, measurement, monitoring, etc.) may be at least as important as the use of results from relevant studies. In fact, in the short run, use of research tools is more important because although we know a lot more about which practice methods are effective than we did ten years ago, empirically tested methods are not available for many practice problems. Therefore, if practitioners are to obtain systematic, empirical data about whether their clients are making progress, they must collect such data themselves.

Medicine provides a useful analogy. Most, if not all, the diagnostic tools used by physicians were originally developed as research tools that were subsequently incorporated into practice. And the pace at which new research tools are applied in medical practice appears to be increasing.

To summarize, over the past decade, we have learned that:

1. With sufficient training, social work practitioners can and many will use research in their practice.
2. Those practitioners who use research techniques in practice do so because they find it useful in helping their clients.
3. The concept of research utilization in social work practice should be expanded to give at least as much emphasis to use of research tools in practice as to the application of the findings of relevant studies.

There are, of course, many unanswered questions about the conduct of research by social workers as part of their practice. Some of the more important questions that need to be studied include: What contextual conditions facilitate use of research techniques by practitioners to evaluate their own practice? What is the relative validity of evaluative research conducted by social workers on their own practice? And are practitioners who evaluate their own effectiveness more effective in helping clients than practitioners who do not?

## *PRACTICE EVALUATION AND ACCREDITATION*

Another potentially important development in practice evaluation during the past decade came with the publication in 1984 by the Council on Social Work Education (CSWE) of new standards for the accreditation of social work education programs (CSWE, 1988). The 1984 standards, the first completely revised set of standards promulgated in several decades, include the following requirements pertaining to practice evaluation by practitioners:

7.15 The content on research should impart scientific methods of building knowledge for practice and of evaluating service delivery in all areas of practice. It should include quantitative and qualitative research methodologies; *designs for the sys-*

*tematic evaluation of the student's own practice;* and the critical appreciation and use of research and of program evaluation. *The plan for teaching research should be explicit in showing how content on research relates to the knowledge base and practice and skills that are included in the curriculum content of social work practice.*

7.16 *The professional foundation content on research should thus provide skills that will take students beyond the role of consumers of research and prepare them to evaluate their own practice systematically.* (CSWE, 1988, p. 127, emphasis added)

The Commission on Accreditation has interpreted the above standards, which apply to BSW and MSW programs, to mean that the tools and methods for evaluating their own practice must be addressed in practice courses as well as in research courses and in the practicum. As a member of the Accreditation Commission when the new standards went into effect and as the current chair of the Commission, I have had an opportunity to observe the impact that this new standard has had on social work education programs. For example, a number of BSW programs that previously relied on offerings in sociology or psychology departments for their foundation research courses, which have not covered methods for practice evaluation, have moved to offer their own research courses, sometimes recruiting new faculty for this purpose. Some MSW programs have added new required courses to cover the necessary material. Some programs have been required to take additional steps to correct inadequate attention to this standard in their programs.

Fraser and his colleagues (Fraser et al., 1988), in a carefully designed study, surveyed all accredited MSW programs to describe the content of research courses in graduate schools of social work and to examine the impact on research curricula of the new accreditation standards regarding preparation of students to evaluate their own practice. A questionnaire was administered by telephone with research sequence chairs. The study findings, which identify four distinct approaches to research curricula, raise a number of important questions for social work educators.

Regarding the impact of the new accreditation standards on research curricula, 86% of the research sequence chairs reported some kind of administrative response or curriculum adjustment (Fraser et al., 1988, p. 21) to the new standards, and 61.5% "reported actual curriculum revisions" (p. 21). Fraser concludes, "across most schools, the guidelines appear to have had a major influence on social work research education" (p. 21).

When asked about their degree of agreement with the new standards, more than 80% of the research sequence chairs said they agreed with the standards either "quite a lot" or "completely." When asked why they agreed with the standards, the dominant theme in the responses was, "a belief that the guidelines support empirically-based practice" (p. 20). However, there was not high consensus about which specific research skills should be taught.

It should be noted that the Fraser study was conducted in 1988, four years after the new accreditation standards were implemented. Since reaccreditation operates on a seven-year cycle and since programs often make modifications in response to new standards as they are preparing for review, Fraser's findings probably understate the extent of the impact of this new standard. In addition, Fraser's research did not investigate the extent to which the new standard has stimulated practice/research integration in practice classes and in the practicum. Nor did Fraser's study include the 360-plus accredited undergraduate social work programs to which the practice evaluation standards also apply.

One additional finding in the Fraser study should be mentioned. The research chairs were asked how new schools, or schools about to be reaccredited, should structure research curricula. The only theme that emerged clearly and consistently was that:

> They (the research sequence chairs) would advise schools to cultivate the practicum as a site in which students might apply their research knowledge and develop their research skills. The chairs admonished new schools of social work to avoid "separating" research from the practicum. (Fraser et al., 1988, p. 22)

This advice makes sense for at least two reasons. First, if developing skills in evaluating one's own practice is to be an objective, then the practicum is a logical place to develop such skills. Second, as countless surveys of graduates by schools of social work have found, the practicum is consistently identified by most graduates as the most important and influential component of their educational experience. If the integration of practice and research is modeled in the practicum, then students probably are more likely to emulate the integration of research and practice in their subsequent practice careers.

What has happened, then, is something that few would have thought possible ten years ago: that is, nearly all social work students are now receiving instruction in how to use research techniques to evaluate systematically their own practice. What will be the effects of this change?

Will there be a significant increase in the amount of practice research conducted by practitioners? It probably is too early to answer that question. If there is an increase, it is not clear where it would find a publication outlet. However, an increase in research conducted by practitioners was only one of the stated objectives of those who ten years ago were advocating what now has happened. A more important objective was to improve practice. Will social workers who systematically evaluate their practice be more effective practitioners than their predecessors who were not taught how to evaluate their practices? We do not know, of course; we need to address that question, but it will not be easy.

But such questions probably are premature. There are more immediate concerns that require attention if the potential benefits of this change in social work education are to be realized. One is the diversity in research instruction across schools of social work that is documented in Fraser's study. This does not come as a surprise to many of us, but Fraser's findings on this point are striking. There appears to be little consensus on what should be taught—whether about research in general or about the evaluation of practice in particular—and there is wide variation in what is taught. There is, of course, value in some diversity, but the extent and character of it give cause for concern about the uneven preparation of students in this area.

Another concern is if social workers do become more research-oriented in their practice, it can be expected that they will look more often to the findings of research studies for solutions to their practice problems. One problem is that the methodologies used in research, and especially the statistical tools, are becoming increasingly sophisticated and obscure to those without advanced training, thus diminishing the capacity of many practitioners to critically and selectively utilize such research. A recent example underscores the importance of this problem. The journal *Social Work* published recently a meta-analysis of social work practice effectiveness with the mentally ill (Videka-Sherman, 1988). This analysis drew conclusions about the most effective approaches to use in serving chronically mentally ill adults in the community. A few months after the meta-analysis appeared, one of the leading researchers in the field of chronic mental illness—who also is a social worker—wrote a detailed, lengthy, and devastating critique of this meta-analysis (Hogarty, 1989). The critique, not yet published, shows that not only were the conclusions of the meta-analysis invalid, but if they are applied by social workers working with the chronic mentally ill, they will have demonstrably deleterious effects on patients and their families. Very few social work practitioners currently are prepared to make the kind of critical analysis of a meta-analytic study required to identify the flaws in this particular application of the technique. We need to find ways to teach practitioners how to interpret and critically evaluate the use of new and advanced statistical tools without necessarily requiring that they undertake the extended study required to learn how to use them.

Until recently, the prevailing view regarding the objective of research instruction in social work education was to prepare students to be well-informed consumers of research findings. As studies of research utilization by social workers have indicated (Rosenblatt, 1968), however, social work education apparently was not very successful in preparing graduates who would use research findings to solve practice problems. Perhaps this failure was due, in part, to the reliance in research curricula on a model, exemplified in the texts used, designed to prepare researchers, not consumers. Education for research consumption should and could be different and more relevant to that objective and, as noted earlier, should give emphasis to research techniques and methods that can be used in social work practice. Thus, more effective education of social workers to be research consumers will require curriculum change and probably expansion of the research component in the curriculum.

## FUTURE DIRECTIONS

What about the future? What are the possibilities for encouraging the further integration of practice and research? There are many possibilities, but I can focus here on only a few that are especially promising.

First, as suggested earlier, part of research instruction — and especially the integration of research skills into practice — should be moved into the field practicum courses. As graduates consistently report, the practicum is the most influential part of the curriculum. If utilization of research tools and findings are taught and modeled in the field, it is likely to increase the probability that students will continue to follow this pattern in their practice careers. To move in this direction would require that schools: (1) provide the necessary training and consultation for agency-based practicum instructors, (2) utilize and cultivate agencies that welcome and support this development, and (3) link research instruction to the practicum. A number of educational programs have taken steps in this direction, some as part of their response to the new accreditation standards.

Second, movement of research skill instruction into the field also would open opportunities to study more closely the organizational obstacles graduates report they encounter when they try to use research tools in their practice, and to identify ways of surmounting these obstacles (Blythe and Briar, 1985).

Third, the efforts made during the past decade to develop tools that make it easier for practitioners to incorporate research into their practice are extremely important. Examples include the collection and creation of outcome measures that practitioners can use (which, in addition, facilitate comparisons across cases and workers) (Hudson, 1982), and the continuing efforts to develop computer programs to support practitioners (Mutschler and Cnann, 1985). Such efforts need to be continued in these and other areas, including, as one example, the development of valid techniques for aggregating outcome results, including outcomes of single-subject design studies.

Finally, perhaps the highest priority needs to be given to the encouragement and support of one of the most important developments of the past decade; the emergence of significant, successful, and useful developmental research efforts designed to discover more effective interventions. There are three examples of such efforts: (1) the impressive work of Hogarty and his colleagues (Schooler and Hogarty, 1987) on how best to provide community-based service to chronic mentally ill adults; (2) the collaborative efforts between Homebuilders and the University of Washington in devising more effective ways of helping families and children at risk of abuse and neglect (Whittaker et al., 1988); and (3) the developmental work of VanDenBerg et al. (1988) on an intensive community support model to serve the most severely disturbed children. All three of these examples are directed to major social problems and have demonstrated dramatically successful results.

While single studies of effectiveness can be extremely useful in providing suggestive guidelines for practitioners and program developers, it usually takes a developmental research effort to refine and adequately test the effectiveness of an intervention model. Such developmental efforts are not easily conducted by solo practitioners working alone, but they cannot be conducted without the active participation of practitioners as research colleagues. Two of the obstacles to the expansion of developmental research to devise more effective interventions are (1) absence of funds, and (2) lack of acceptance by some research funding agencies of the methodologies used in developmental research. Concerted efforts are needed to educate funding agencies about the importance of investing in developmental research for the social services.

Clearly, the foundation for empirically based practice is more firmly established and accepted than it was a decade ago. With this foundation, the profession is in a stronger position to demonstrate that social work can make significant contributions to the reduction of major social and human problems.

# REFERENCES

Blythe, B. J. (1983). An examination of practice evaluation among social workers. Unpublished doctoral dissertation, University of Washington.

Blythe, B. J., & Briar, S. (1985). Agency support for evaluating the outcomes of social work services. *Administration in Social Work, 9*(2), 25-36.

Briar, S. (1980). Toward the integration of practice and research. In D. Fanshel (Ed.), *Future of social work research* (pp. 31-37). Washington, DC: National Association of Social Workers.

Briar, S., Weissman, H., & Rubin, A. (eds.) (1981). *Research Utilization in Social Work Education.* New York: Council on Social Work Education.

Council on Social Work Education, Commission on Accreditation. (1984). *Handbook of accreditation standards and procedures*: Washington, DC: Council on Social Work Education.

Council on Social Work Education, Commission on Accreditation. (1988). *Handbook of accreditation standards and procedures*: Washington, DC: National Association of Social Workers.

Fraser, M. W., Lewis, R. E., & Norman, J. L. (1988, March). Research education in M.S.W. programs: Four competing perspectives. Paper presented at the Annual Program Meeting of the Council on Social Work Education, Chicago.

Gingerich, W. J. (1982, March). Teaching students to use single-case evaluation methods: Enhancing generalization from classroom to practice setting. Paper presented at the Annual Program Meeting of the Council on Social Work Education, New York.

Hogarty, G. E. (1989). The meta-analysis of social work practice effects with the chronic mentally ill: A critique and reappraisal of the literature. Unpublished manuscript.

Hudson, W. W. (1982). *The clinical measurement package: A field manual.* Homewood, IL: Dorsey Press.

Kolevzon, M. A. (1975). Integrational teaching modalities in social work education: Promise as pretense? *Journal of Education for Social Work, 11*(2), 60-67.

Morelock, M., Connaway, R. S., & Gentry, M. E. (1981, March). Evaluation of the effects of research content on social work practice activities. Paper presented at the Annual Program Meeting of the Council on Social Work Education, Louisville.

Mutschler, E., & Cnann, R. (1985). Success and failure of computerized information systems: Two case studies in human service agencies. *Administration in Social Work, 9*(1), 67-69.

Rosenblatt, A. (1968). The Practitioners Use and Evaluation of Research. *Social Work,* 13, 53-59.

Schooler, N. R., & Hogarty, G. E. (1987). Medication and psychosocial strategies in the treatment of schizophrenia. In Meltzer, Bunny, Coyle et al. (Eds.), *Psychopharmacology: The third generation of progress* (pp. 1111-1119). New York: Raven Press.

Siegel, D. H. (1982). A study of the integration of research and practice in social work education. Unpublished doctoral dissertation, University of Chicago.

Thomas, E. J. (1978). Research and service in single-case experimentation: Conflicts and choices. *Social Work Research and Abstracts, 14*(4), 20-31.

VanDenBerg, J. Born, D. G., & Risley, T. R. (1988). Status report: The Alaska youth initiative. Juneau, AK: Department of Health and Social Services.

Videka-Sherman, L. (1988). Meta-analysis of research on social work practice in mental health. *Social Work, 33*, 325-338.

Welch, G. J., & Granwold, D. (1980, March). Does it work? Training students to evaluate their casework practice. Paper presented at the Annual Program Meeting of the Council on Social Work Education, Los Angeles.

Whittaker, J. K., Kinney, J., Tracy, B. M., & Booth, C. (Eds.). (1988). *Improving practice technology for work with high risk families: Lessons from the "Homebuilders" social work education project.* Seattle, WA: Center for Social Welfare Research, School of Social Work, University of Washington.

# Creating Tools for Intervention: The Convergence of Research Methodologies

### Jack Rothman

The organizers of the conference have asked me to peer over my shoulder to note changes and developments that have occurred with the R&D model over the last ten years. Keenly aware of what happened to Lot's wife when she looked back, I will, nevertheless, play intrepid historian, stoically awaiting the forthcoming critical shakedown by my caustic colleagues. Actually, my gaze will span a 20-year time period since I began this type of research activity in 1968, and published the basic formulation of the Research and Development Model in 1974 (Rothman, 1974). My reflections will be of two types: conceptual ruminations on the model itself and observations related to its implementation.

## *INTERVENTION DESIGN AND DEVELOPMENT AS AN OVERARCHING CONCEPT*

An important realization that has crystallized for me over time is that research and development is but one branch of a broader school of problem-solving research endeavor, having the goal of producing innovative intervention technology that addresses practice and policy deficiencies. In addition to Social R&D (Rothman, 1980), it includes Thomas' (1978a) developmental research, Fairweather's (1967) experimental social innovation, the behavioral community assessment approach of Fawcett and his associates (1980), and the educational R&D school (Baker and Schultz, 1971). Recent works by Reid (1987), Whittaker et al. (1989), and Mullen (1989), among others, have been influenced by this perspective.

The umbrella term "Intervention Design and Development" (ID&D) has been devised recently by Rothman and Thomas to encompass their work as well as similar modalities. Although no single phrase is able to capture the complexity in the process and the nuances of difference, ID&D seems to be a serviceable cognitive handle, which, in Herbert Simon's pragmatic wording, should be "satisficing" for immediate purposes.

Intervention design and development commonly entails a particular series of sequential and interconnected activities that culminate in the creation of innovative intervention tools. I have previously delineated these steps as follows (Rothman, 1989):

1. Identify critical practice-related issues/problems;
2. Retrieve pertinent existing research findings, practical/practice information, and related particular or situational knowledge on the subject;
3. Synthesize existing empirical research knowledge and formulate supportable scientific generalizations;
4. Aggregate relevant situational information, including proposed solutions, policies, and programs from knowledgeable professionals, civic leaders, clients, and other sources including social indicators, agency records, and professional practice journals;
5. Design intervention modalities derived from the varied knowledge sources;
6. Field test these programs in pilot sites and establish a working model of the intervention for more advanced development;
7. Conduct developmental research of implementation of the intervention in additional field sites — operationalization, proceduralization, and evaluation of the intervention;
8. Package positively evaluated and adequately developed programs in appropriate user-ready form (handbooks, posters, and videotapes) for use by professionals in the community;
9. Use trainers and dissemination processes to widely diffuse developed program packages to agencies and professionals. This research regimen can be applied equally to creating micro and macro practice methods, both within each of the branches of

ID&D as well as collectively in the overarching evolving school.

The core sequential components may not be accepted by all researchers in precisely this language or configuration, but the listing indicates the essential thrust of the developmental approach and approximates a common framework. Advantages of acknowledging the commonality include optimizing conceptual advancement through drawing forth the strongest elements from each branch, and promoting enhancement by building a critical mass of scholarship sufficient to have an impact on various social sciences and social professions. Presently, each of the separate efforts is small and isolated within its discipline, and is therefore somewhat encapsulated intellectually. The maxim about unity conferring strength aptly applies here. There is a danger, however, of premature closure, which might hinder promising avenues of exploration within each branch. However, the existence of a common rubric and conceptual orientation should not be perceived as discouraging continuation of concurrent work within each of these scholarly thrusts.

The need to advance this area of endeavor is evident. Because it explicitly aims to create, expand, and enhance the tools of a professional practice, ID&D is the most relevant research methodology currently available for social work and the other social professions. The central omission of these professional fields is to make beneficial changes in society, employing reliable, knowledge-driven methods of intervention. ID&D has as its central mission the production of such intervention instrumentalities for use in practice. The match between these missions is clear and compelling.

## *RECENT DEVELOPMENTS*

Several newer conceptual and methodological refinements in ID&D have emerged recently. Also, some key problems and issues have been sharpened.

### Complexity and Multiple Method Character

It has become clear that ID&D is a complex process that entails a series of different interlocked research tasks and methods. The early stage may involve needs assessment techniques and procedures of library science and meta-analysis. The middle stage is characterized by field experiment methods and evaluation research. The final stage requires diffusion studies and marketing research. This diversity or multiplicity of research methods and traditions joined together sequentially in one holistic research endeavor, may be one reason that it is difficult to communicate the nature of ID&D to uninitiated colleagues and to implement the paradigm. ID&D may be conceived as a meta-research methodology. It has a distinct methodological character, but this involves incorporation of a number of already existing methods that are in common use, such as needs assessment, clinical trials, experimental field study, evaluation research, and others. It is the configuration of these various methods and the aim to which they are directed that gives ID&D its particular quality.

### Producing Practice Technology
### vs. Producing Practice Knowledge

A fundamental purpose of ID&D, as stated earlier, is to set forth the procedures of reliable intervention. It is research *for* practice, not *about* practice. Without the output of practice aids the method in any particular case can be said not to have reached its objective. However, research procedures are employed at every stage, and systematic data are gathered. Thus, there are incipient or potential knowledge products available at each stage. Any development project experiences tension between these two goals (Thomas 1978b). For example, a needs assessment or meta-analysis near the onset conducted as a practical activity to lead into the next stage can readily yield a paper or article if the researcher undertakes to exploit that data toward that end. Indeed, based on the work of our research team in the Community Intervention Project, one or more books materialized from the knowledge retrieval and synthesis stage (Rothman 1974), the pilot testing and development stage (Rothman et al., 1976; Rothman et al., 1977), and the diffusion stage (Rothman et al.,

1983). Substantial academic contributions have been made by other proponents and experimenters as an aspect of pursuing pragmatic ends. Knowledge contributions are an option or a discretionary result, similar to the situation in industrial R&D. There, new scientific knowledge is generated (as in Bell Labs or the space program) in some cases; in other instances new consumer products alone suffice and the team pushes on to the next pragmatic venture.

The issue of knowledge product versus practice product has also preoccupied the field of educational R&D. Borg (1969) states that the most prominent question of strategy in that field has been: "What should be the relative balance in an R&D program between research and evaluation on the one hand and development on the other?" (p. 5). Without providing a precise formula, he indicates that in his work he decided upon, "testing at least one or two important research hypotheses during the development of each mini-course" (p. 11). Other educational developers state: "Every phase of development can serve as a highly heuristic source of expanding the limits of elegant and sophisticated educational research" (Baker and Schultz, 1971, p. xx).

It may be assumed that when ID&D is carried out under the sponsorship of or in the context of a university structure, as is likely in the period ahead, the knowledge component needs to be included as a co-product. This provides the justification for university involvement. It also provides both the justification for faculty researcher involvement and the payoff in scholarship that enables the researcher to enjoy academic career advancement concomitant to this activity.

### Institutional Base

Intervention research is a complex, multidisciplinary, multifunctional process, requiring a relatively long time-frame for full implementation. For this reason, it is probably not useful to conceive of it in the traditional terms of the solo entrepreneurial researcher. For maximum effectiveness it needs to be situated in an institutional base that provides an enabling environment. This environment may offer resources (facilities, staff, equipment), funding, legitimation, "clout" in dealing with community agencies, and continuity over time. The base could be a professional school or a relevant subunit, such as a research center within the school. In my own case, after proceeding slowly through all the phases of this research process over almost a decade, formulating and refining the model and piloting the method itself along the way, it became obvious that further development would require a substantial structural home.

The analogue is industrial R&D, which is conducted typically through a lab, a center, or mission-oriented independent organization. Accordingly, at UCLA we established the Center for Child and Family Policy Studies to fulfill this purpose. Intervention design and development exists as a specialized unit, the R&D Program, within the Center. Without that structural support the work would have been impeded, or it would have taken a different form with less collaborative interplay with local agencies aimed at critical community-based problems. Fairweather (1967) devotes a considerable portion of his analysis to this structural issue in his discussion of "forming the research team" and building an organizational platform as a requirement for implementing this type of research activity.

The rationale for an academic unit supporting this approach, from a dean's point of view, has been articulated as follows:

> Professional education of the highest quality requires mechanisms to link research and practice, to assure that research is directed to the solution of practice-relevant problems, and that attention is given to the diffusion and utilization of research findings.

> To make this possible, a laboratory environment is required to allow faculty and students to develop, test, and practice the profession's methods at the most advanced state of the art. Pilot and demonstration projects are needed to test new ideas, to increase the range and excitement of field learning opportunities, and to place faculty and students at the cutting edge of new and innovative developments in service delivery . . .

> The R&D approach supplies us with the methodology to use in such a laboratory environment. It translates existing social sci-

ence research into practical action principles that can be applied to the delivery of social services . . .

Expanded collaboration with colleagues in practice will enrich our course offerings and help to keep our scholarship focused on practice-relevant issues. (Schneiderman, 1986, p. 2)

## *Interinstitutional Relations*

Given an institutional base, field research in community agencies can be conceptualized as interinstitutional relations. Fairweather and Tornatzky (1977) give a great deal of emphasis to such collaborative arrangements, referring to them as "interorganizational agreements." They speak of the need to negotiate a contract for "providing the research team with the social conditions under which (ID&D) experiments can be carried out" (p. 123). In their view, such agreements should be formal, in writing, and before-the-fact. Some areas they note as requiring specification include: funding, control of access to staff and clients, sampling procedures, publication rights, roles and relationships of personnel, news releases and publicity, and stability of the intervention design or program. While stressing the importance of promulgating such pre-established agreements, the authors also acknowledge the unstable nature of the ID&D environment. Each operational problem that has "ostensibly been 'solved' by developing a pre-experimental agreement, is likely to emerge again when the research action begins." Thus, the ID&D researcher should realize that "the organizational glue holding these agreements together is thin," and it is wise to "avoid a feeling of overconfidence" (p. 148).

Strategies for optimizing the possibilities for productive work in agency settings can benefit from theory and research from the field of interorganizational analysis. The value of this approach is illustrated in a paper by Hasenfeld and Furman (1989) who point out that this type of research engagement can usefully be approached from the exchange theory standpoint. Each organization (the school and the agency) has something to offer the other and something to gain from the other (research capability, knowledge, student aid, and credibility on the one hand, and access to clients, staff, interesting problematic situations, and funding on the other). When these sets of factors balance off relatively evenly, the optimal conditions are brought about for agency-centered research. The advantage of an institutional base is that it brings substantial potency to negotiating the exchange relationship beyond what the independent researcher has available, thus buttressing the researcher's claims in seeking a favorable research climate.

In this type of arrangement we have found it helpful to symbolize and formalize the institutional connection by having the agreements concluded at the highest organizational level. This has meant that the "contract" governing project work is made by the chief executive officers of both organizations; the dean or research center director and the agency director. Ongoing project activity is at the level of the program directors and line staff, but all policy issues and major operational problems are "bumped" up to the top for resolution. Sometimes we have done this when it was not essential in order to reinforce the interinstitutional association and the formal basis for that linkage. Final reports, feedback meetings, and public dissemination of findings, likewise, are occasions for involving the organizational heads. These events are viewed as opportunities for institutional reinforcement rather than as bureaucratic hurdles impeding the research process.

## Amalgam Between Problem Solving and Research Processes

ID&D is at its core a *problem-solving process*, out of which specifically targeted intervention techniques are created to confront presenting difficulties. R&D specialists Andreasen and Hein (1987) indicate that a basic "description of development activities is General Problem Solving" (p. 117). However, this is *research-rooted problem solving*. It involves a slower, more deliberate, rational, and controlled approach to problem solving than could occur or be used normally in the practice environment. This connection between problem solving and empirical study symbolizes the wedding of research and practice inherent in ID&D. It also suggests that this mode of research will probably not be adopted widely by the social science disciplines. It is, rather, a methodology of greater relevance to researchers in the social professions, for whom practice should be a fundamental concern.

Problem solving as a metaphor for the process also relates back to the initiating impulse for any intervention research undertaking. In my original diagrammatic depiction of the Social R&D Model in 1974, basic social research knowledge was the stated starting point of the process. Later experience has indicated that while R&D can emanate out of a push from new knowledge, the more typical mode is through initial concern over a problematic condition. The model has been revised to reflect the more usual pattern. This analysis applies in similar fashion to industrial R&D where a demand from consumers or a new scientific or technological breakthrough can be the impetus for a development undertaking. The typical impetus, however, is from actual or potential demand from consumers.

### Multiple Discipline Contributions

There is growing recognition of the value of perspectives from various disciplines as useful knowledge sources for advancing ID&D. There is high potential in certain tendencies within community psychology and sociological practice, operations research and evaluation research. The policy sciences are another useful resource. Illustratively, policy sciences offer techniques for problem analysis, and evaluation research provides methods of process evaluation and utilization-focused evaluation. My own work in social R&D has drawn heavily on engineering and industrial research and development, and Thomas' developmental research has drawn on applied behavioral assessment, as has Fawcett's endeavors. It can be argued that these are not conflicting perspectives, but rather each offers different and compatible grounding for ID&D development.

### Multiple Information Sources

In the early phases of the ID&D process, information about the focal problem can be sought from a number of different knowledge areas. In addition to (1) *empirical research knowledge*, there are (2) *general professional practice experience and knowledge*, as reported in journals, books, conference papers, etc., and (3) *particular/situational information* from relevant knowledgeable individuals in the local study setting: clients, professionals, citizens, activists, etc. The information configuration that is constructed depends on the problem under study and the availability of different information resources. This aspect of the work can entail retrieval of existing information, or gathering original data.

Because of a long-standing interest in research utilization, my associates and I originally placed a great deal of emphasis on using existing empirical research findings to inform intervention design. This has involved a meta-analysis methodology employing systematic research synthesis, and has been applied to numerous subject areas, such as community change (Rothman, 1974); ideology of planners (Rothman and Hugentobler 1986); culturally based family intervention (Rothman et al., 1985); serving runaway and homeless youth (Rothman with David, 1986); and case management for the chronically mentally ill (Rothman, 1987). The approach that has evolved entails a methodology of conceptual integration of research findings rather than a quantitative common metric (Rothman, Damron and Shenassa, 1989). The approach is particularly suited to the ID&D context because of its shorter time frame and emphasis on application.

I believe the pool of existing empirical knowledge should be a major input to ID&D, but that view may be a matter of style or belief. In the fledgling field of research for intervention design and development, there are as yet no clear data to indicate which are the most useful knowledge sources for novel applications, generally or in particular cases. This suggests more research and experience, as well as openness to a wide range of sources including, as suggested by Thomas, allied technology, applied research, legal policy, etc. (Thomas, 1984).

### Design and Pilot Testing Overlay

Project experience has shown that the pilot testing stage is highly interactive with the design stage that precedes it. Feedback here may be frequent to the point that intervention testing and design construction in some ways blend into one another. Bacon and Butler (1981), speaking of this process in the industrial sphere, state: "Several iterations may be necessary . . . before a suitable product is developed'' (p. 176). In other situations the demarcation between the two phases may be more distinct. In some cases the design stage per se may require field exploration. This will likely occur where the intervention is complex and available knowledge is sparse. For example, in developing a procedural pattern for carrying out the case management role, we delineated from a literature search 15 different functions having varying possible relationships to one another. Rather than speculating *a priori* on the patterned relationship among the functions, the design effort involved a field survey of case managers on their views of the sequencing and relationships of the functions. We followed this with a small scale pilot implementation of the functions in practice in order to sharpen the design (Rothman 1987, 1988).

## *Scope of Coverage*

Several different emphases have been brought to bear in the amalgam comprising ID&D. One is the *research utilization* emphasis, which is concerned about specific means by which empirical knowledge created in the social sciences can be made to influence professionals and other applied people. Some typical work along these lines has examined the mechanisms by which research is used by policy makers and public officials (Weiss and Bucavalas, 1980). The point of departure is research findings, and the objective is to examine ways to put them to use. Another emphasis is *empirically based practice*, where the point of departure is enhancing the effectiveness of professional helpers and change agents. Research findings and methods are drawn upon heavily to achieve this purpose (Briar, 1973). A third emphasis is concerned with the *diffusion of innovations*, focusing on widescale impact on problem conditions through broad utilization of knowledge (Glaser et al., 1983). The point of departure is new ideas and practices, and the objective is to stimulate their spread through relevant systems.

A question may be raised as to whether ID&D should encompass all of these perspectives and objectives or limit its scope within the range. In particular, there is the issue as to whether diffusion ought to be incorporated as a basic component. It can be argued that the work should concentrate on intervention development, with diffusion as a related but external factor. In industrial R&D, for example, R&D personnel keep their sights on the creation of the product, and then pass it on to separate branches of manufacturing, marketing, and sales.

During the present emergence of ID&D such an organic division of labor does not exist. The ID&D team needs to oversee both manufacturing (production of a handbook, manual, visual aids, etc.) and dissemination, if utilization is a serious consideration. There are no built-in instrumentalities to pick up sequential tasks down the line. In his work, Fairweather directed almost as much effort to disseminating his lodge treatment model among mental health organizations as in devising the intervention (Fairweather et al., 1974). Mathews and Fawcett (1985) gave concerted attention to the dissemination of a job-finding skills guide they developed. In our Community Intervention Project, substantial effort went into diffusing a handbook on community outreach techniques to community mental health professionals (Rothman et al., 1983).

These examples from projects in the field suggest both that including diffusion as a phase is a rather common practice in this research area, and that it may be necessary given the constraints of the current situation. In addition, the diffusion stage affords opportunities for important research on how to reach and motivate potential users of the practice innovations that are developed. In the Community Intervention Project we were able to study and evaluate such theoretical/practical issues as workshop versus mass communications approaches, the level at which to enter a target organization, internal versus external workshop leadership, and types of reference group appeals to potential users. The Fairweather team, likewise, combined the dissemination of the "lodge model" with substantive research on fostering utilization in organizations.

## SOME PROBLEMS AND ISSUES

Probably a much longer list of problems than developments could be compiled. Only a few that seem particularly salient will be introduced here.

## Labs vs. Agency Setting

What are the benefits and disadvantages of using project-directed laboratory settings for pilot testing versus using more open agency situations? Each approach has different benefits to offer, best characterized in terms of control of variables as contrasted with manipulation of a naturalistic environment that is equivalent to ultimate implementation setting. In work conducted by ID&D researchers, both approaches have been employed, with the naturalistic predominating. As yet no "smoking gun" of proof regarding superiority has been discovered, but it is evident that employment of the intervention in the intended end-user situation is essential at some time before the development phase has been completed.

## Procedural Completeness of the Intervention

What degree of specificity and completeness is useful in the procedural descriptiveness of an intervention (Thomas et al., 1987)? Do all possibly discernible details of implementation need to be delineated? Can there be alternative patterns of implementation in carrying out a given basic intervention design? How much room should be left for practitioner discretion? How much for reinvention during the diffusion/adoption period? Is reinvention a beneficial occurrence or a confounding difficulty?

## Character of the Focal Problem

How does the selection of an initial problem by an agency affect the intervention research process? There may be central versus peripheral problems on the agency's agenda, and problems related to organizational politics versus professional service goals (Hasenfeld and Furman, 1989). In our work with a county child serving department, the issue of runaway and homeless youth was selected by agency representatives for attention. In part this was because the runaway issue had created a great deal of turmoil in the community and there was an obvious gap in available programs. But at the same time this was an area out of the mainstream of child welfare professional concern, with its heavy emphasis on child protective services, adoption and foster placement for young children. Our research team produced visible results through a research and development approach. The methodology was not generalized for application in the core service areas (Rothman with David, 1986; Rothman et al., 1989).

In another instance, our Center was asked to deal with the question of proper caseload size for staff. It surfaced very quickly that the main motivation was not to arrive at an optimal arrangement in terms of service provision. The concern, rather, had a more political aspect. There was a high degree of conflict in the organization about numbers of clients carried in the caseload, with different views being advocated by the staff union, administrative and supervisory personnel, an advisory citizens group, and the county board of supervisors. The director's objective in approaching the University was to quell dissention and arrive at some kind of compromise that carried with it legitimation and an aura of objectivity. The aim, in a sense, was to "bury the issue" as an organizational irritant. How would this kind of atmosphere affect the viability and validity of the research?

### Slow Growth

There are difficulties, as stated previously, in conveying the ID&D concept to colleagues in the research community. The result has been a slow rate of dissemination of the methodology and halting advancement, conceptually and methodologically. Recognition of this circumstance has led to some attention to the diffusion issue. At the suggestion of a group of doctoral students, we organized at UCLA a specialized national conference on the subject. As an outgrowth of that event, there potentially may emerge a network of ID&D researchers, including scholars from diverse disciplines who are already involved in intervention research, particularly psychology, sociology, psychiatry, and educational R&D, as a way of expanding the base of participation. Another approach my colleagues and I have taken is to conduct a varied set of studies involving community intervention, problems of runaway and homeless youth, case management for the chronically mentally ill, and health promotion for inner-city minority communities, geared to demonstrate the reality of this approach as a research modality and the different forms it may take. The cumulative mass of studies overall in the field, however, is still quite small.

## Academic Constraints

A number of practical problems exist for intervention research scholars around such matters as promotions, tenure, funding, status, acquiring agency research sites, etc. These have contributed to the slow diffusion noted above. As with any innovative idea or technology, there are resistances and misunderstandings to be overcome. Some approaches to this will be discussed in the next section.

## THE NEXT STEPS

It is obvious that the next steps in intervention research ought to include concerted examination of the problem areas just described. These alone constitute a considerable agenda and will require work over an extended time. Some other issues, however, also compete for attention.

There is a need for a book of case illustrations of intervention research so that the process is made clearer, more concrete, and reality-based for those who have had no involvement. Currently, a number of researchers who are potential appliers perceive an abstract and amorphous set of ideas that they do not know how to begin to use. The case illustration compendium would concretize the methodology and might stimulate more widely distributed efforts.

Along the same lines, there is a need for a methodology textbook that sets forth in detail and in systematic fashion the procedural steps for doing design and development. The absence of such a resource is analogous in conventional basic research to having available concepts and bits and pieces of methodology in scattered articles and general analytical and expository books, but no standard "how to" textbooks. This area sorely needs such a resource as a platform for further development.

On an even more pragmatic level, those new to intervention research and younger faculty members have expressed a need for a professional survival manual for coping with academic impediments. The nature of the research is not understood among colleagues, resulting in blocks to gaining tenure promotion and acceptance for dissertation projects. Outside of the university, difficulties are experienced in obtaining entré to agencies and maintaining sustained collaborative relationships. Acquiring funding for studies is also a particular burden because grant-providing organizations almost uniformly evaluate study proposals from the perspective of traditional research methodology. A survival manual with practical advice, examples of successful tactics, information resources to call upon, and such would be a welcome document for those undaunted scholars wanting to enter into this uncertain realm.

As an example, the previous discussion on creating research products versus technical products brought forth the notion that research can and should accompany effort toward such practice enhancement objectives as composing practitioner manuals. It also indicated that such research products are feasible at each successive stage, not only at the terminal point of this rather protracted process. Such perspectives offer both guidance and encouragement for proceeding with research endeavors, while addressing necessary academic considerations and career imperatives.

Overall, there is a need for more activity and more projects of varying types in order to provide cumulative experience which can be used to further both methodology and conceptual underpinnings. If this can be done with close communication and collaboration of colleagues in various disciplines, a more extensive foundation for analysis will accrue.

## BIBLIOGRAPHY

Andreasen, M., and L. Hein. (1987). *Integrated Product Development*. Berlin: Springer-Verlag.

Bacon, F. R. Jr., and T. W. Butler, Jr. (1981). *Planned Innovation*. Ann Arbor: University of Michigan.

Baker, R. L., and R. E. Schultz. (1971). *Instructional Product Development*. New York: Von Nostrand Reinhold Co.

Borg, W. R. (1969). "The Balance Between Educational Research and Development: A Question of Strategy," *Educational Technology*, 5(7):5-11.

Briar, S. (1973). "Effective Social Work Intervention in Direct Practice: Implications for Education." In *Facing the Challenge*. New York: Council on Social Work Education.

Fairweather, G. W. (1967). *Methods for Experimental Social Innovation*. New York: John Wiley & Sons.

Fairweather, G., and L. G. Tornatzky. (1977). *Experimental Methods for Social Policy Research*. New York: Pergamon Press.

Fairweather, G. W., D. H. Sanders, and L. G. Tornatzky. (1974). *Creating Change in Mental Health Organizations*. New York: Pergamon Press.

Fawcett, S. B., R. M. Mathews, and R. K. Fletcher. (1980). "Some Promising Dimensions for Behavioral Community Technology," *Journal of Applied Behavioral Analysis*, (13)3.

Glaser, E.M., H. H. Abelson, and K. N. Garrison. (1983). *Putting Knowledge To Use*. San Francisco: Jossey-Bass.

Hasenfeld, Y., and W. Furman. (1989). "Social Research and Development as an Interorganizational Exchange." Paper presented at the National Conference on Intervention Research, Los Angeles, School of Social Welfare, Center for Child and Family Policy Studies California, University of California, Los Angeles, March 19-21, 1989.

Hedge, D. M., and J. W. Mok. (1989). "The Research Values of Policy Analysts." *Knowledge in Society: The International Journal of Knowledge Transfer*, 2(1):21-41.

Mathews, R. M., and S. B. Fawcett. (1985). "Assisting in the Job Search: A Behavioral Assessment and Training Strategy." *Journal of Rehabilitation*, 51(2):31-35.

Mullen, E. J. (1989). "Designing Intervention Strategies: Methods and Issues." Paper presented at the National Conference on Intervention Research, Los Angeles, School of Social Welfare, Center for Child and Family Policy Studies, University of California, Los Angeles, March 19-21, 1989.

Reid, W. J. (1987). "Evaluating and Intervention in Developmental Research," *Journal of Social Service Research*, 11(1):17-36.

Reid, W. J. (1987). "Research in Social Work." *Encyclopedia of Social Work* (pp. 474-487), (18th Ed.). Silver Spring, MD: National Association of Social Workers.

Rothman, J. (1989). "Intervention Research: Application to Runaway and Homeless Youths," *Social Work Research and Abstracts*, 25(1):13-18.

Rothman, J. (1988). "An Empirically-Based Model of Case Management: Results of a Field Study," Los Angeles, California, School of Social Welfare, Center for Child and Family Policy Studies, University of California, Los Angeles.

Rothman, J. (1987). "Case Management Action Guidelines: A Synthesis of Social Research," Los Angeles, California, School of Social Welfare, Center for Child and Family Policy Studies, University of California, Los Angeles.

Rothman, J. (1987). "The Practice of Case Management: A Study of Case Managers' Experiences and Views," Los Angeles, California, School of Social

Welfare, Center for Child and Family Policy Studies, University of California, Los Angeles.

Rothman, J. (1980). *Social R&D: Research and Development in the Human Services*. Englewood Cliffs, NJ: Prentice-Hall.

Rothman, J. (1974). *Planning and Organizing for Social Change: Action Principles from Social Science Research*. New York: Columbia University Press.

Rothman, J., J. Damron, and E. Shenassa. (1989). "Systematic Research Synthesis: An Alternative Approach to Metaanalysis." Paper presented at the Intervention Research Conference, UCLA Center for Child and Family Policy Studies, March 19-21, 1989.

Rothman, J. with T. David. (1986). "Status Offenders in Los Angeles County, Focus on Runaway and Homeless Youth: A Study and Policy Recommendations," Los Angeles, California, School of Social Welfare, Bush Program in Child and Family Policy, University of California, Los Angeles.

Rothman, J., J. L. Erlich, and J. G. Teresa. (1976). *Promoting Innovation and Change in Organizations and Communities: A Planning Manual*. New York: John Wiley & Sons.

Rothman, J., and W. Furman. (1987). "An Interim Evaluation of the Runaway Adolescent Pilot Program," Los Angeles, California, School of Social Welfare, Center for Child and Family Policy Studies, University of California, Los Angeles.

Rothman, J., W. Furman, and J. Weber. (1988). "Aiding Runaway and Homeless Youths: Evaluation of the Department of Children's Services' Strategy," Los Angeles, California, School of Social Welfare, Center for Child and Family Policy Studies, University of California, Los Angeles.

Rothman, J., L. M. Gant, and A. A. Hnat. (1985). "Mexican-American Family Culture." *Social Service Review*, 59(2):197-215.

Rothman, J., and M. Hugentobler. (1986). "Planning Theory and Planning Practice: Roles and Attitudes of Planners." In M. J. Dluhy and K. Chen (Eds.), *Interdisciplinary Planning: A Perspective for the Future*. New Brunswick, NJ: Center for Urban Policy Research, Rutgers, the State University of New Jersey.

Rothman, J., J. G. Teresa, and J. L. Erlich. (1977). *Developing Effective Strategies for Social Intervention: A Research and Development Methodology*, Springfield, VA: National Technical Information Service.

Rothman, J., J. G. Teresa, and J. L. Erlich. (1983). *Marketing Human Service Innovations*, Beverly Hills, CA: Sage Publications.

Schneiderman, L. (1986). "Dean's Message," *UCLA Social Welfare*, 2(1):2.

Thomas, E. J. (1985). "Design and Development Validity and Related Concepts in Developmental Research." *Social Work Research and Abstracts*, 21(2):50-55.

Thomas, E. J. (1984). *Designing Interventions for the Helping Professions*. Beverly Hills, CA: Sage Publications.

Thomas, E. J., et al. (1987). "Assessing Procedural Descriptiveness: Rationale and Illustrative Study," *Behavioral Assessment*, (a):43-56.

Thomas, E. J. (1978a). "Generating Innovation in Social Work: The Paradigm of Developmental Research." *Journal of Social Service Research*, 2(1):95-116.

Thomas, E. J. (1978b). "Research and Service in Single-Case Experimentation Conflicts and Choices." *Social Work Research and Abstracts*, 14(4):20-31.

Weiss, C. H., and M. J. Bucavalas. (1980). *Social Science Research and Decision-making*. New York: Columbia University Press.

Whittaker, J. K., E. M. Tracy, and M. Marckworth. (1989). *Family Support Project: Identifying Informal Support Resources for High Risk Families*. University of Washington School of Social Work and Behavioral Sciences Institute of Federal Way, Washington.

# The Design and Development Model of Practice Research

Edwin J. Thomas

It has been over a decade now since developmental research and related approaches to design and development were introduced to social work and social welfare (e.g., see Thomas, 1978a, 1978b, 1980; Mullen, 1978, 1981; Reid, 1979, 1980, 1983b; Rothman, 1974, 1978, 1980). In this period, design and development (D&D) has moved from initial frameworks and proposals to a model with a rapidly emerging methodology. Research with a D&D emphasis is increasingly being taught, written about, funded, and carried out in one form or another by researchers, practitioners and others in and outside of social work and other areas of human service. Although considerable work remains to be done, developmental research and related approaches have clearly arrived on the scene.

D&D approaches presently have a variety of names in addition to developmental research (e.g., social R&D, programmatic research, problem solving research, experimental social innovation, technique building research, model building research, and, more recently, intervention research). Although they are not all the same, they address one or another aspect of interventional innovation and, hence, are included here as part of the D&D model. It is beyond the scope of this chapter to describe the many contributions of these diverse approaches to the D&D model or to contrast their similarities and differences. For these details, the reader is referred elsewhere (e.g., Thomas, 1980, 1984, 1985, 1987) and particularly to the contributions of others cited below. In the pages that follow, "developmental research" will be used to illustrate the D&D model and occasionally will be referred to interchangeably with D&D.

## OVERVIEW OF THE DEVELOPMENTAL
## RESEARCH APPROACH TO D&D

Inasmuch as the introduction of developmental research represents a conceptual shift for the field, an overview of the rationale
for and conception of this approach is summarized below, based
upon selected theses taken from earlier, more detailed presentations
(Thomas, 1978a, 1978b).

### Rationale

Among the points to be made to indicate the need and justification for developmental research are the following:

1. Social technology is a primary means by which social work
   and social welfare accomplish their objectives. For example,
   intervention methods, one form of social technology in social
   work, are a major means social workers use to try to help
   individuals and families function more effectively.
2. There is a continuing need to generate new social technology
   in social work and social welfare. Most interventions are generally used only briefly, particularly those that are found wanting or that are supplanted by alternative approaches judged to
   be superior. There are frequent changes in resources, priorities, and social objectives that provide impetus for changing
   the goals, tasks, and methods of human service. Information
   from the behavioral sciences, human service professions, and
   other related areas that can be applied to improve social work
   intervention pours forth continuously and at an increasingly
   rapid rate.
3. The conventional research methodologies of behavioral science and of social work are ill-suited to the task of developing
   new social technology. Although behavioral science research
   contributes a methodology for assisting in the evaluation of
   existing interventions, behavioral science has no methodology
   for developing interventional innovations.
4. Enough is known to begin to formulate the main activities,
   such as the phases and steps, of developmental research.
5. Developmental research may be the single most appropriate

model of research for social work and human service because it consists of methods directed explicitly toward the analysis, design, development, and evaluation of the very technical means by which social work and human service objectives are achieved.

## A Working Conception of the Developmental Approach

The following quotation brings together several of the important features of the developmental approach (Thomas, in press).

In contrast to traditional research methods in the behavioral and social sciences and in social work in which the focus of inquiry is on contributing to knowledge about human behavior, the developmental approach emphasizes one or another of the means by which innovations in the human services may be developed. The outcomes of developmental research are likewise different from those of traditional research. Instead of yielding findings that shed light on some aspect of human behavior, the outcomes of developmental research are "products" that are the technical means of achieving social work and social welfare objectives. Among the more familiar types of social technology in social work are assessment methods, intervention methods, service programs, organizational structures for delivering service, service systems, and social welfare policy. Less often thought of in this context, although equally relevant, are physical structures, such as the architecture of a residential facility for the aged, electromechanical devices, and information systems.

The developmental approach also has a distinctive set of phases. Developmental research proper may be thought to consist of four phases of activity: analysis, design, development, and evaluation which, when followed by the additional phases of diffusion and adoption, may be thought of as developmental research and utilization (DR&U) (see Figure 1). The methods and techniques employed in the developmental approach derive from a variety of fields and often have application to other types of inquiry. However, their application in developmental research is distinctive. The author has previ-

FIGURE 1. Developmental Research and Utilization (DR&U). From E. J. Thomas, 1984, p. 140. Reprinted by permission.

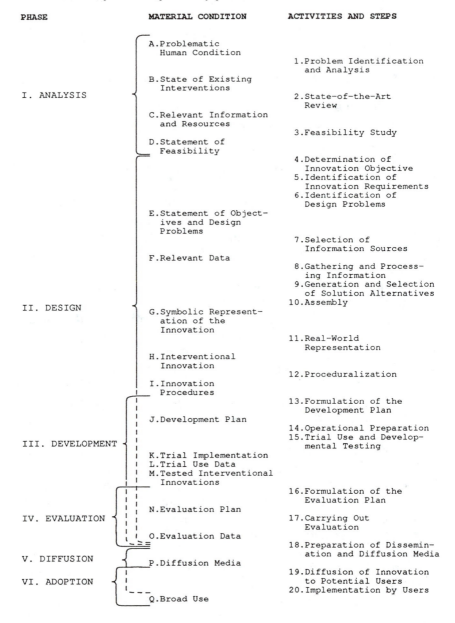

| PHASE | MATERIAL CONDITION | ACTIVITIES AND STEPS |
|---|---|---|
| I. ANALYSIS | A. Problematic Human Condition | 1. Problem Identification and Analysis |
| | B. State of Existing Interventions | 2. State-of-the-Art Review |
| | C. Relevant Information and Resources | 3. Feasibility Study |
| | D. Statement of Feasibility | 4. Determination of Innovation Objective<br>5. Identification of Innovation Requirements<br>6. Identification of Design Problems |
| | E. Statement of Objectives and Design Problems | 7. Selection of Information Sources |
| | F. Relevant Data | 8. Gathering and Processing Information<br>9. Generation and Selection of Solution Alternatives<br>10. Assembly |
| II. DESIGN | G. Symbolic Representation of the Innovation | 11. Real-World Representation |
| | H. Interventional Innovation | 12. Proceduralization |
| | I. Innovation Procedures | 13. Formulation of the Development Plan |
| | J. Development Plan | 14. Operational Preparation<br>15. Trial Use and Developmental Testing |
| III. DEVELOPMENT | K. Trial Implementation<br>L. Trial Use Data<br>M. Tested Interventional Innovations | 16. Formulation of the Evaluation Plan |
| IV. EVALUATION | N. Evaluation Plan | 17. Carrying Out Evaluation |
| | O. Evaluation Data | 18. Preparation of Dissemination and Diffusion Media |
| V. DIFFUSION | P. Diffusion Media | 19. Diffusion of Innovation to Potential Users |
| VI. ADOPTION | Q. Broad Use | 20. Implementation by Users |

ously provided a framework for developmental research (e.g., see Thomas, 1978a, 1978b, 1980, 1981, 1984, 1985, 1987). Other authors who have written on one or another particular aspect of the developmental research process include Azrin (1977), Baer, Wolf, and Risley (1987); Benn (1981); Barlow and Hersen (1984); Bloom and Fischer (1982); Briar (1973, 1980); Briar, Weissman, and Rubin (1981); Epstein and Tripodi (1977); Fairweather (1967); Fischer (1978); Fischer and Hudson (1983); Grinnell (1981, 1984); Gottman and Markman (1978); Guterman, Hodges, Bronson and Blythe (in press); Havelock (1973); Jayaratne and Levy (1979); Paine, Bellamy and Wilcox (1984); Poertner and Rapp (1987); Mullen (1978, 1981, 1983); Reid (1979, 1980, 1983a); Risley (1982); Robinson, Bronson, and Blythe (1988); Rose (1988); Rothman (1974, 1980); Taber (1987); Tripodi (1983); Tripodi and Epstein (1978); Tripodi and Epstein (1980); Tripodi, Fellin and Epstein (1971); Tripodi, Fellin, and Meyer (1983); and Wortman (1983). (Thomas, 1984, p. 140)

## *AREAS OF WORK AND PROGRESS IN D&D*

Although from the outset developmental research was justifiable as a distinctive approach with its own objectives, its methodology, as indicated earlier, was just emerging. A great deal of work needed to be done. Methods and techniques from related fields had to be identified, explicated, and applied to the tasks of D&D, contributions from diverse sources needed to be synthesized and made relevant to the objectives of D&D, and exemplars of D&D had to be identified and made available for review by researchers, practitioners, and others. Progress has been made in addressing these tasks. In addition to articles, contributions have been made available in the form of books on evaluation research and social work research, and, in particular, books devoted exclusively to D&D concepts and methods (e.g., Paine, Bellamy, and Wilcox, 1984; Rothman, 1980; Thomas, 1984). However, there have been relatively few publications in the last ten years in developmental research proper. In a recent review of advances in developmental research during the last decade, I found that most of the contributions during that period came from more mature methodologies such as conventional research methods, evaluation research, social and psychological assessment, and systems engineering (Thomas, in press). The methodology of developmental research presently consists of many techniques and methods from other fields and disciplines that have been or may be adapted to the objectives and tasks of D&D.

For a mature methodology of developmental research to evolve, work must address conceptual and methodological problems in a number of areas. Some of the major areas of work are indicated below. For each area, selected contributions are briefly noted; space precludes a more detailed summary. Advancement in the areas has varied, with some being farther along than others, and with most areas needing much more work.

### What Developmental Research Produces

The products of developmental research consist of innovative social technology for human service, as was indicated. The product most commonly thought of in this context is new intervention methods, and rightly so since it is largely by means of the intervention methods that human service is provided. However, there are other important types of social technology related to intervention methods which are also the products of developmental research: assessment methods, service programs, organizational structures, service systems, social welfare policy, physical structures, electromechanical devices, and information systems. For further details concerning these nine types of social technology, the reader is referred elsewhere (Thomas, 1978a, 1984).

Although not its primary product, developmental research can and does produce knowledge of human behavior as a by-product. For example, in our development and evaluation of unilateral family therapy for alcohol abuse (Thomas and Santa, 1982; Thomas and Yoshioka, 1989; Thomas, Santa, Bronson, and Oyserman, 1987), my associates and I have recently developed a theory of spouse enabling. The theory evolved from the work on a Spouse Enabling Inventory and the design of a treatment module directed toward reducing particular enabling behaviors of the spouses of uncooperative alcohol abusers (Thomas, Yoshioka, Ager and Cun-

ningham, 1988). In the theory, two types and two modes of enabling are distinguished, as are "wet" and "dry" enabling. In
addition to its relevance in the unilateral approach and to understanding codependency, the theory has application to the enabling
of many other problems.

## What Is an Innovation?

To qualify as an "innovation," the change need not be entirely
new (e.g., see Pelz and Munson, 1982; Rice and Rogers, 1980).
The innovation may range from an invention of novel technology,
through adaptation by alteration of existing technology, to novel
application for different purposes of existing technology (often
called technological transfer), to adoption of existing technology by
a different user group (Thomas, 1984). Further, the use and implementation of an innovation may involve "reinvention" in which the
innovation or its use is changed to fit with the conditions and context in which it is to be employed (Rice and Rogers, 1980). Reinvention is an important aspect of the D&D process that presently
is not well understood.

## What Is Designed and Developed

It appeared that the components of a helping strategy that could
be subject to D&D had not been identified in the literature. Although considerable attention has been given to selected components (e.g., assessment and intervention methods), little work had
been done on some (e.g., intervention theory in contrast to behavior
theory), and no one had distinguished, explicated, and brought together all the diverse components. I studied the problem and came
up with 17 distinctive components. Names of these components are
listed in the last column of Figure 2, and are described and illustrated elsewhere (Thomas, 1984). All are important parts of the
anatomy of the helping strategy and any component or set of them
could be the focus of D&D.

There are two additional features to what is designed and developed in D&D. One is the connectedness of the components of the
helping strategy. For example, an innovative intervention method
generally presupposes a means of assessment appropriate to it. My

FIGURE 2. Relationship between particular sources of information and generation processes, all as they relate to components of the helping strategy. From E. J. Thomas, 1984, p. 130. Reprinted by permission.

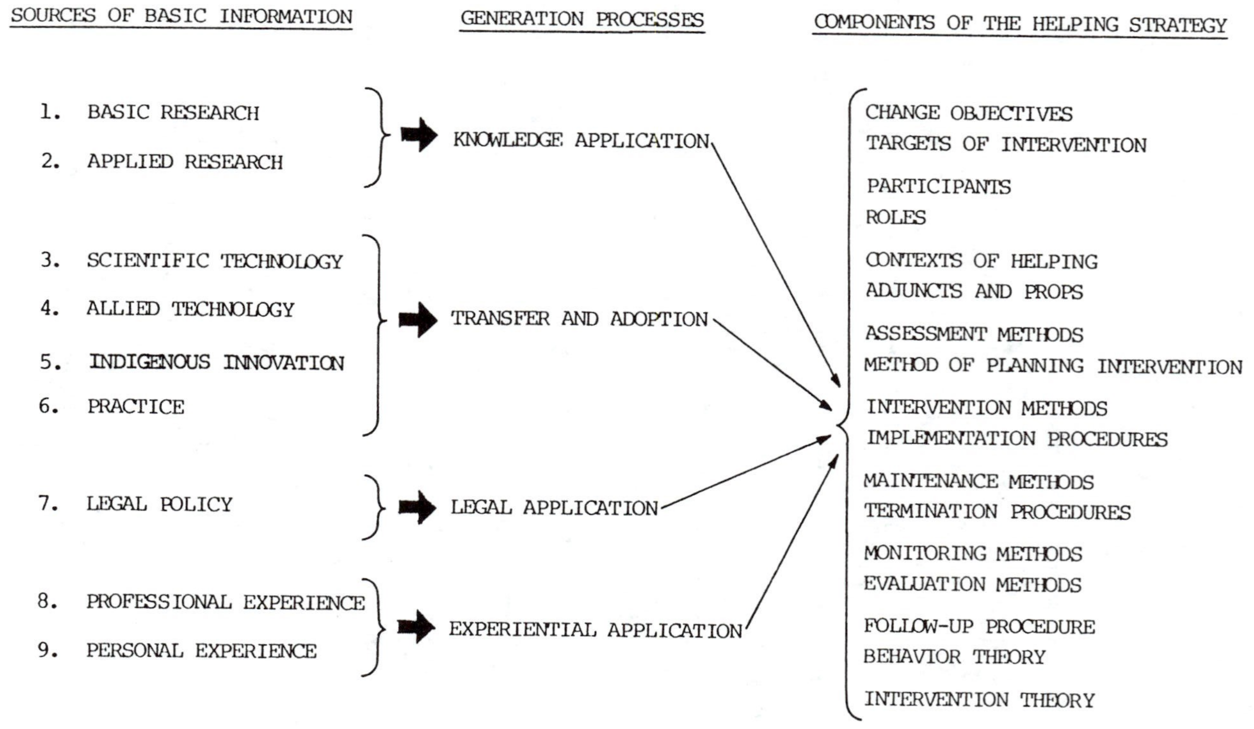

SOURCES OF BASIC INFORMATION

1. BASIC RESEARCH
2. APPLIED RESEARCH

3. SCIENTIFIC TECHNOLOGY
4. ALLIED TECHNOLOGY
5. INDIGENOUS INNOVATION
6. PRACTICE

7. LEGAL POLICY

8. PROFESSIONAL EXPERIENCE
9. PERSONAL EXPERIENCE

GENERATION PROCESSES

KNOWLEDGE APPLICATION

TRANSFER AND ADOPTION

LEGAL APPLICATION

EXPERIENTIAL APPLICATION

COMPONENTS OF THE HELPING STRATEGY

CHANGE OBJECTIVES
TARGETS OF INTERVENTION
PARTICIPANTS
ROLES
CONTEXTS OF HELPING
ADJUNCTS AND PROPS
ASSESSMENT METHODS
METHOD OF PLANNING INTERVENTION
INTERVENTION METHODS
IMPLEMENTATION PROCEDURES
MAINTENANCE METHODS
TERMINATION PROCEDURES
MONITORING METHODS
EVALUATION METHODS
FOLLOW-UP PROCEDURE
BEHAVIOR THEORY
INTERVENTION THEORY

associates and I found that it was necessary to develop a method to assess spouse enabling of the partner's alcohol abuse as part of designing and developing a treatment module of unilateral family therapy for alcohol abuse to reduce the enabling. The Spouse Enabling Inventory, already mentioned, was then developed as an important part of the method to assess spouse enabling. Most, if not all, of the helping strategy components are thus interrelated.

A second feature is the connectedness of what is being designed and developed with its organizational and agency context. Consider a management information system (MIS). Grasso and Epstein (1987) have indicated, as have others, that a MIS can have important implications for the functioning of an organization of which it is a part. In discussing the Boysville Management Information System they helped develop and implement, these authors have described some of the requirements of an integrated MIS that is directly connected with the management and social service delivery of the organization as well as with the functions of research and training. More generally, the helping strategy and service delivery system may be thought of as interrelated aspects of what Munson and Pelz (1982) have called the "technical" component of an organization viewed as a sociotechnical system. The technical subsystem, in turn, is related to other aspects of the organizational and service context (e.g., see Hasenfeld, 1983), all of which are subject to D&D (e.g., see Munson and Pelz, 1982; Thomas, 1988).

## The Characteristics of a Good Intervention

The criterion of effectiveness has been employed to appraise interventions for several decades. This criterion clearly can help shape the selection and design of interventions (e.g., see Fischer, 1978; Hanrahan and Reid, 1984) and the methods for evaluating them (e.g., see Bloom and Fischer, 1982; Jayaratne and Levy, 1979). More generally, the effectiveness and other characteristics of what is considered a good intervention set standards that have great importance in guiding the design, development, and evaluation of interventional innovations, for appraising them at each step in the D&D process, and for their adoption and use.

Although there are as yet no generally agreed upon assessment criteria, examination of the literature has indicated that more and more criteria are being seriously invoked for appraising interventions. I came up with four sets of criteria (Thomas, 1984) indicating that the intervention should have (1) objective capability consisting of effectiveness and efficiency; (2) ethical suitability; (3) adequacy, as indicated by the validity of the informational and research basis for the intervention, the completeness, specificity, and correctness of the procedure, and the extent to which it guides the behavior of those who use it; and (4) useability, as reflected in whether the intervention is relevant to the task, codified, simple, flexible, modular, inexpensive, satisfactory to consumers, sustainable in a host environment, and compatible in its social and environmental context. To these criteria can be added a fifth type, the social desirability of the innovation (e.g., see Sarason, 1984; Thomas, in press). Most of these criteria are relatively new and can have important and very different implications for the innovations subject to D&D. What it means to design for effectiveness or efficiency or for any other appraisal criterion has yet to be worked through.

### Sources of Information for Innovation

Developmental research derives its data and resources for technological development from a large number of sources. These include basic research and applied research, customary sources in social R&D and literature retrieval models of development (e.g., see Mullen, 1978; Rothman, 1974, 1980), as well as scientific technology, allied technology, legal policy, indigenous innovation, practice, personal experience, and professional experience (for further details see Thomas, 1978a, 1984). (Names for these sources are listed in the first column of Figure 2.)

### Generation Processes for Innovation

Information from the different sources comes in raw form and generally cannot be used without some transformation and specific application. The changes required to transform and apply basic information from one or more sources into results or products that may be used more directly in the design and development of innovative interventions are referred to as the generation processes of intervention design. For example, in the generation process of knowledge application, there is the transformation of the research findings into relevant empirical generalizations and the deduction of appropriate practice guidelines from the generalizations, followed by the operationalization of guidelines in real-world terms. In addition to knowledge application, four additional generation processes have been identified and described. These are technology transfer and adoption, legal application, and experiential application, as listed in the middle column of Figure 2. For further details, see Thomas (1980, 1984). Considerable prior work has been done on knowledge utilization which has helped to illuminate the processes involved in the application of basic and applied research (e.g., see Bloom, 1975; Fischer, 1978; Glaser, 1981; Havelock, 1973; Mullen, 1978, 1981; Rothman, 1974, 1978; Tripodi et al., 1969; Thomas, 1964). However, much more work remains to be done on all of the generation processes.

## Phases

The ordered phases of developmental research are intended to embrace the main activities and conditions involved in the development human service technology. These were described earlier and are given in Figure 1. There have been advances relating to each of these phases. For example, there are new methods of data aggregation and synthesis, such as meta-analysis (e.g., see Fiske, 1983; Light, 1987), that have application in the analysis phase of developmental research. A concept of design validity (Thomas, 1985) has been proposed which is relevant to the design phase. Techniques of developmental testing, such as proceduralization (Thomas, 1984; Schafer, 1985), developmental logs (e.g., see Guterman et al., in press; Rothman, 1974; Yaffe, 1987), critical incidents (e.g., Reid and Davis, 1987; Thomas et al., 1987), and failure analysis (e.g., see Foa and Emmelkamp, 1983; Barlow, Hayes, and Nelson, 1984) are relevant to the development phase. Concepts for treatment integrity (Yeaton and Sechrest, 1981), procedural reliability (Billingsley, White, and Munson, 1980), and shift in intervention procedure (McMahon, 1987) have been put forward that have important implications for the assessment of whether the intervention in the evaluation phase was implemented as intended. Developments relating to the dissemination phase include advances in the methodology of dissemination, such as designing for useability from the outset of D&D and actively programming the utilization of the D&D product (e.g., see Backer, Liberman, and Kuehnel, 1986; Paine, 1984). For a more detailed review of advances, the reader is referred elsewhere (Thomas, in press).

## Concepts

The concepts of design and of development are of course central to the D&D approach. Additional concepts have been introduced to assist researchers and practitioners to identify what is important and to describe relevant processes and activities in developmental research. For example, in recognition that innovations can vary greatly in the extent to which they have been tried, tested, and suitably revised before having been introduced to potential users, a concept of developmental validity has been proposed. Developmental validity has thus been defined as ". . . the extent to which innovations have been adequately used on a trial basis and have been tested developmentally. . . . Interventions that have developmental validity have been evolved by means of developmental processes that increase the likelihood that the innovations will be reliable and will not have to be redesigned to achieve the objectives of the intervention" (Thomas, 1985, pp. 54-55). Other concepts include the domain of design, the validity of design, sampling for developmental relevance, and developmental practice (Thomas, 1984, 1985). As more is learned and understood about the D&D process, additional concepts will inevitably be needed.

## Methods

As the major activities that may be carried out to attain particular D&D objectives, methods are important aspects of the D&D methodology. The methods include a state-of-the-art review and feasibility study for the phase of problem analysis, proceduralization for the phase of design, trial use and developmental testing for the development phase, and the formulation of an evaluation plan (e.g., a treatment experiment with an experimental control-group design) for the evaluation phase. Because the methods have application largely at one or selected points in the D&D sequence, they may also be thought of as operational steps (see Figure 1). Again, the reader is referred elsewhere for details (e.g., Paine et al., 1984; Rothman, 1980; Thomas, 1984).

In the last decade, there has been an increase in the number of methods identified and described. Using my own work in this area as a case in point, I came up with 11 activities and operational steps in 1978 (Thomas, 1978a), 15 in 1981 (Thomas, 1981), and the 20 given in Figure 1 in 1984 (Thomas, 1984). I could now come up with some five more. It is the increase and not the particular numbers that is relevant here. In addition to the work that has been done, additional inquiry is needed to explicate further the methods already known and to identify possible additions. From the outset, the identification and systematization of the methods of D&D have been the central tasks to be accomplished, and the job is far from finished.

## Techniques

In addition to the methods, there are also many techniques that have diverse and specialized application in developmental research. Task analysis, for example, is a technique that may be employed to analyze behavioral repertoires to isolate the constituent behavioral components required to accomplish given objectives (Resnick and Ford, 1978; Zemke and Kramlinger, 1982). Among other tools are the critical incident technique, needs assessment, flow charting, latticing, decision tables, information retrieval and review, and selected practice techniques (for details, see Thomas, 1984).

A concluding comment I made earlier on the operational steps and phases of DR&U is still relevant: "This framework is subject to possible extension and revision as the methodology of developmental research becomes more sophisticated and systematic" (Thomas, 1978b, p. 473). From the outset, the identification and systematization of the developmental research methodology has been one of the central tasks to be accomplished.

## D&D AND PRACTICE

Much has been written in recent years on the relationship between practice and research, but little attention has been given to the question of the relationship between practice and D&D. Clearly, the innovations deriving from D&D may make important contributions to the field of practice. And practice may be used as a medium in particular D&D endeavors (e.g., to deliver a new treatment program in an evaluation study). What is less obvious is that now that a D&D model is available, practice may be used not only as a medium but also as a tool for D&D. Without a D&D perspective, the use of practice as a tool for D&D is hard to imagine; and without a D&D methodology, conventional practice methods would be a most uncertain means to attain D&D goals.

A genuine interface between practice and D&D can now be envisioned. By interface is meant that practice can now be carried out to achieve practice objectives and outcomes through the use of selected methods of practice, *and* it can also be directed toward achieving D&D objectives and outcomes through the use of selected D&D methods. This interface can be realized in the form of developmental practice (Thomas, 1984, 1985), as is indicated in more detail in the excerpt quoted below.

> *Developmental practice* is conceived as a mode of practice in which the practitioner is also a developer of interventions, practice is a medium and a principal instrument of development, and the practitioner makes systematic use of selected methods of developmental research to achieve the D&D objectives pursued in the practice. In contrast to conventional practice, developmental practice has D&D objectives in addition to those of service; selects cases that fall within a domain of D&D by the criterion of developmental relevance; provides service within the domain of D&D using practice methods appropriate to that domain, including research findings, behavior and intervention theory, state-of-the-art in practice and the intervention or model subject to D&D; gathers, monitors, and evaluates data on service outcomes and innovation-related results using systematic evaluation methods, including time

series and single-case experiments; addresses potential design problems and the D&D aspects of practice in general using the methods of developmental research, including developmental testing; and, in addition to results involving service outcomes, produces innovative interventions or models of intervention along with related evaluation data. (Thomas, 1988, August, p. 7-8)

Developmental practice has several applications in D&D and in practice. In D&D proper, it could be used as a major tool of development and, in a service agency, it could be employed in a selective fashion as a distinctive mode of practice to address those aspects of service identified as requiring D&D, such as evolving interventions or programs in new areas. Further, one can learn more generally about the process of D&D itself through solving specific practice and/or D&D problems in conducting developmental practice, in reflecting on what was done and why, and then endeavoring to conceptualize the results. My associates and I continue to learn a great deal by this means.

## D&D AND RESEARCH UTILIZATION

Although D&D is not a model of research utilization, properly speaking, it has roots in several precursor developments that place strong emphasis on research utilization. Many of the contemporary approaches to D&D grew directly out of an awareness of the lack of utilization of research findings and the absence of a viable methodology for putting useful contributions in the hands of practitioners and others in human service. Most writers who have advocated D&D and related approaches have recommended them as promising to be more effective means of achieving utilization and of bridging the gap between research and practice. It is therefore most appropriate to examine the ways in which D&D relates to utilization. There are at least four different aspects worthy of note.

The first involves what might be called "resource utilization" — i.e., the extent to which research, information, related technology, and other resources are drawn on and used. An important difference between the earlier research utilization models and the developmental research approach to D&D is the extent to which resources other than basic and applied research are systematically made use of in the D&D process. As indicated earlier, developmental research derives its information and resources for technological development from a number of sources. In addition to basic and applied research, these include scientific and allied technology along with social innovation, practice, legal policy, and professional and personal experience (see list of sources in Figure 2). Each of these sources can make a distinctive and important contribution to D&D, depending on the problem addressed and the richness of the resources that may be derived from a given source (Thomas, 1978b, 1981, 1984).

A second aspect consists of the "utilization processes" by which the resources are transformed and applied. These have been referred to above as generation processes. As indicated earlier, they include knowledge application, the mainstay of most of the earlier approaches that focused largely on research and knowledge utilization, along with technological transfer and adoption, legal application, and experiential application mentioned earlier. Each process is different and calls for very different ways of proceeding in D&D (for details, see Thomas, 1981, 1984).

A third aspect of utilization is the extent to which the products and other results of D&D are useable, (i.e., have "product useability"). As indicated above, the innovations of D&D are themselves aspects of social technology, such as interventions and practice methods, rather than being "pretechnological," such as behavioral science theory or research findings that require some transformation before they can be utilized. As technology, the products of D&D may be readily applied, depending in part on the extent to which the innovations were designed and developed with practitioner and other consumer use in mind.

A fourth aspect is the extent to which D&D contains a methodology for designing and developing utilization itself (has "utilization D&D," as it were). For too many years now in many of the approaches to the utilization problem, there has been no D&D for utilization. Rather, in such approaches utilization typically has been hoped for, its absence lamented, implications of the contributions to be utilized highlighted, and practitioners and others exhorted to utilize the contributions in question. Instead, in D&D for utilization, the particular utilization events, processes, and outcomes themselves would be specified and conceptualized as problems for D&D, and they would then be designed and developed using the D&D methodology. It is thus that utilization would be programmed in D&D. Further, the reader is reminded that in the sequence of phases of D&D, one begins with problem analysis and moves on through to adoption of the innovation. Thus, if the phases of D&D are carried out in sequence, the products should not only be useable, as indicated above, but adopted. For relevant D&D methods and examples, the reader is referred elsewhere (e.g., Backer, Liberman, and Kuehnel, 1986; Paine, Bellamy, and Wilcox, 1984).

Considering these four aspects of utilization — resource utilization, utilization processes, product utilization, and utilization D&D — it should be evident that there is a great deal of utilization made possible in and through D&D. Inasmuch as the D&D model consists of an interrelated set of methods and processes that involve these different aspects of utilization and serves to make possible a high degree of potential utilization, the D&D model may be thought of as one Grand Utilization Machine. Clearly, adoption of D&D should go a long way toward facilitating the utilization of research findings and other contributions to human service.

## D&D AND THE FUTURE

Research to generate innovative human service needs to be conducted which is guided by the perspective and methods of developmental research. D&D has many applications in and outside of the social service agency that have yet to be realized. One is to conduct developmental practice in which service has D&D objectives and in which selected methods of developmental research are employed. D&D methods should be at least coequals with the more conventional research methods taught in social work (Thomas, 1978b). Research projects and dissertations should be oriented toward evolving new models of intervention and human service (Reid, 1979; Rose, 1988; Thomas, 1978b). And finally, because it is relatively new, scholars and researchers should give high priority to strengthening and extending the methodology of D&D to accelerate its own development. Some of the main areas in which work has

been accomplished were briefly reviewed here along with directions
for further effort.

## REFERENCES

Azrin, N. H. (1977). A strategy for applied research: Learning based but outcome
oriented. *American Psychologist, 32*, 140-149.
Backer, T. E., Liberman, R. P., & Kuehnel, T. G. (1986). Dissemination and
adoption of innovating psychosocial interventions. *Journal of Consulting and
Clinical Psychology, 54*, 111-118.
Baer, D. M., Wolf, M. M., & Risley, T. R. (1987). Some still current dimen-
sions of applied behavior analysis. *Journal of Applied Behavior Analysis, 20*,
313-329.
Barlow, D. H., & Hersen, M. (1984). *Single-case experimental designs: Strate-
gies for studying behavior change* (2nd ed.). New York: Pergamon.
Barlow, D. H., Hayes, S. C., & Nelson, R. O. (1984). *The scientist practitioner:
Research and accountability in clinical and educational settings*. New York:
Pergamon.
Benn, C. (1981). *Attacking poverty through participation*. Melbourne, Australia:
Preston Institute of Technology Press.
Billingsley, F., White, O. R., & Munson, R. (1980). Procedural reliability: A
rationale and an example. *Behavioral Assessment, 3*, 229-243.
Bloom, M. (1975). *The paradox of helping: Introduction of the philosophy of
scientific practice*. New York: John Wiley.
Bloom, M. & Fischer, J. (1982). *Evaluating practice: A guide for helping profes-
sionals*. Englewood Cliffs, NJ: Prentice-Hall.
Briar, S. (1980). Toward the integration of practice and research. In D. Fanshel
(Ed.), *Future of social work research*. Washington, DC: National Association
of Social Workers, Inc.
Briar, S. (1973). Effective social work intervention in direct practice: Implica-
tions for education. In *Facing the challenge*. New York: Council on Social
Work Education.
Briar, S., Weissman, H., & Rubin, A. (Eds.) (1981). *Research utilization in
social work education*. New York: Council on Social Work Education.
Epstein, I., & Tripodi, T. (1977). Research techniques for program planning,
monitoring and evaluation. New York: Columbia University Press.
Fairweather, G. (1967). *Methods for experimental social innovation*. New York:
John Wiley & Sons.
Fischer, J. (1978). *Effective casework practice: An eclectic approach*. New York:
McGraw-Hill Book Co.
Fischer, J., & Hudson, W. W. (1983). Measurement of client problems for im-
proved practice. In A. Rosenblatt & D. Waldfogel (Eds.), *Handbook of clini-
cal social work*. San Francisco, CA: Jossey-Bass.

Fiske, D. W. (1983). The metanalytic revolution in outcome research. *Journal of Consulting and Clinical Psychology, 51,* 65-71.

Foa, E. B., & Emmelkamp, P. M. (1983). *Failures in behavior therapy.* New York: Wiley.

Glaser, E. M. (1981). Durability of innovations in human service organizations: A case-study analysis. *Knowledge, 3,* 167-185.

Gottman, J. M., & Markman, H. J. (1978). Experimental designs in psychotherapy research. In S. L. Garfield & A. E. Bergin (Eds.), *Handbook of psychotherapy and behavior change* (2nd ed.). New York: John Wiley & Sons.

Grasso, A. J. and Epstein, I. (1987). Management by Measurement: Organizational Dilemmas and Opportunities. *Administration in Social Work,* 11 (3/4) 89-100.

Grinnell, R. M. (Ed.). (1981). *Social work research and evaluation.* Itasca, IL: F. E. Peacock.

Grinnell, R. M. (Ed.). (1985). *Social work research and evaluation,* (2nd ed.). Itasca, IL: F. E. Peacock.

Guterman, N., Hodges, V., Bronson, D., & Blythe, B. (In press). Using developmental research to design social work interventions. *Child Welfare.*

Hanrahan, P., & Reid, W. J. (1984). Choosing effective interventions. *Social Service Review, 58,* 244-258.

Hasenfeld, Y. (1983). *Human Services Organizations.* Englewood Cliffs, NJ.

Havelock, R. G. (1973). *Planning for innovations through dissemination and utilization of knowledge.* Ann Arbor: Institute for Social Research, University of Michigan.

Jayaratne, S., & Levy, R. (1979). *Empirical clinical practice.* New York: Columbia University Press.

Light, R. J. (1987). Six evaluation issues that synthesis can resolve better than single studies. In D. S. Cordray & M. W. Lipsey (Eds.), *Evaluation Studies Annual Review, 11,* 703-719.

McMahon, P. M. (1987). Shifts in intervention procedures: A problem in evaluating human service interventions. *Social Work Research and Abstracts, 23,* 13-18.

Mullen E. J. (1978). The construction of personal models for effective practice: A method for utilizing research findings to guide social interventions. *Journal of Social Service Research, 2,* 45-65.

Mullen, E. J. (1981). Development of personal intervention models. In R. M. Grinnell (Ed.), *Social Work Research and Evaluation.* Itasca, IL: F. E. Peacock.

Mullen, E. J. (1983). Personal practice models. In A. Rosenblatt & D. Waldfogel (Eds.), *Handbook of clinical social work.* San Francisco, CA: Jossey-Bass.

Munson, F. C., & Pelz, D. C. (1982). *Innovating in organizations: A conceptual framework.* Ann Arbor, MI: Institute for Social Research, University of Michigan.

Paine, S. C. (1984). Models revisited. In S. C. Paine, G. T. Bellamy, & B. L.

Wilcox (Eds.), *Human services that work: From innovation to standard practice*. Baltimore, MD: Paul H. Brookes.

Pelz, D. C., & Munson, F. C. (1982). Originality level and the innovating process in organizations. *Human Systems Management*, *3*, 173-187.

Paine, S. C., Bellamy, G. T., & Wilcox, B. (1984). *Human services that work: From innovation to standard practice*. Baltimore, MD: Paul H. Brookes.

Poertner, J., & Rapp, C. A. (1987). Designing social work management information systems: The case for performance guidance systems. *Administration in Social Work*, *11*, 177-191.

Reid, W. J. (1979). The model development dissertation. *Journal of Social Service Research*, *3*, 215-225.

Reid, W. J. (1980). Research strategies for improving individualized services. In D. Fanshel (Ed.), *Future of social work research*. Washington, DC: National Association of Social Workers.

Reid, W. J. (1983a). Developing intervention methods through experimental designs. In A. Rosenblatt & D. Waldfogel (Eds.), *Handbook of clinical social work*. San Francisco, CA: Jossey-Bass.

Reid, W. J. (1983b). Research developments. In S. Briar (Ed.), *1983-84 Supplement to the encyclopedia of social work*, 17th ed. New York: National Association of Social Workers.

Reid, W. J., & Davis, I. P. (1987). Qualitative methods in single-subject research. In N. Gottlieb, Ishisaka, H. A., Kopp, J., Richey, C. A., & Tolson, E. R. *Perspectives in direct practice research, Monograph 5*. Seattle, WA: Center for Social Welfare Research, School of Social Work, University or Washington.

Resnick, L. B., & Ford, W. W. (1978). The analysis of tasks for instruction: An information-processing approach. In A. C. Catania & T. A. Brigham (Eds.), *Handbook of applied behavioral analysis: Social and instructional processes*. New York: Irvington Publishers.

Rice, R. E., & Rogers, E. M. (1980). Re-invention in the innovation process. *Knowledge: Creation, Diffusion, Utilization, 1*, 449-515.

Risley, T. (1982). *Behavorial design for residential programs*. Paper presented at the annual convention of the Australian Behavior Modification Association, Surfers Paradise, Australia, May.

Robinson, E. A. R., Bronson, D. E., & Blythe, B. J. (1988). An analysis of the implementation of single-case evaluation by practitioners. *Social Service Review*, *62*, 285-301.

Rose, S.D. (1988). Practice experiments for doctoral dissertations: Research training and knowledge building. *Journal of Social Work Education*, *24*, 115-122.

Rothman, J. (1974). *Planning and organizing for social change: Action principles from social science research*. New York: Columbia University Press.

Rothman, J. (1978). Conversion and design in the research utilization process. *Journal of Social Service Research, 2*, 117-131.

Rothman, J. (1980). *Social R & D: Research and development in the human services*. Englewood Cliffs, NJ: Prentice-Hall.

Sarason, S. B. (1984). If it can be studied or developed, should it be? *American Psychologist, 39*, 477-485.

Schafer, A. (March/April 1985). Commentary on "The randomized clinical trial: For whose benefit?" *IRB*, Vol. 7, No. 2, 4-6.

Taber, M. A. (1987). A theory of accountability for the human services and the implications for social program design. *Administration in Social Work, 11*, 115-127.

Thomas, E. J. (1964). Selecting knowledge from behavioral science. *In building social work knowledge: Report of a conference*. New York: National Association of Social Workers.

Thomas, E. J. (1978a). Generating innovation in social work: The paradigm of developmental research. *Journal of Social Service Research, 2*, 95-116.

Thomas, E. J. (1978b). Mousetraps, developmental research, and social work education. *Social Service Review, 52*, 468-483.

Thomas, E. J. (1980). Beyond knowledge utilization in generating human service technology. In D. Fanshel (Ed.), *Future of social work research*. Washington, DC: National Association of Social Workers, 91-103.

Thomas, E. J. (1981). Developmental research: A model for interventional innovation. In R. M. Grinnell (Ed.), *Social Work Research and Evaluation*. Itasca, IL: F. E. Peacock.

Thomas, E. J. (1984). *Designing interventions for the helping professions*. Beverly Hills, CA: Sage.

Thomas, E. J. (1985). Design and development validity and related concepts in developmental research. *Social Work Research and Abstracts, 21*, 50-58.

Thomas, E. J. (1987). Developmental approach to research. *Encyclopedia of social work* (18th ed.). Silver Spring, MD: National Association of Social Workers.

Thomas, E. J. (in press). Advances in developmental research. *Social Service Review*.

Thomas, E. J. (1988, August). *Modes of practice in developmental research*. Paper presented at the conference on Empiricism in Clinical Practice: Present and Future, Center for Social Work Practice Research of the School of Social Welfare, State University of New York at Albany, Albany, NY.

Thomas, E. J., & Santa, C. (1982). Unilateral family therapy for alcohol abuse: A working conception. *The American Journal of Family Therapy, 10*, 49-58.

Thomas, E. J., & Yoshioka, M. (1989). Spouse interventive confrontations in unilateral family therapy for alcohol abuse. *Social Casework, 70*, 340-347.

Thomas, E. J., Bastien, J., Stuebe, D. R., Bronson, D. E., & Yaffe, J. (1987). Assessing procedural descriptiveness: Rationale and illustrative study. *Behavioral Assessment, 9*, 43-56.

Thomas, E. J., Santa, C., Bronson, D., & Oyserman, D. (1987). Unilateral family therapy with the spouses of alcoholics. *Journal of Social Service Research, 10*, 145-163.

Thomas, E. J., Yoshioka, M., Ager, R., & Cunningham, J. (1988, November). *Spouse enabling: Concept and measurement.* 50th Annual Conference Program, National Council on Family Relations, Philadelphia, PA.

Tripodi, T. (1983). *Evaluative research for social workers.* Englewood Cliffs, NJ: Prentice-Hall.

Tripodi, T., & Epstein, I. (1978). Incorporating knowledge of research methodology into social work practice. *Journal of Social Service Research, 2,* 65-79.

Tripodi, T., & Epstein, I. (1980). *Research techniques for clinical social workers.* New York: Columbia University Press.

Tripodi, T., Fellin, P., & Meyer, H. J. (1969). *The assessment of social research: Guidelines for the use of research in social work and social science,* Itasca, IL: F. E. Peacock.

Tripodi, T., Fellin, P., & Meyer, H. J. (1983). *The assessment of social research* (2nd ed.). Itasca, IL: Peacock.

Tripodi, T., Fellin, P., & Epstein, I. (1971). *Social program evaluation: Guidelines for health, education, and welfare administrators.* Itasca, IL: F. E. Peacock.

Tripodi, T. (1983). *Evaluative research for social workers.* Englewood Cliffs, NJ: Prentice-Hall.

Wortman, P. M. (1983). Evaluation research: A methodological perspective. In M. W. Rosenzweig & L. W. Porter (Eds.), *Annual Review of Psychology,* Vol. *34,* Palo Alto, CA: Annual Reviews, Inc.

Yaffe, J. (1987). *The developmental log: A method for assisting in the development of innovations.* Unpublished doctoral dissertation, University of Michigan, Ann Arbor, MI.

Yeaton, W. H., & Sechrest, L. (1981). Critical dimensions in the choice and maintenance of successful treatments: Strengths, integrity and effectiveness. *Journal of Consulting and Clinical Psychology, 49,* 156-168.

Zemke, R., & Kramlinger, T. (1982). *Figuring things out: A trainer's guide to needs and task analysis.* Reading, MA: Addison-Wesley.

# INTRODUCTION TO SECTION II

# Research Utilization
# in Interpersonal Practice

## Martin Bloom

This section deals with interpersonal practice in social work, that is, interventions focusing on individuals, families, and small groups. In addition, ethical issues related to the integration of research and practice are introduced.

The authors are all distinguished scholars in social work. William Reid has made several major contributions to the social work literature and profession, including his early research on short-term versus long-term practice (with Anne Shyne) which led to a significant series of conceptual and programmatic research studies (with Laura Epstein and others) under the title of task-centered casework. His co-author, Anne Fortune, a professor of research and practice, has written a book on task-centered group work and is currently editor of the *Journal of Social Work Education*. Both are presently at the State University of New York at Albany.

The Reid and Fortune chapter begins with a clarification of the forms that research utilization may take. One does not have to hit clients over the head with a full-fledged experimental/control group design from the esoteric pages of a journal in order to be said to be using research to guide practice; there are gentler and kinder ways.

Reid and Fortune suggest that in addition to the instrumental use of research results, practitioners may also make use of conceptual and methodological understanding, as well as indirect uses of all of the above. Each of these is an important source of utilization of the researchers' results. Together, they are beginning to make an impact on direct practice in social work. The authors explore this impact in social work education, with particular reference to research-based practice methods and single-case methodology.

Contributors generally accepted the new categories of meaning involving the utilization of research, although some wondered what in practice was not at least indirectly related to research. But as to the new advances in social work theory and research, some commentators noted that the initial optimism of single-case designs dissolves in the face of huge social problems like the epidemic of drugs, AIDS, and the like. It may be enough that we make some progress on skills acquisition in specific cases through research-based technology, while others seek to address structural dimensions of social problems. It was also noted that researchers need to customize models from social work theory and research to fit the environment of agency practice.

Harold Lewis is Dean of the School of Social Work at Hunter College, and brings an unmatched depth of experience and insight into the intellectual bases of social work practice. Dean Lewis' contribution is all too rare in these research conferences. He writes about the pervasive ethical implications of the many conflicting aspects of research and practice. He correctly points out that whenever we entertain, as part of our study's objectives, how we are going to use the results, we must accept the ethical obligations involving the application of "truth" to practice. He chastises researchers in social work for hardly confronting the ethical issues of applying the knowledge derived from research to practice.

Members of the Conference did battle with Dean Lewis' challenge. One response suggested that social work researchers are always concerned with values, to which Dean Lewis replied that this was exactly the problem; values (preferences in means and ends of action) are not the same as ethics (the rules for priorities in attaining valued objectives). Another response suggested that single-case evaluation, as contrasted with research, may involve clients directly in identifying goals, selecting means, monitoring changes and evaluating outcomes, which means that ethical considerations are very closely related to this form of empirically based practice. Overall, the ethical challenge remains a persisting obligation to social work researchers and evaluators, just as it does to practitioners.

Sheldon Rose is not only a prolific writer in the area of group work, but is also persistent and systematic in the development of his particular model, a cognitive-behavioral approach. His paper is an important record, not merely for its documentation of the process of aiding the widespread dissemination of the research he and his colleagues have done over the past decade, but it is also a personal document of the struggles that effective dissemination of research requires. He presently teaches at the University of Wisconsin, Madison.

Professor Rose's chapter presents a number of principles of promoting research utilization, each generated out of his experience with the planned campaign to disseminate his innovation in group work practice. Some of these principles potentially involve researchers in areas in which they may be neither familiar nor comfortable. But the facts of life regarding utilization of research innovations require us to consider these activities or join with others who can perform them. Professor Rose suggests, for example, that researchers must consider creating manuals that translate the research into practice terms. He also suggests that tools for evaluating practice should be part of every treatment package, and that all dissertations have a utilization section as a basic part of this scholarly endeavor.

A chapter by Hamilton McCubbin and Marilyn McCubbin is included in this section, although the authors were not present at the conference itself. The McCubbins are at the University of Wisconsin-Madison, and have been centrally involved in studies of family treatment for many years. Their chapter reviews a wide range of research and theory in relationship to social work practice with families.

This chapter considers five major developments over the past 20 years: (1) The question of effectiveness of family systems interventions. (Results are encouraging; specific modes of family-based interventions for particular types of problems are being identified.)

(2) Research on family stress. (Results are encouraging; studies are focusing on family strengths and family processes regarding the resistance to hardships.) (3) The development of family typologies. (A major breakthrough for family research as these typologies bridge the gap among research, theory, and practice.) (4) Developments in marital and family strengths. (These developments lead the way to preventive and promotive services for families.) (5) Developments in assessment methods for research, practice, and program evaluation. (There is enough advance in this area; this is a major challenge for the future.) Overall, there is much to be encouraged about, except that the past two decades have not produced any new or dramatic developments in family treatment per se. The McCubbins point to the need to integrate theory, research, and practice in the family treatment field.

The Chair of this session introduces another concept and challenge. Although the topic of discussion is research utilization, meaning roughly how much of our precious research contributions practitioners are able or willing to use in their practice, there was little discussion of a parallel concept, practice utilization. This concept points to how much of the important problems and contributions by practitioners and clients are systematically incorporated into research, rather than letting researchers call the shots by defining all problems, creating methods and designs, and interpreting results. Empirically based practice is obviously a two-way interactive street. At the Conference there were only two administrators present and no front-line practitioners. Until philosophers (theorists, researchers) become kings (administrators, practitioners), or kings become philosophers, we may continue to hold conferences where we essentially talk to ourselves.

# Research Utilization
# in Direct Social Work Practice

William J. Reid
Anne E. Fortune

The focus of this chapter is research utilization in direct social work services to individuals and families. We shall offer a perspective on research utilization in direct practice, review developments in this area of utilization, and suggest some directions for the future.

It is customary to emphasize the nonutilization of research in the direct services. The familiar complaint is that practitioners do not read research and if they do, they do not use it. This grim assessment, which has changed little since the dawn of a research presence in social work a half-century ago, has been based on the narrow concept of instrumental utilization. A broader and more differentiated view permits a more discriminating and, we argue, accurate assessment of the status of research utilization.

## A PERSPECTIVE ON UTILIZATION

In earlier times research utilization in direct social work practice was considered a relatively straightforward process. Studies were conducted and their results disseminated to "program people" who then found ways to use them in their work with clients. Although some research utilization did in fact occur this way, contemporary views suggest that the utilization process is far more varied, complex, and indirect. Weiss and Bucavalas' (1980:312) observation about social science research states our argument well: "Our understanding of research utilization has to go beyond the explicit adoption of research conclusions in discrete decisions to encompass the assimilation of social science information, generalizations, and ideas into agency perspectives as a basis for making sense of problems and providing strategies of action.''

Dissatisfaction with the narrow notion of utilization as direct application of findings to programs and practice has led utilization researchers to different types of utilization (Pelz, 1978; Rich, 1977; Beyer and Trice, 1982). A key distinction is between "instrumental utilization" — specific uses of research "for decision-making or problem-solving purposes" — and "conceptual utilization" — "influencing thinking about an issue without putting information to any specific documentable use" (Rich, 1977:200). Instrumental utilization preserves the classic, "strict constructionist" notion of utilization. In conceptual utilization a user's decisions may draw on some combination of their own beliefs and research findings. This form of utilization can also be extended to use of terms, constructs, and other "conceptual knowledge" imbedded in research reports (Tripodi, Fellin, and Meyer, 1983:95). A third type of utilization referred to by Leviton and Hughes (1981:528) as "persuasive" utilization involves "drawing on . . . evidence to support a position." Advocates, lobbyists, policy makers, and agency executives who marshall scientific findings to promote a cause or a program are making persuasive use of research.

Two additional types are especially relevant to direct social work practice. A fourth category is *methodological utilization*, or use of research tools such as single-case designs or standardized tests (Tripodi, Fellin, and Meyer, 1983). A social work practitioner who employs the Generalized Contentment Scale (Hudson, 1990) to trace changes in client depression over the course of treatment is engaged in methodological utilization. The final category is *indirect utilization* which, as we use the term, involves use of theories, practice models, or procedures that are themselves *products* of research. Thus the practitioner who employs a form of social skills training that was itself shaped by a research process is utilizing research, albeit indirectly. Unlike other forms of utilization, indirect utilization requires no direct exposure to research. The practitioner's interface is not with the research itself but with the practice approach based on it.

In direct social work practice, these different forms of utilization interact over time to produce effects that are difficult to trace precisely. The dynamics can be best understood if one adopts a systemic view of the direct practice community, a community consisting of line practitioners, supervisors, program administrators, agency executives, researchers, educators, consultants, students, and so on, who interact through such media as publications, conferences, workshops, committee meetings, classes, consultations, and supervisory sessions.

This system draws on the broad domain of research and research-based practice methods in the social sciences and the helping professions. Although little is known about how this system processes these research products, we suggest that conceptual and indirect modes of utilization are the prevalent forms. It may be true that practitioners seldom turn to research studies to inform their practice, but their practice may be more influenced by research than is commonly thought — through what they learned in graduate school, through their use of empirical practice methods, through books and articles that draw on research, through program directors and supervisors who themselves are influenced by such literature, and through data generated by their agencies.

It is our thesis that these forms of utilization, often indirect and secondary, are cumulative and *in toto* are beginning to make an imprint on direct social work services, modest as that imprint may yet be. As might be imagined, self-serving and other distortions of the truth are commonplace in these processes, and it is difficult to separate good from bad utilization. We must understand this complex processing, however, if we are to comprehend how research is utilized in direct practice.

We have not only overemphasized instrumental utilization but we have also tended to overlook evidence of its occurrence, perhaps because so little evidence has been found in studies of research consumption by practicing social workers (for reviews see Kirk, 1979, 1990). Here we may be blinded by our own expectations. Hoping to find much more instrumental utilization than occurs, we have tended to equate little utilization with none at all. It may be more instructive to use a zero rate of instrumental utilization as our point of reference. In fact, this was probably close to the actual rate in the earlier years when there was little research to utilize. Against this reference point, any evidence of instrumental utilization is of interest. This prompts reinterpretation of some older studies. For example, Rosenblatt's (1968) survey has been widely and appropriately cited as evidence that social workers largely ignore research in their practice. Yet even in the discouraging findings of this study, *some* of his respondents, on the order of 10%, were making *some* use of research. Such small minorities of utilizers should perhaps be identified and studied more intensively. More generally there is need to study the occurrence of instrumental utilization as a means of building knowledge that will enable us to increase existing low rates. There is ample research to suggest that instrumental utilization does occur often enough in the human services to justify this kind of knowledge-building effort (Glaser and Taylor, 1973; Rich, 1977; Leviton and Boruch, 1980; Weiss and Bucavalas, 1980; Beyer and Trice, 1982; Velasquez, Kuechler, and White, 1986).

We argue that conditions have become more favorable for research utilization of all kinds in direct social work practice and that utilization is, in fact, increasing, albeit slowly. Using the perspective just presented we outline certain developments relating to such research utilization in direct social work practice over the past quarter century. These include changes among social work educators, developments in teaching practice and research, a shift in locus and substance of research, and a change in the agency environment. Because of the slow rate of change, it is necessary to take a long view in order to discern trends.

## RESEARCH UTILIZATION: SOCIAL WORK EDUCATION

Schools of social work affect research utilization in many ways, for example, through the education of masters and doctoral students, through the scholarly work of faculty and students, and through providing research expertise to agencies. Since the 1960s, schools of social work have become increasingly research oriented. Proportions of faculty with doctorates have risen steadily. According to most recent statistics, well over half the faculty members in schools of social work hold doctorates (Hildalgo and Spaulding, 1987) and the majority of schools expect a doctorate of new faculty (Feld, 1988; Harrison, Sowers-Hoag, and Postley, in press). Although having a doctorate is by no means equivalent to research interests or competence, faculty members with doctorates are more likely to do research, to be skilled at it, and to use it in teaching than those without doctorates (Kirk and Rosenblatt, 1984). Moreover, criteria for promotion and tenure indicate a growing expectation that all faculty members produce research and scholarship (Euster and Weinbach, 1983).

### Teaching Behavior and Practice

These developments are creating direct practice faculties that are much more research oriented than faculties of an earlier era. Direct practice faculties consequently are more likely to embrace and teach an empirical perspective toward human behavior and social treatment, which includes teaching research-based practice methods as well as single-case methodology for practice evaluation. Moreover, they draw on practice texts that espouse an empirical orientation (e.g., Fischer, 1978; Gambrill, 1983; Hepworth and Larsen, 1986; Barth, 1983). A recent survey of direct practice teaching in the first year of graduate education found that "action-oriented and task-centered methods are increasingly being used to teach social work practice" (LeCroy and Goodwin, 1988:42). The authors attribute this trend to the increased emphasis on social work practice outcomes — an indirect utilization of effectiveness research, we might add. Moreover, methods covered in one of the more widely used texts (Hepworth and Larsen, 1986) include such research-based approaches as relaxation training, cognitive restructuring, stress inoculation, and communication of empathy, with citations of relevant research. On the other hand, LeCroy and Goodwin (1988) also lament the lack of attention in practice courses paid to published research. As practice teachers, we are not surprised at this finding. The need to cover a wide range of practice methods in these courses precludes much reading of individual research studies. The distinction between direct and indirect utilization is critical here. As the variety of empirical methods grows, there may be in fact less *direct* but more *indirect* utilization of research in the practice classroom.

While the impact beyond the classroom is hard to gauge, there is little doubt that the new look in teaching human behavior and practice has resulted in research utilization by students, especially conceptual and indirect utilization. Through the education of students, schools over time exert influence on practice itself, as the psychodynamic casework movement of the 1950s and 1960s demonstrated.

## Teaching Research

From the standpoint of research utilization, the major developments in research teaching include classroom integration of practice and research teaching (Siegel, 1985; Richey, Blythe, and Berlin, 1987), introduction of single case methodology for student evaluations of their own practices (Gingerich, 1984), and approaches to enable students to use research to develop their own personal practice models (Mullen, 1983). The one that has attracted the most attention is the single case design. The single case movement gives students relevant, comprehensible research that fits well with the case study traditions of student learning. It also gives them a range of methods for evaluating their own cases, from full-scale controlled designs to devices for monitoring client progress during treatment. There is evidence that this methodology is well-received by students (Siegel, 1985) who use it in the field in conjunction with practice and research courses (Welch, 1983; Gingerich, 1984, Simons, 1987; Richey, Blythe, and Berlin, 1987). Whether they continue to use single case methodology after leaving school is another issue to be dealt with subsequently, but we would like to note here that student practice in field agencies *is* practice.

## Faculty Research

In the past quarter century, research based in schools of social work has become increasingly dominant over agency-based research. For example, the proportion of research articles authored by academic (versus agency) researchers in social work journals has increased over time (Grinnell and Royer, 1983); by the mid-1980s academics were the authors of over three-quarters of research articles (Reid, 1987). Much of this research activity concerned the development and testing of empirical models for doing and teaching social work practice. For example, most recent experimental tests of social work practice models have been conducted in academic settings or by academics (Reid and Hanrahan, 1982; Rubin, 1985; Rose, 1988). Behavioral contracting, social skills training, and task-centered approaches have been among those tested. Moreover, numerous experiments on the effectiveness of teaching practice skills have been conducted in schools of social work (Sowers-Hoag and Thyer, 1985).

Most of the practice and educational models tested underwent a developmental process (Thomas, 1987, 1984) in which the results of a preliminary trial are used to revise the model for the next trial. This is instrumental use of one's own research. The product of this research, a practice or educational model, is a form of "research-hardened" technology. When practitioners use the model, they are indirectly engaging in research utilization.

## RESEARCH UTILIZATION: THE AGENCY WORLD

In direct social work service, the bottom line for research utilization is drawn in the field. The critical question is: "How (and how much) is practice influenced by research?"

Probably the major impact of research on individualized services in social agencies is the same empirical practice movement that so influenced social work education (Fischer, 1981). As we know, the leading proponents of this movement have been academics who promote their views through writing, research, workshops, and student education. However, the social work educational establishment is only one medium for the spread of empirical approaches in agency social work. Psychology, psychiatry, and education, among other disciplines, are influenced by behavioral and other forms of empirical practice. This influence has an important impact on service programs in various settings in which social workers practice, especially mental health, child welfare, schools, and corrections.

In a national survey of clinical social workers, Jayaratne (1982) found the great majority (84%) to be eclectic in their orientations to practice. Of these workers, almost 30% cited some use of a behavioral approach and 17% indicated it was one of their two most used orientations. Of more significance was the greater use of a behavioral approach at the expense of a more traditional (and less empirical) psychodynamic orientation among more recent graduates.

The indirect utilization of research embedded in empirical practice approaches has been accompanied by increased methodological utilization. As discussed earlier, students in graduate educational programs use single case evaluations in their field agencies. But, do students use these methods after they leave school? Two surveys of graduates taught single case methodology show appreciable use of a variety of measurement techniques including specifying goals in measurable terms, use of client self-monitoring, and use of standardized instruments (Richey, Blythe and Berlin, 1987; Gingerich, 1984). Graduates made little application of single system research *designs* to assess the effectiveness of their work, but some use was reported — 12% of the respondents in one study (Richey, Blythe, and Berlin, 1987). Such results can be viewed pessimistically as the failure of single system methodology to survive the hurly-burly of the practice world, or they can be legitimately viewed as indications of tangible progress in use of elements of this methodology. Again if we accept a zero baseline as a starting point, this development reflects encouraging results. It is unrealistic to expect a large-scale and faithful application in the agency world of *any* method we teach, whether practice or research.

The empirical practice movement and accompanying case-evaluation methodologies represent one strand of research utilization in service programs. Another strand is an increasing emphasis in agencies on operations research. Included here is the development of accountability systems including quality assurance programs, of management information systems, of evaluation research capabilities, and of computer applications.

The purpose of operations research is to guide decision-making in agency contexts rather than to produce generalizable knowledge. Information systems that routinely collect, store and retrieve client and service data are a major feature of such operations research. Although most information systems are oriented to the needs of managers rather than direct practitioners, management decisions that affect direct practice programs are a form of secondary utilization by practitioners if data from information systems influenced the decisions. Recently there has been a push toward information systems more directly relevant to the needs of both managers and practitioners (Mutchsler and Hasenfeld, 1986). Among recent examples of such systems is the Management Information and Program Evaluation System at Boysville, Michigan (Grasso and Epstein, 1987). This system routinely provides direct service professionals with information on client problems and change and can also generate program evaluations with direct practice implications.

The Boysville example is part of a trend toward more service-relevant information systems in child welfare agencies generally, a trend accentuated by federal legislation (PL 96-272) requiring states to use information systems in planning for the substitute care of children. One study indicates that use of such systems does have an impact, although as yet limited, on case planning at the agency level (McMurtry, 1985).

Hospital social work provides another example of the growth of information systems related to direct service (Volland, 1976, 1980; Spano, Kiresuk, and Lund, 1977; Coulton, 1984; Wimberly, 1988). While these systems focus on accountability and performance measures, they also provide ways of defining and profiling patient problems and practitioner activities that are useful at the direct service level.

Of course, modern information systems rely heavily on the computer and probably include the best developed examples of computer applications in social work. However, numerous other uses have emerged in what Finnegan, Ivanoff and Smyth (1988) have called the "computer applications explosion." In fact, there is now a journal, *Computer Applications in Social Work and Allied Professions,* devoted exclusively to reports of work in this burgeoning field. Two developments are particularly relevant to direct practice: one is the use of expert systems and matching programs to assist practitioners in decision making (Mullen and Schuerman, 1990; Schuerman, 1987; Schuerman and Vogel, 1986; Schwab, Bruce and McRoy, 1986). A second is the creation of computer programs to enable practitioners to store, retrieve, and manipulate case data, such as the scores of standardized tests or observational measurements obtained by the practitioner (Hudson, 1990; Bronson and Blythe, 1987). The capability of such programs to generate graphs and compute statistics facilitates single case evaluations. What is more, such programs can provide practitioners with data to guide decision making during the course of a case.

We have far discussed forms of research utilization that hardly existed a quarter century ago. But what of the old-fashioned utilization that researchers hoped for but seldom achieved: the application to agency programs of the *findings* of practice research? We suggest utilization of this kind does occur but not in the way thought of, and looked for, by earlier researchers. This can be illustrated by an example from the first author's experience.

In the late 1960s Reid with Anne Shyne published the results of a field experiment in which planned brief service did somewhat better than a much longer extended service (Reid and Shyne, 1969). The results were a surprise not only to the authors but to the staff of the agency, which was a national leader in direct casework services and committed to a long-term treatment model. Planned brief treatment was definitely an ancillary service.

So what effect did the startling findings have on the agency itself? As it happened the use of short-term treatment did increase, but most of the increase took place *prior* to completion of the study and long before the findings were known. A few dramatic successes at the beginning of the service phase of the experiment were made known in the agency by the project caseworkers. These successes supported the beliefs of key agency staff who then encouraged greater use of short-term treatment. From a researcher's point of view the staff were jumping the gun in their conclusions about the effectiveness of the short-term service in the absence of any real data, yet the final results supported their judgment. This is an example of conceptual utilization. In this case there was no systematic implementation of short-term service due to final results, the response researchers traditionally look for. Instead, conceptual utilization led to gradual, spontaneous change, if technically premature. We would argue this example is by no means atypical. Similar processes are often seen in agency demonstration projects in which staff may reach their conclusions about success or failure well before the final results appear on paper.

Outside the agency, another nontraditional pattern of apparent utilization occurred. Reid was invited to give workshops at various agencies by executives or program managers who were favorably disposed toward short-term treatment. The workshops, which were of course also favorable to short-term treatment, were then used to whip up enthusiasm for the approach, perhaps reflecting a blend of conceptual and persuasive utilization.

In still other instances known to the first author, the Reid-Shyne study was directly influential in practitioners or agencies trying short-term service — examples of instrumental utilization. Even in these examples, however, the one study probably was not the deciding factor. Rather, practitioners and agencies were reacting to a study in the context of an increasingly favorable climate of opinion about brief treatment, fostered not only by numerous favorable studies but also by a burgeoning practice literature on short-term methods.

The mixture of conceptual, persuasive, and instrumental utilization of short-term treatment research is, we think, typical of the way research is influential in direct social work practice. The original empirical base may be service experiments, demonstration projects, behavioral research, or some combination thereof. This base may serve as a springboard for advocacy for new approaches by opinion leaders through media such as articles, books, conference presentations, or agency in-service training. The innovations that prosper are usually those that strike decision makers as reasonable, needed, or exciting in the light of their own experiences or sources of information. As Leviton and Hughes (1981:543) put it, "the direction of the findings interact with the position taken by potential users."

Examples of this process can be found in a number of approaches in social work that have gained currency in recent years. In child welfare, tests of experimental programs in permanency planning (Emlen et al., 1978; Stein, Gambrill, and Wiltse, 1978) and decision making (Stein and Rzepnicki, 1984) led to large-scale training and dissemination efforts and to the development of field manuals for child welfare staff (Stein and Rzepnicki, 1983). The staffs of child welfare agencies in at least five states are currently using training materials and manuals emanating from these research efforts (Stein, 1989: personal communication).

In mental health, research on expressed emotion (Vaughn and Leff, 1976) was used as a basis for developing experimental psychoeducation programs for families of the mentally ill. Evaluations of these programs, which have been quite positive (Anderson, 1983), have been a factor in their growing use.

In services to the aging, research on perceived control (Kuypers, 1972) and the deleterious effects of relocation (Lieberman, Prock, and Tobin, 1968) have stimulated initiatives to reduce the negative relocation effects (Hunt and Roll, 1987) and to promote self-help models for elderly in residential settings (Berkowitz, Waxman, and Yaffe, 1988).

In these examples, and others could be cited, it is difficult to connect specific studies to specific program developments. Instead, we are dealing with a complex force field in which research is one of many forces. To trace the effects of research in any of these examples would itself require a major study.

## SOME DIRECTIONS

Thus, if one takes a long and broad view of research utilization in direct social work practice, it is possible to see that progress has been made over the past quarter century on a number of fronts. What is more, in both schools and agencies infrastructures are developing that should result in some acceleration of progress in the next decades. However, much more needs to be done before ordinary social work practice can be considered scientifically based in any real sense. Among the possible directions to pursue, two appear particularly promising: the generation of useful practice technology and the development and application of methods of diffusion and implementation.

### Useful Methods

As we have argued, advances in research utilization in recent years have occurred in large measure through the creation of research-based technology which has included practice approaches, methods of single case study, information systems, and computer applications. Methods of this kind have resulted in important advances in indirect and methodological utilization.

However, to be utilized the methods must be useful, and by that we mean defined as useful by agency program people. The continued development and testing of practice models is central to the generation of useful methods and may well be the single most important kind of contribution that research can make to practice. But it is not enough for researcher/developers to produce practice models. The models need to go through a process of testing, evaluation, and revision with the kind of practitioners and clients for which they are intended. Adaptations for particular types of settings need to be tried out. Practice protocols need to be sufficiently detailed, comprehensible, and flexible to provide realistic guidance for practitioners who use them. Models that have been shaped by this process have attained what Thomas (1985) has called developmental validity, a critical requirement for a useful practice model.

The same thinking applies to methodological utilization. Gingerich (1990) has argued for the need to assess the utility of single case methodology as a means of discovering if, and how, it may be useful to practitioners. More generally, the notion of treatment utility (Hayes, Nelson, and Jarrett, 1987) can be applied to any type of methodological utilization. For example, what benefits do practitioners perceive from using Hudson's (1990) computerized clinical assessment package or from receiving data on client change from the information system at Boysville (Grasso and Epstein, 1987)? What difference does this information make in terms of intervention processes and outcomes? The primary purpose of such studies would not be to demonstrate how valuable all this methodology was in practice, although some benefits would be documented, it is hoped. Rather they would be designed to discover how the utility of this methodology could be improved.

### Methodology of Diffusion and Implementation

No matter how potentially useful they may be, neither practice methods nor research findings will be adequately used unless we develop better methods of diffusion and implementation. That is, we need to find more effective ways to acquaint practice personnel with research products (diffusion) and to get such personnel to actually use them (implementation) (Robinson, Bronson, and Blythe, 1988). Traditionally, a principal means of diffusion is published articles, which, as has been well documented, practitioners pass over (Kirk, 1990).

Perhaps practitioners would be more inclined to read research if the articles were written for them instead of for researchers. Researchers may think they are writing for practitioners if they publish in journals such as *Social Work* or *Social Casework* and if they go light on methodology and stress implications. But, as Schilling, Schenke, and Gilchrist (1985) argue, reaching practitioners requires a radically different format that emphasizes practice methods or knowledge rather than research methodology. Furthermore, practitioner-oriented articles that summarize and interpret existing research in particular areas is needed. Unlike conventional reviews, these articles would feature useful knowledge and methods and would illustrate potential applications. In general, research-based information should be presented with boldness, as Schilling, Schenke, and Gilchrist (1985) have observed. In research terms, the primary concern should be to avoid withholding possible useful information (Type II error) rather than making interpretations that might be wrong (Type I error). Obviously the two types of errors must be balanced but in the practice arena in which decisions are often made on the basis of a metaphorical flip of a coin, a metaphorical Type I error rate of 20 or 30% may be worth the risk if the margin of error is made clear (Reid and Smith, 1989).

The academic establishment needs to provide more, and more sophisticated, initiatives in respect to implementation of research-based technology. One-shot workshops or consultations are inadequate. In-service training projects in which staff help shape the technology to their own purposes and in which trainees are provided feedback about actual case applications are required. Such projects are reported by Mutschler (1984), Rothman (1980), Rooney (1988), and Toseland and Reid (1985). Such training and adaptations should be informed by the growing literature on utilization [for example, Beyer and Trice (1982), Munson and Pelz (1982), and Paine, Bellamy, and Wilcox (1984)]. Social workers themselves must continue to contribute to that literature (Rothman, 1980; Weinbach, 1984; Robinson, Bronson, and Blythe, 1988). Both agency and academic establishments must provide better rewards for these activities, otherwise few will be undertaken.

In conclusion, new ways of thinking about and studying research utilization processes in direct social work services are needed. Traditional reviews of research utilization are discouraging and will continue to be so because they neglect the realities of how knowledge — research or otherwise — gets incorporated into what social workers and social agencies actually do.

## REFERENCES

Anderson, C.M. 1983. "A Psychoeducational Program for Families of Patients with Schizophrenia." In W.R. McFarlane (Ed.), *Family Therapy in Schizophrenia*. New York: Guilford Press.

Barth, R.P. 1983. "Professional Self-Change Projects: Bridging the Clinical-Research and Classroom-Agency Gaps." *Journal of Education for Social Work*, 13-19.

Berkowitz, M.W., R. Waxman, and L. Yaffee. 1988. "The Effects of a Resident Self-Help Model on Control, Social Involvement and Self-Esteem Among the Elderly." *The Gerontologist*, 28(5):620-24.

Beyer, J.M. and H.M. Trice. 1982. "The Utilization Process: A Conceptual Framework and Synthesis of Empirical Findings." *Administrative Science Quarterly*, 27:591-622.

Bronson, D.E. and B.J. Blythe. 1987. "Computer Support for Single-Case Evaluation of Practice." *Social Work Research and Abstracts*, 23(3):10-13.

Coulton, C. 1984. "Confronting Prospective Payment: Requirements for an Information System." *Health and Social Work*, 9:13-24.

Emlen, A. et al. 1978. *Overcoming Barriers to Planning for Children in Foster Care*. Portland, OR: Regional Research Institute for Human Services, Portland State University.

Euster, G.L. and R.W. Weinbach, 1983. "University Rewards for Faculty Community Service." *Journal of Education for Social Work*, 19:108-14.

Feld, S. 1988. "The Academic Marketplace in Social Work." *Journal of Social Work Education*, 24:201-10.

Finnegan, D.J., A. Ivanoff, and N.J. Smyth. 1988. "The Computer Explosion: What Practitioners and Managers Need to Know." School of Social Welfare, State University at Albany, New York. Manuscript.

Fischer, J. 1978. *Effective Casework Practice: An Eclectic Approach*. New York: McGraw-Hill Books.

_____. 1981. "The Social Work Revolution." *Social Work*, 26(3):199-207.

Gambrill, E. 1983. *Casework: A Competency-based Approach*. Englewood Cliffs, NJ: Prentice-Hall.

Gingerich, W.J. 1984. "Generalizing Single-Case Evaluation from Classroom to Practice." *Journal of Education for Social Work*, 20(1):74-82.

_____. (1990). "Rethinking Single-Case Evaluation." In L. Videka-Sherman and W.J. Reid (Eds.) *Advances in Clinical Social Work Research.* Washington, DC: National Association of Social Workers.

Glaser, E.M. and S.H. Taylor. 1973. "Factors Influencing the Success of Applied Research." *American Psychologist*, 28(2):140-46.

Grasso, A.J. and I. Epstein. 1987. "Management by Measurement: Organizational Dilemmas and Opportunities." *Administration in Social Work*, 11(3/4): 89-100.

Grinnell, R.M. Jr. and M.L. Royer. 1983. "Authors of Articles in Social Work Journals." *Journal of Social Service Research*, 6(3/4):147-54.

Harrison, D.F., K. Sowers-Hoag, and B.J. Postley. In press. "Faculty Hiring in Social Work: Dilemmas for Education or Job Candidates." *Journal of Social Work Education*.

Hayes, S.C., R.D. Nelson and R.B. Jarrett. 1987. "The Treatment Utility of Assessment." *American Psychologist*, 42:63-74.

Hepworth, D.H., and J. Larsen. 1986. *Direct Social Work Practice: Theory and Skills*, 2nd ed. Homewood, IL: Dorsey Press.

Hildalgo, J. and E.C. Spaulding, (Eds.) 1987. *Statistics on Social Work Education in the U.S.: 1986.* Washington DC: Council on Social Work Education.

Hudson, W.W. 1990. "Computer-based Clinical Practice: Present Status and Future Possibilities." In L. Videka-Sherman and W.J. Reid (Eds.) *Advances in Clinical Social Work Research.* Washington, DC: National Association of Social Workers.

Hunt, M.E. and M.K. Roll. 1987. "Simulation in Familiarizing Older People with an Unknown Building." *The Gerontologist*, 27(2):169-75.

Jayaratne, S. 1982. "Characteristics and Theoretical Orientations of Clinical Social Workers: A National Survey." *Journal of Social Service Research*, 4:17-29.

Kirk, S.A. and A. Rosenblatt. 1984. "The Contribution of Women Faculty to Social Work Journals." *Social Work*, 29(1):67-69.

Kirk, S.A. 1990. "Research Utilization: A Friendly Revisit." In L. Videka-Sherman and W.J. Reid (Eds.) *Advances in Clinical Social Work Research.* Washington, DC: National Association of Social Workers.

_____. 1979. "Understanding Research Utilization in Social Work" in A. Rubin and A. Rosenblatt (Eds.) *Sourcebook on Research Utilization.* New York: Council on Social Work Education.

Kuypers, J. 1972. "Internal-External Locus of Control, Ego Functioning, and Personal Characteristics in Old Age." *The Gerontologist*, 12:168-73.

LeCroy, C.W. and C.C. Goodwin. 1988. "New Directions in Teaching Social Work Methods: A Content Analysis of Course Outlines." *Journal of Social Work Education*, 24(1):43-49.

Leviton, L.C. and E.F. Hughes. 1981. "Research on the Utilization of Evaluations: A Review and Synthesis." *Evaluation Review*, 5(4):525-48.

Leviton, L.C. and R.F. Boruch. 1980. "Illustrative Case Studies." In R.F. Boruch and D.S. Cordray, (Eds.). *An Appraisal of Educational Program Eval-*

*uations: Federal, State, and Local Levels.* Washington, DC: U.S. Department of Education.

Lieberman, M.A., V. Prock, and S. Tobin. 1968. "Psychological Effects of Institutionalization." *Journal of Gerontology*, 23:343-53.

McMurtry, S.L. 1985. "Automated Information Management in Substitute Care for Children: A Study of Contributions to Planning, Review, and Case Outcomes." Doctoral Dissertation, University of Wisconsin, Madison.

Mullen, E.J. 1983. "Personal Practice Models." In A. Rosenblatt and D. Waldfogel (Eds.) *Handbook of Clinical Social Work*. San Francisco: Jossey-Bass.

Mullen, E.J. and J. Schuerman. 1990. "Expert Systems and the Development of Knowledge in Social Welfare." In L. Videka-Sherman and W.J. Reid (Eds.) *Advances in Clinical Social Work Research*, Washington, DC: National Association of Social Workers.

Munson, F.C. and D.C. Pelz. 1982. *Innovating in Organizations: A Conceptual Framework.* Ann Arbor: University of Michigan, Institute for Social Research.

Mutschler, E. 1984. "Evaluating Practice: A Study of Research Utilization by Practitioners." *Social Work*, 29:332-37.

Mutschler, E. and Y. Hasenfeld. 1986. "Integrated Information Systems for Social Work Practice." *Social Work*, 31:345-49.

Paine, S.C., B.T. Bellamy, and B. Wilcox. 1984. *Human Services That Work: From Innovation to Standard Practice.* Beverly Hills, CA: Sage.

Pelz, D.C. 1978. "Some Expanded Perspectives on Use of Social Science in Public Policy." In M. Yinger and S.J. Cutler, (Eds.) *Major Social Issues: A Multidisciplinary View*, pp. 346-57. New York: Free Press.

Reid, W.J. and A. Shyne. 1969. *Brief and Extended Casework.* New York: Columbia University Press.

Reid, W.J. and A.D. Smith. 1989. *Research in Social Work*, 2nd ed. New York: Columbia University Press.

Reid, W.J. and P. Hanrahan. 1982. "Recent Evaluations of Social Work: Grounds for Optimism." *Social Work*, 27:328-40.

Reid, W.J. 1987. "Research in Social Work." In Ann Minahan (Ed.), *Encyclopedia of Social Work*, 18th ed. New York: NASW.

Rich, R.F. 1977. "Uses of Social Science Information by Federal Bureaucrats: Knowledge for Action versus Knowledge for Understanding." In C.H. Weiss (Ed.) *Using Social Research in Public Policy Making*, Lexington, MA: Lexington Books.

Richey, C.A., B.J. Blythe, and S.B. Berlin. 1987, "Do Social Workers Evaluate Their Practice." *Social Work Research and Abstracts*, 23(2):14-20.

Robinson, E.A.R., D.E. Bronson, and B.J. Blythe. 1988. "An Analysis of the Implementation of Single-Case Evaluation by Practitioners." *Social Service Review*, 62(2):285-301.

Rooney, R.H. 1988. "Measuring Task-Centered Training Effects on Practice: Results of an Audiotape Study in a Public Agency." *Journal of Continuing Social Work Education*, 42(4):2-7.

Rose, S.D. 1988. "Practice Experiments for Doctoral Dissertations: Research

Training and Knowledge Building." *Journal of Social Work Education*, 24(2):115-22.

Rosenblatt, A. 1968. "The Practitioner's Use and Evaluation of Research," *Social Work*, 15, 53-59.

Rothman, J. 1980. *Social R&D: Research and Development in the Human Services*. Englewood Cliffs, NJ: Prentice-Hall.

Rubin, A. 1985. "Practice Effectiveness: More Grounds for Optimism." *Journal of the National Association of Social Workers*, 30:469-76.

Schilling, R.F., S.P. Schenke, and L.D. Gilchrist. 1985. "Utilization of Social Work Research: Reaching the Practitioner." *Journal of the National Association of Social Workers*, 30(6):527-29.

Schuerman, J.R. 1987. "Expert Consulting Systems in Social Welfare." *Social Work Research and Abstracts*, 23(3):14-18.

Schuerman, J.R. and L.H. Vogel. 1986. "Computer Support of Placement Planning: The Use of Expert Systems in Child Welfare." *Child Welfare*, 65(7): 531-43.

Schwab, A.T. Jr., M.E. Bruce, and R.G. McRoy. 1986. "Using Computer Technology in Child Placement Decisions." *Social Casework: The Journal of Contemporary Social Work*, 67(7):359-68.

Siegel, D.H. 1985. "Effective Teaching of Empirically Based Practice." *Social Work Research and Abstracts*, 21(1):40-48.

Simons, R.L. 1987. "The Impact of Training for Empirically Based Practice." *Journal of Social Work Education*, 23(1):24-30.

Sowers-Hoag, K. and B. Thyer. 1985. "Community Planning and Organization in an Era of Retrenchment: Structural and Educational Approaches to Serving Human Needs." *Journal of Social Work Education*, 21(3):5-15.

Spano, R., T. Kiresuk and S. Lund. 1977. "An Operational Model to Achieve Accountability for Social Work in Health Care." *Social Work in Health Care*, 3:367-76.

Stein, T.J. and T.L. Rzepnicki. 1984. *Decision Making in Child Welfare Services*. Boston: Kluwer-Nijhoff.

_____. 1983. *Decision Making at Child Welfare Intake: A Handbook for Social Workers*. New York: Child Welfare League of America.

Stein, T.J., E.D. Gambrill, and K.T. Wiltse. 1978. *Children in Foster Homes: Achieving Continuity in Care*. New York: Praeger.

Thomas, E.J. 1985. "The Validity of Design and Development and Related Concepts in Developmental Research." *Social Work Research and Abstracts*, 21(2):50-55.

_____. 1987. "Assessing Procedural Descriptiveness: Rationale and Illustrative Study." *Behavioral Assessment*, 9:43-56.

_____. 1984. *Designing Interventions for the Helping Professions*. Beverly Hills, CA: Sage.

Toseland, R.W. and W.J. Reid. 1985. "Using Rapid Assessment Instruments in a Family Service Agency." *Social Casework*, 66:547-55.

Tripodi, T., P. Fellin and H.J. Meyer, 1983. *The Assessment of Social Research*, 2nd ed. Itasca, IL: Peacock.

Vaughn, C. and J. Leff. 1976. "The Measurement of Expressed Emotion in the Families of Psychiatric Patients." *British Journal of Social and Clinical Psychology*, 15:157-65.

Velasquez, J.S., D.F. Kuechler, and M.S. White. 1986. "Use of Formative Evaluation in a Human Service Department." *Administration in Social Work*, 10(2):67-77.

Volland, P. 1976. "Social Work Information and Accountability System in a Hospital Setting." *Social Work in Health Care*, 1:277-85.

———. 1980. "Costing for Social Work Services." *Social Work in Health Care*, 6:73-87.

Weinbach, R.W. 1984. "Implementing Change: Insights and Strategies for the Supervisor." *Social Work*, 29(3):282-86.

Weiss, C.H. and M.J. Bucavalas. 1980. Truth Tests and Utility Tests: Decision-Makers' Frames of Reference for Social Science Research. *American Sociological Review*, 45:302-13.

Welch, G.J. 1983. "Will Graduates Use Single-Subject Designs to Evaluate Their Casework Practice?" *Journal of Education for Social Work*, 19:42-47.

Wimberly, E.T. 1988. "Using Productivity Measures to Avoid Reductions in Force." *Social Work*, 33(1):60-61.

# The Ethics and the Utilization of Interpersonal Practice Research

## Harold Lewis

One facet of scholarly interest in the relationship of knowledge to action is the problem one encounters when promoting the utilization in practice of knowledge derived from scientific studies. This chapter focuses on ethical issues that accompany such efforts. It assumes that when one entertains the potential for utilization in practice of a study's process and findings as part of the formulation of a study's objectives, one also assumes obligations and duties that transcend the standards of science. In such instances one meets the principles of ethical behavior that govern relationships involving applications of the "truths of science" (Jonas, 1976). Despite an awareness on the part of researchers that ethical dilemmas frequently occur in utilization efforts, rarely do their reports address such issues in depth. If, as some report (Constable, 1985), "There is little influence of practitioner's conception of practice on what they actually say they would prefer to do, and little skill among practitioners in conducting an ethical analysis," the omission in study reports is matched by a similar omission in descriptions of practice. These omissions do not necessarily represent a failure on the part of researchers and practitioners to address ethical issues in their work, but they do represent the relative importance assigned to such issues.

There is disagreement among social work researchers as to whether their charge includes the linking of knowledge to action and assuring the utilization of their research findings in practice. There have always been those who stress the need to protect and perfect the methods of the social sciences from the contaminating influence of action-oriented special interest groups. These researchers argue that more benefits will accrue to society if the findings of their studies are viewed as free of bias, having been validated by methods that meet the most rigorous tests of science. They believe it is the responsibility of the practitioner to develop and apply the means whereby the findings of research are incorporated into their practice. Others have deplored the lack of relevance of findings generated by these social scientists. Among these are some who doubt that an objective, value-free science is possible, holding to the view that the true test of the validity of findings will be found in their application.

For the greater part of the 20th century there have been social work researchers who have viewed social work research as a form of social action. They have pursued the development of study designs and methods which together alter what is studied in order to penetrate beyond the appearances of social phenomena and understand their essence. These researchers believe that research tools are most revealing when incorporated into practice as part of the interventions intended to achieve specific ends. Ideally, they would have the researcher and practitioner in one person, a "scholarly practitioner." In this chapter the ethical issues discussed can arise in the research work of adherents to any of the above perspectives, though each perspective generates issues of special interest to its adherents.

## DEFINITION

For our purposes the professional ethics we will refer to are those principles that are intended to define the rights and responsibilities of researchers and practitioners in social work in their relationship with each other and with other parties including employers, research subjects, clients, and students (Chalk, 1980).

I will assume that the social work practitioner and the social work researcher share a common concern for the well-being of the recipients of social services. I expect that both subscribe to the prevalent set of imperatives that are used to frame ethical issues in clinical research and practice. These imperatives include:

1. "Respect for Persons: This principle recognizes the autonomy of the individual, the rights of persons to decide for themselves what course of action they choose to pursue. The right to privacy and the requirement for informed consent derive their legitimacy from this principle."
2. "The Harm Principle: Consideration of harm places limitations on the individuals' freedom of action. In medicine (read 'Social Work,' chapter author) it obligates the physician (read 'social worker,' or 'researcher,' chapter author) when possible to avoid doing harm."
3. "Beneficence: This principle requires that actions be based on considerations of the interest and welfare of others—both individuals and the community. It demands balancing potential benefits against potential risks and adopting the course of action believed to have the most favorable risk to benefit ratio."
4. "Justice: This principle requires an equitable distribution of benefits and burdens" (Meyers and Dunton, 1986).

Given this framework of ethical principles (imperatives), the following prerequisites are acceptable to researchers and practitioners for evaluating the ethical components of a research program in interpersonal practice.

1. "The purpose of the research must be ethically acceptable; e.g., to promote the well being of the service recipient."
2. "The means used in the research practice and the intended use of the information must be appropriate for accomplishing the purpose."
3. "Qualified personnel (research and practice) must be used."
4. "Recipients must be informed that research will take place."
5. "Individuals who receive the service have a right to know the assessment of their condition by the practitioner; how they will be affected by the research design, and the results of the study."
6. "Confidentiality of the recipient must be protected" (Meyers and Dunton, 1988).

Assuming this framework and these prerequisite conditions, this chapter will first identify differences in function and role in the work of practitioners and researchers, then, all too briefly, relevant epistemological concerns. Some current ethical issues confronting researchers in interpersonal practice will be addressed. The end result of this analysis, it is hoped, will be a more explicit appreciation of the complexity of "doing ethics" in this area of intellectual work. Finally, recommendations for collective actions that could possibly make such "doing" less demanding for the individual researcher and practitioner will be proposed.

## FUNCTION AND ROLE

The researcher's function differs from the practitioner's in ways that are critical to an evaluation of ethical issues. Research seeks to add to knowledge, to pursue truth, and to affirm existing knowledge claims. Research also seeks to demonstrate new uses of knowledge. The researcher employs methods appropriate to the study of interpersonal practice, including the context of such practice. The logic of such methods cautions against unwarranted assumptions. For this reason the researcher will favor maximizing doubt and minimizing certainties. The researcher's preference is for Type 1 error: to reject as false what may be true, rather than risk the error of accepting as true what may be false.

In carrying out the research function, the research worker may be called upon to enact a variety of roles. Depending on the location and auspice of the study, s/he may be an academic scholar, consultant, agency employee, entrepreneurial problem-solving expert, etc. In each role the ethical virtues may be represented by a similar set of behaviors, but obligations and duties incurred, and the common good pursued, will vary. For example, as agency employee, the role is that of service provider. When viewed as a service, research work takes on the obligations that inhere in any professional interpersonal practice. The contract as employee may call for obligations that limit the dissemination of findings, more so than what an academic scholar would find tolerable. When viewed in light of function and role, the research worker is found to be enmeshed in a variety of situations that involve choices and judgments and is necessarily affected by ethical issues germane to such work.

The practitioner is not primarily committed to adding to knowledge. S/he pursues the service process with intentions to do good, defined in terms of the benefits to be derived by the recipient. For the practitioner, the recipient is not a means to an end, as is true for the researcher. Employing methods appropriate to helping functions, the practitioner accepts the profession's Code of Ethics as a set of guiding imperatives to be followed in seeking to implement the service transaction. The logic of these methods dictates caution lest s/he miss opportunities to effect desired changes. Thus, in contrast to the researcher, the practitioner seeks to maximize certainties and minimize doubts, since the practice function promotes "doing," in contrast to "knowing." The practitioner's preference is for error Type 2. S/he would risk assuming to be true what in fact may be false rather than, in error, rejecting an opportunity to exercise a positive influence.

In carrying out the practitioner function, the worker may be called upon to enact a variety of roles. Depending on the setting and auspice of the service, the practitioner may be helper/therapist/educator/counselor/problem solver, etc., and may be a private practitioner, consultant, agency employee, etc. In each role different obligations and duties may be incurred. The common good to be pursued may vary, as will the emphasis given to one or more of the ethical virtues. As does the researcher, so too does the practitioner get enmeshed in a variety of situations that involve choices and judgments and that are necessarily affected by ethical issues germane to such work.

While both researcher and practitioner may subscribe to a similar ethical framework and may agree on similar prerequisites for ethical practice, the differences in functions and roles inherent in their work militate against a facile blending of both functions. The possibility of sequencing these functions so as to avoid the concurrent contradictory demands they make is problematic. Unhappily, the difficulties arising out of these dual functions do not disappear by simply separating contradictory expectations in time. In rendering the service, the worker is the participant whose process helps generate the data to be observed. Separating the functions in time may be theoretically plausible but practically unachievable if one considers the mental and emotional demands on the worker. "Feeling" and "being" are less amenable to partialization on a time continuum than is "doing." The wish to locate both functions in one person, as some propose, needs critical evaluation if for no other reason than to resolve the ethical conundrums that are inherent in such a merger.

## EPISTEMOLOGICAL CONSIDERATIONS

Means and ends, in practice, are inseparable, though mental categorizing of both is common. For a professional practice, which necessarily is influenced by intentions, goals and objectives reflect commitments that must be accounted for in any conceptualization of its guiding practice principles. Formulating the knowledge claims of a professional practice and concurrently incorporating its ethical commitments into such formulations is an intellectual challenge. Clearly, distinctions that highlight the is/ought knowledge/value duality are useful, but insufficient.

It is helpful to approach the task of welding the propositional statement to the ethical component as an essential step in formulating practice science generalizations. Unlike the "laws" that are the products of theoretical science, the practice principles of a practice science are time- and place-specific and heavily burdened by contingent variables. This characteristic of practice principle generalizations (or practice prescriptions, as some prefer to call them) enhance their utility to practitioners, while serving to inform and direct interventions that are necessarily probabilistic in nature (Wedenoja, 1988). Propositions from the disciplines and from experiential reports are useful in building practice science generalizations. However, it is essential that these propositions be welded to ethical commendations usually expressed as "ought," "will," "should," and "must" if the principles are to command, as well as direct, worker actions. It is no accident that rule-governed behavior plays so large a role in guiding professional interventions. Such rules are crucial to the technological maturation of a profession, serving to both direct and command the behavior of the worker. Heavily dependent on the practice principles used to generate them, rules provide some assurance of a principled practice. Thus, at the level of practice principle and rule, the ethical commendation is joined to the propositional statement. When reporting findings from research, formulating the results in terms of practice principles and derivative rules will make them far more useful to the practitioner, than simple affirming or denying hypotheses stated in propositional terms.

Moreover, on the knowledge side, utilization requires, at a minimum, knowledge elicitation, knowledge formalization, and knowledge representation—elements identified in expert systems construction, now so popular among "knowledge engineers" (Barnett, 1988). Each of these elements involves choices shaped by intentions of those soliciting, organizing, and presenting the knowledge, hopefully in a user-friendly format. Given the difficulty in perceiving ourselves as simultaneously both observers and participants in a system, and the imprecise and common sense knowledge and reasoning under conditions of uncertainty that characterize the practice we observe, we need to make explicit what are the criteria for selecting acceptable sources of knowledge that warrant our close observation.

The prime ethical concern confronting practice research is the requisite that the practice being observed is itself principled, and that it justifies its interventions on ethical grounds. Can research based on unethical practice meet the criteria used to evaluate ethical research? Further, can the findings of such research be treated as neutral to ethical concerns, and therefore useful for constructive purposes? In relation to the use of human fetal tissue derived from an aborted fetus, and in relation to medical findings based on research conducted on concentration camp victims by Nazi physicians, this issue has been raised, with contending views remaining unresolved. The crucial assumption in these debates is that, "The overlap between the categories of therapy and research, in predicted benefit of outcome and indeed in uncertainty of prediction, is too great to allow the distinction of the categories for ethical purpose," (Freedman, 1988).

It is often not easy to be sure whether an intervention should be regarded as a treatment undertaken only in the patients' best interest, or whether it is guided also by an intent to gain scientific knowledge (Miller, 1988). Although it is generally accepted that the decision of whether a research intent is present in the service is a determination to be made by the service provider (Miller, 1988), this is not always a simple matter. Often the intervention is itself experimental, representing an innovation in practice. In such instances it is argued that such interventions may be viewed as preliminary studies and should be subject to the same ethical judgments that apply to all research protocols (Miller, 1988).

Let us assume that the researcher and practitioner agree on a program that they believe is in the recipients' interest. Both should be able to assure the recipients that they will be receiving the best available service known. This is particularly important in a random assignment where the recipient may be provided with no service (placebo) other than inclusion in the program. Since in typical instances the research is usually prompted by some evidence, though not necessarily scientifically validated, that one intervention holds promise of achieving results not otherwise achievable, it is problematic to provide the assurance that meets the standard of ethical justification noted above. If, in order to attract and hold a sample, less than full disclosure is considered, the ethical dilemma is posed: which shall prevail, benefit to recipient or benefit to society (Schafer, 1985)?

As noted earlier, the practitioner is impelled by a primary commitment to the well-being of the recipient whose personal welfare is the basic objective of their relationship. The researcher's primary commitment is to add to knowledge, placing the societal welfare as the prime objective of their relationship. While these differing obligations can separate the two, they need not be mutually exclusive. In most situations a rational process that treats these different purposes as an instance of dialectic can be pursued, with an outcome acceptable to all concerned.

Consider, for example, how the differences in objectives noted affect differences in the interpersonal exchange posed by these questions:

1. Who initiates and terminates the exchange and who decides on parties to be included?

2. Whose needs are addressed? Whose goals are worked on?
3. Who determines the process? Who controls its development?
4. What information is sought and in what manner expressed?
5. What obligations are assumed by parties to the transaction?

In each of these aspects of the exchange the researcher may have different interests than the clinician stemming from differences in purpose and intention. Preferences, ethically commended, will vary, with considerable overlap. Resolving the ethical ambiguities and dilemmas requires a mix of epistemological and axiological analysis. The process is necessarily ongoing, dynamic, and specific to the exchange involved. Unacceptable from an ethical perspective is a copping-out alternative, such as ignoring the ethical issues or reducing them to polarities of a mechanistic mode where choices are so limited that any possibility of resolution of differences is excluded.

Does the practitioner's treatment purpose free him/her from the usual human subject restraints exercised in IRB (Internal Review Boards) procedures governing research protocols? For example, if it is experimental treatment, should the requirements of human subject research be met? Given the fuzzy knowledge we are dealing with in the practice being observed, one can argue that most interpersonal interventions are uncertain in outcome to a degree that warrants their being considered innovations. Another view considers that the practitioner's application of the best knowledge available in the field of practice meets the ethical imperative to act on that condition. The danger in knowingly or unknowingly masking a research purpose in the guise of a clinical intervention and thus avoiding an IRB review must be noted. As far as I can determine, this rarely occurs where the research design includes a specified intervention. It can occur more readily where one defines the research intervention as the treatment, so that the choice of categorizing the practice as experimental is more likely to be based on convenience.

In our own profession, the issue of justifications for practicing deceptions in research and for failing to obtain informed consent of subjects has recently surfaced as an ethical problem. At issue is the ethics of a study by William M. Epstein of the policies of social work journals which he hypothesized amount to "prior censorship" of academic research. John Schuerman notes that in certain kinds of social science research, investigators must deceive subjects or at least not fully inform them about the purpose of an experiment. To determine when deception is necessary, the costs and benefits of the research should be taken into account in making judgments about the legitimacy of deception and the failure to obtain informed consent. In the case of Epstein's study, Schuerman argues that the deception was unjustified and that the author violated the professional association's (NASW) Code of Ethics. Schuerman utilizes consequentialist criteria in challenging the justification of deception. If this were a therapeutic intervention affecting the welfare of a service recipient, the recipient's right to know and not to know would require that the harm principle, respect for persons principle, and beneficence principle all be demonstrated. That less demanding criteria are acceptable in research than would be in practice is debatable (Coughlin, 1988).[1]

Nevertheless, it is necessary to deal with the different ethical positions of researcher and practitioner in more detail. When the practitioner decides not to fully inform the recipient, s/he does so based on a clinical judgment that withholding the information is for the recipient's own good. In short, the right to know that is crucial to respect of persons is sacrificed, with the intention of benefiting the person whose "right" is sacrificed. The paternalistic aspects of such choices have been extensively discussed in the literature. When the researcher does not fully inform or uses a deception, it is for the good of the study goal (i.e., to benefit society). The recipient's right to know is here sacrificed for a potential future good, not necessarily to benefit the recipient whose right is sacrificed. At the very least, a much more rigorous justification of this latter sacrifice of recipient's "rights" is required. Where deliberate deception is involved, a consequentialist ethical analysis is necessary but insufficient. Two rights may be in conflict, i.e., the right of the researcher to pursue truth using means which allow for obtaining crucial data, and the right of the recipient to be dealt with in a manner that respects his/her person. If this is the case, a lexical ordering of rights is required. While some effort should be made to weight the extent of harm that can result, not merely the benefits that are entailed, such calculations are often difficult and muddied. But the admonition to "avoid doing harm" is an absolute one, regardless of how much harm may be involved. This imperative can be overridden by another, such as to save a life. Not surprisingly, how to take into account both the teleological and deontological approaches to ethical analysis is a much debated issue.

Still another ethical issue in utilization of research findings is related to the time and nature of the report. Because research on practice is never neutral to the concurrent social and psychological process in the surround, the impact of findings and the reception they will receive often threaten the bond of trust that prompted participation in the study by those observed. If one is insensitive to context, the negative fallout of untimely and inappropriate release of findings may mitigate against their utilization, but even more significant, may cut off future access to the population involved, closing the door for other studies by other researchers. The scientist is taught very early in his/her career not to conduct a study in a manner that would deny future scientists an opportunity to replicate it. To this imperative we might add not reporting the findings in an untimely and inappropriate manner, for similar reasons. Yet this imperative can corrupt the knowledge building process where an unpopular finding is deliberately suppressed. In such situations time may be a crucial variable, with time postponed representing opportunity lost. The ethical issues entailed are applicable to all phases of the research process, but surfaced most dramatically at the point where findings are presented for action by the recipients of the report.

The issue here is whether the researcher is responsible for what goes on up to the conclusion of the study and the report of findings. Is what is done with the findings beyond his/her control and hence not his/her responsibility? Recent research on AIDS patients has sharpened our awareness of how the lack of appropriate ethical concern for privacy and autonomy of persons in timely reports of findings can produce undesirable fallout. In interpersonal practice, the effects on individuals, groups, and communities of untimely reporting of findings are significant. Often studies never get off the ground because some funding group anticipates such untimely publication of what may be negative results. Our profession has also experienced instances where findings were buried. I need only recall one of the guidelines proposed by the Hamovitch Committee in 1958 to illustrate how important this issue has been to social work research practitioners:

> Researchers have responsibility for anticipating and correcting improper use of research findings. If experience has shown that certain professional organizations or individual social workers persist in distorting social work research findings for their own purposes, either research service should be withheld or public statements should be issued. (Hamovitch, 1957; Lewis, 1961)

Arthur Vidich observed long ago:

> that the obligation to do scientific justice to one's findings quite often conflicts with the social obligation to please all objects of research. One can accept a "scientific ethic" or a "social contractual ethic." It is not easy to accept both. (1960)

I do not believe the picture in social work research is as bleak as Vidich suggests. I suspect that the "social obligation" is a variable one, subject to the influence of professional skill in helping. Principles wedded to competence and the virtues courage and imagination are necessary if the ethics of the practitioner are to live productively together with the ethics of the researcher.

From the discussion thus far a number of practical suggestions can be extracted. To recapitulate, an ethical framework derived from the experience of IRBs, and the analyses conducted by a variety of ethicists working in human subject areas, was assumed. Differences in function and role were identified. The need for an epistemological framework compatible with an ethical framework was stressed, emphasizing the importance of practice principles. These three foci suggest the following: in any research conducted on practice involving interpersonal interventions, the ethical framework, the function and roles, and the epistemological frame should be made explicit at the outset. Although no minor undertaking, clarity in these areas early in the study process can help avoid misunderstandings and resolve ethical dilemmas that can later hinder the utilization of findings. Recognizing the difficulties inherent in efforts to meld the research and practice goals and objectives, particularly where an "observing participant" role is anticipated, developing a strategy for dealing with these difficulties early in the study process can be helpful.

Our discussion then turned to specific issues currently of interest to researchers in human subject disciplines. Conflicts between "rights" and "good," two or more rights, or multiple goods are unavoidable where the subject of study is interpersonal interventions. The need to utilize both teleological (consequentialist) and deontological analyses in dealing with such conflicts suggests the need for persons skilled in conducting ethical assessments. It is possible for researchers and practitioners to develop some competence in conducting such assessments, but experience seems to indicate a function and role for specialists in this area. If such skill is sought and available it should be utilized early in the study process; be on call during the process and brought back in, if the need is indicated, at the conclusion of the study.

## CONTEXT

Next, attention will be given to the importance of context in dealing with ethical issues. Earlier I looked at the variety of settings in which the research function is housed and the variety of settings in which the practice observed can occur. I noted that these variations could be of considerable ethical significance, particularly when seeking to resolve dilemmas arising from the intrusion of the interests of the setting into the relationships of researcher and practitioner.

It seems to me unlikely that a practice can be neutral to the context in which it occurs. Nor, I believe, can a research design successfully insulate the study process from the setting. Rather than defend these assertions, I'll take them as givens, which if proven false, could nullify what follows.

Context influences process in a number of ways, of which I will consider only two: the selection of goals and objectives, and the setting of limits to what can be studied and how study results can be utilized.

## Goals and Objectives

Goals are value based, often reflecting ideological preferences. Objectives are steps along the way leading to the achievement of goals; they are much more related to ethical imperatives which operationalize values. Goal-directed research is more likely to seek evidence of effectiveness and objective oriented studies seek evidence of effect. While it is likely that one can successfully accomplish objectives yet not achieve the intended goal, it is a certainty that an ethically sound performance will sustain the values that justify the imperatives that in turn guide the performance. Thus, the goals and objectives to be pursued in a study should be agreed on early in the study process, lest conflicting values and inoperable ethical imperatives distort the study process. For this reason, early attention to an ethical framework can be a useful tool in seeking to clarify objectives and goals at the outset of the study process. For example, if early on the sponsor of the study, the researcher, and the practitioner agree on the beneficence and justice principles, it can justify sample selection and various techniques to be employed in the study. But more important, it can sustain commitment to questioning objectives and goals, when conclusions from the study are not in the direction anticipated.

## Setting of Limits

Setting limits to what can be studied and how study results can be utilized calls for reconciliation of feasibility of means, and timeliness and appropriateness of ends. The fact that something can be done does not mean it should be done. Context influences decisions in both areas. What can be done is not merely a question of technical competence, but also depends on access and funding. Context also sets parameters affecting the sponsorship, location, staffing and period to be covered by the study. Evaluation of contingent factors, such as relevant historical precedence, concurrent happenings in the surround, and readiness of decision makers to entertain the potential findings of the study, are all contextual influences that set limits to what can be studied and how study results can or will be utilized. In the process of setting limits, duties and obligations are incurred, thereby establishing ethical constraints on the behavior of parties to agreements reached.

Some additional suggestions, which may be useful:

1. Ethics Review Committees in social agencies are needed. Such committees do not substitute for the judgments of staff, but can provide sounding boards for staff seeking advice on critical ethical dilemmas. They can, through their experience over time, accumulate a body of practice wisdom and ethical guidance to be drawn upon as a rich resource for both new and seasoned staff. Most important, they can suggest measures to be taken by the agency to strengthen adherence to practice principles in the delivery of its services.
2. Research workers and research sponsors can benefit from case studies involving ethical issues in research practice. The research journals might consider incorporating such studies as a regular feature.
3. Effort should be made to encourage schools of social work, and to incorporate content on ethical issues and the "how" of their resolution in research courses. This is in addition to the necessary content on ethics prescribed by the new curriculum policy statement and accreditation standards.

If implemented, these modest innovations should heighten our sensitivity to ethical issues, and generate empirical data which are necessary for more systematic study of these issues.

## ENDNOTE

1. Chronicle of Higher Education (February 3, 1988) Daniel Goleman, "Test of Journals is Criticized as Unethical." *The New York Times* (September 27, 1988), science section; Laurence Feinberg, "Social Researcher's Ethics Challenged." *The Washington Post* (October 22, 1988); Ellen K. Coughlin "Scholar Who Submitted Bogus Article to Journals May be Disciplined." *The Chronicle of Higher Education* (November 2, 1988).

"Editorial," *Social Service Review* 62, No.3 (September 1988): 351-52 and Vol. 63 No. 1 (March 1989) pp 1-4; John R. Schuerman, *Memo* to Editors of Journals (October 4, 1988): Suzanne Dworak-Peck, *Letter to John R. Schuerman* (March 20, 1989) re: Action of NASW National Committee on Inquiry re: Schuerman vs. Epstein; Daniel Goleman, "Charge Dropped on Bogus Work," *The New*

*York Times* (April 4, 1989), science section; Charles Levy, "Mutuality of Responsibility in Social Work Ethics," *Social Work,* 34 (May 1989) p. 268 and William M. Epstein's reply to Charles Levy in *Social Work* "Letters" 35 (November 1990) p. 571.

# REFERENCES

Barnett, Peter. "Computing in Philosophical Research." *Communications.* CUNY University, Vol. 14, Nov.-Dec. 1988, pg. 75.

Chalk, Rosemary, Frankel, Marks, Chafer, Sallie B. AAAS Committee on Scientific Freedom and Responsibility, AAAS Professional Ethics Project. Washington, DC, 1980, pg. 6.

Constable, Robert, Managhan, Thomas, Cocozelli, Carmelo. "An Exploration of the Influence of Values and Theory on Practitioner Decision Making." Mimeo. 1985.

Coughlin, Ellen K. "Scholar Who Submitted Bogus Article To Journals May Be Disciplined." *The Chronicle of Higher Education.* Nov. 2, 1988-A7.

Freedman, Benjamin "The Ethics of Using Fetal Tissue." IRB, Vol. 10, No. 6, Nov.-Dec. 1988, pg. 1.

Hamovitch, Maurice B. "Report of The Committee on Standards for the Professional Behavior and Agency Practices in Social Work Research." Social Work Research Section, NASW. April 1957, pg. 4-5.

Jonas, Hans. "Freedom of Scientific Inquiry and The Public Interest: the Accountability of Science as an Agent of Social Action." HCR, August 1976, Vol. 6, No. 4, pg. 15-17.

Lewis, Harold. "Can One Code of Ethics Cover All Specialties?" Paper presented at meeting of Maryland Chapter, NASW, November 1961.

Meyers, K. and Dunton, D. W. "Applying an Ethical Framework to a Proposed HIV Antibody Screening Program." *IRB*, Vol. 10, No. 1, Jan/Feb 1988, pg. 6. Framework adapted from Bayer, R., Levine C., Wolf, S. "HIV antibody screening. An ethical framework for evaluating proposed programs." *JAMA*. 1986, Vol. 256, pg. 1268-74. A useful discussion of ethical issues frequently encountered in *IRB* reviews can be found in Levine, Robert L., *Ethics and Regulation of Clinical Research*. Urban and Schwarzenberg, Baltimore, 1981.

Miller, Judith. "Towards an International Ethic for Research with Human Beings." *IRB*, Vol. 10, No. 6, Nov/Dec. 1988, pg. 9-10.

Schafer, Arthur. Commentary on "The Randomized Clinical Trial: For Whose Benefit?" *IRB*, Vol. 7, No. 2, March/April 1985, pg. 4-6.

Vidich, Arthur. "Fundamental Responsibility in Research." *Human Organization*, Spring 1960.

Wedenoja, Marilyn, Nuvius, Paula S., Tripodi, Tony. "Enhancing Mindfulness in Practice Prescriptive Thinking." *Social Casework*, Vol. 69, No. 7, Sept. 1988, pg. 427-433.

# Utilization of Research in Group Work Practice: An Example

Sheldon D. Rose

## RESEARCH IN GROUP WORK

It is strange that group work and research have not developed a closer relationship in recent years. On the one hand, much of empirical social psychological research was developed in the 1950s and 1960s around the small group. In the 1960s some schools of social work (see in particular the work of Vinter and his associates, 1974) turned to the findings of the group dynamics scholars (e.g., as summarized in the anthologies of Cartwright and Zander, 1968) for their practice generalizations. Many social work research scholars have come out of a group work background. On the other hand, group dynamics rarely looked at individual outcomes as a function of group process; moreover, it focused more on the work group and the laboratory group than on the kind of groups in which social workers were interested. As a result, after its great initial surge, research on lab groups began to lose the interest of the group work audience.

Throughout the 1970s a number of social work scholars used observational systems to examine group process. These findings did not seem to have much of an effect on the field because of the cumbersome nature of the observational systems and the absence of group process implications for outcome. Other instrumentation that a few group worker authors (e.g., Anderson, 1986) have advocated incorporated into their practice (but no one reports that actual incorporation has taken place) have been various self-disclosure, leadership, helpfulness, and amount of influence scales. For the most part, neither the findings nor the instrumentation of process-only research have been utilized by practitioners.

There are several areas of interest to group work practitioners for which bodies of research do exist and of which there appear to be some utilization by practitioners: group therapy and encounter groups, self-help groups, caregiver groups, children social skills groups, and cognitive behavioral groups for adults. Lieberman, Yalom, and Miles (1973) suggested that 9.6% of all participants in encounter and similar types of insight group therapy had major psychological breakdowns that could be directly attributed to the group experience. In spite of the fact that later studies showed a much lower breakdown rate, these data seemed to mark the beginning of the end of rapid expansion of the encounter movement in social work and in other treatment professions as well, although other forms of group therapy appear to be continuing unabated.

Social work has shown increasing interest in self-help groups. Lieberman and Borman (1979) report on a number of studies in which researchers carried out retrospective consumer research with members from a variety of self-help groups. These descriptive data provided the field information about what members said they valued in such groups. This gave impetus to the greater employment of self-help groups under the auspices of social agencies, although no experimental research has come out of it. In social work similar retrospective research on a specific type of self-help group, the recently divorced, has been carried out by Bell, Charping, and Strecker (1989); the research lends support to the approach. Toro et al. (1988) found that professionals in self-help groups favorably influenced the group climate as well as the behavior of participants. The implication for practitioners was that there was a place for them in self-help groups.

Experimental research with groups of caregivers has been recently carried out by several sets of authors. Lovett and Gallagher (1988) studied the effect of pscyhoeducational intervention strategies on the self-efficacy of family caregivers. Toseland, Rossiter, and Labrecque (1988) compared peer led training groups for caregivers to similar groups with professional leaders. Haley, Lane, Brown, and Levine (1987) examined the effects of support group intervention for caregivers of elderly schizophrenics on life satisfaction, coping skills, depression and social support of the caregivers, but found no differences between the treatment and wait list control groups. The impact of this research on group work practice with caregiver groups is not yet known, although it promises to be of use to a mainstream movement in group work practice.

Since the late 1970s a wealth of research by social work scholars and some psychologists has been carried out on social skill training in groups. Most of the results have been positive although not overwhelmingly so. The impact of this research has been primarily on the role of school social workers, many of whom are using the strategies but rarely the data collection strategies in their practice with children.

Although there has been little development of group process research, there has been a growing interest in outcome research. In fact, in the classic meta-analysis of Smith, Glass, and Miller (1980), a review of over 400 treatment studies (most in psychology journals) suggested that the group was the context of over half the studies, but almost none of these referred to any process concern. Most of the outcome studies on groups that had positive outcomes were behavioral or cognitive-behavioral in orientation. Since that time there has been an explosion of cognitive-behavioral group work and group therapy experiments, most of which had positive results. Unfortunately, few of these studies make any reference to process variables that might impinge on outcome. Even in the absence of process findings, the results of experimental outcome studies have stimulated greater utilization of variations of the program than the earlier process-only research. Moreover, some researchers have been beginning to use some descriptive measures to get at some elements of process, even though it is not manipulated in the experiments. In social work agencies groups of highly focused groups appear to be growing daily as research support begins to accrue for this type of approach and as funding begins to fade for long-term treatment.

Although there has been increased use of the results and sometimes the instruments used in the groups mentioned above, the vast majority of group workers, group counselors, and group therapists for the most part not only fail to draw on models of group work which have an empirical foundation, but they rarely use any of the research tools, observation instruments, role play tests, or paper and pencil inventories and tests. This may be due in part to the fact that there is so little research of quality to draw on and most models of group work practice are basically normative approaches, the work of convincing and charismatic leaders. Moreover, these models tend to have vague and general goals which rarely lend themselves to systematic evaluation (with the exception of task-centered, problem solving and cognitive-behavioral group work). Neither the leadership of the organization nor its membership appear to be interested in utilizing the findings of research. Yet all is not grim. Research articles in social work journals on group work have increased from 4% in 1966 to 10% in 1986 (Feldman, 1986). Nevertheless, the vast majority of articles in the group work literature are descriptive or traditional statements of principles. There is also little encouragement for research from many of the group work leadership. Major speakers at group work conferences have often been highly critical of empirical approaches to group work practice. Workshops and papers on research in group work are poorly attended at such conferences.

In summary, there has been an extremely modest increase of research and research utilization in group work over the past ten years. Group workers have drawn from the research of social workers as well as non-social worker scholars for instrumentation and in some cases systematic descriptions of practice. Though increasing, the rate of utilization is probably still extremely low. Research has not generated interest in either the practicing group workers or the leaders of the profession. The question must be raised as to the cause of this disinterest and lack of use.

### If Not, Why Not?

First, much of the research presently being carried out is not directly related to the interests of the group worker. In the exceptional cases of self-help group and more recently caregiver research, there is a population of group workers who are interested, and research in these areas should stimulate further research and utilization. Second, the quality of the limited research is not always very high.

Third, the norms of the leadership of group work practice are not proresearch.

The second question that should be raised is: what can we do to stimulate greater interest in utilizing available group work research or research from allied fields applicable to groups? Obviously increasing research would be of major importance. I suggest that merely a greater quantity of research projects is not enough. One way is to develop along with any research plan a concrete utilization plan. The principles of developing such a plan are discussed in the following section. But first let us describe briefly the ways in which practitioners can utilize research.

## How Practitioners Can Use Research

Practitioners can make use of or engage in practice research in many different ways. First, the practitioners can use the evaluation tools developed by researchers to evaluate their own practices. Of particular interest to the group worker are various process measures, post-session questionnaires, personality inventories, behavior checklists, and roleplay or analog tests, all of which have been used in recent group work research. Second, practitioners can utilize clinical programs which have an empirical foundation. Reid (this volume) refers to this as indirect utilization. This type of research permits the group worker to test the implication of the original research findings for his or her own unique conditions. The purpose of the second half of this chapter is to describe how investigators, having carried out an extensive research program to evaluate a group work approach, simultaneously developed a program to enhance utilization of their empirically supported program in social work agencies. Since the research program has been described elsewhere (Rose et al., 1986), only the utilization enhancement program will be described here. It is sufficient to state that we attempted through a series of experiments to establish an empirical foundation for a cognitive-behavioral approach to group work. To a large degree the utility of the approach was supported by our research and that of others.

### Principles of Planning for Research Utilization

Without a plan for enhancing utilization, practice research on group treatment or other clinical programs may have little or no impact on the field. Research scholars have for years attempted unsuccessfully to rely solely on the practitioners to develop the skills of reading research and using the best available research as the basis of their practice. Several surveys have assured us that not only do practitioners rarely read research articles, those few who read them do not do so critically or with sufficient skill to evaluate the significance of the article. Moreover, practice approaches are shaped not by research outcomes but by the testimonials of charismatic leaders. Therefore, researchers must make an effort not only to carry out their research as well as possible but to endeavor to reach the ear of those who actually apply the clinical programs that have been previously developed and evaluated. Therefore it remains to the researcher to present the program and its research in such a way that the findings will be given serious consideration and that data collection strategies that impinge on practice will be carried out as part of that approach.

## PRINCIPLES OF ENHANCING RESEARCH UTILIZATION

In our experience a number of principles have guided us in developing a program to enhance utilization of our research findings. These principles include developing an explicit utilization plan, selecting a topic relevant to practitioner interest, instituting a multistudy program of research, defining the method in terms of both data collection and intervention strategies, training practitioners in the use of data and intervention strategies, promoting utilization through workshops and courses, developing practitioner handbooks, and investing resources for the promotion of utilization. These principles are discussed in the section below.

### Selecting Topics Relevant to Practitioner Interest

If the researcher expects his or her research to be used by practitioners, a topic of practice must be selected of current interest to a given sector of the practice community. If this research overlaps with a burning interest of the investigator, so much the better. The very title of the research must contain a topic that would attract the practitioner. Either a survey of community interests or requests from represented members of the treatment community might suffice to answer the question whether such a population exists. In our example we selected group treatment from a cognitive-behavioral orientation as the topic of research. Group treatment was selected because (in addition to the interest of the investigator) group therapy was broadly used at that time throughout the country. A survey that we had conducted suggested that almost 50% of practicing behaviorists (members of the Association for the Advancement of Behavior Therapy) were using groups, but that few if any were leading groups with a behavioral orientation (Rose et al., 1979). In social work we discovered that behavioral strategies were of growing interest at that time, but few people had applied the principles of behavioral intervention in such a way as to adapt them to the group. Finally, clinical articles describing a behavioral and cognitive-behavioral group work program were well responded to. At group work conferences we discovered that some in the group work community were dissatisfied with the vague precepts of practice and were looking for a reasonable alternatives. Also some earlier steps made to systematize group work practice had attracted a number of practitioners and scholars. We concluded that there was a potential audience.

## Instituting a Multi-Study Program of Research

Because any single small study will probably be given little attention, one isolated study is unlikely to result in a significant level of utilization. A single study receives limited publicity and, even with significant findings in support of the approach, lends only limited support for the efficacy of the approach being evaluated. This is especially important where small samples are used, as in most of our experiments. If the researcher wants credence to be lent to his findings by practitioners, it is necessary to develop a program of research over time. Of course a program of research runs the risk of inconclusive or mixed findings which make a proposed utilization program a moot point. After a large number of studies, it may be possible to do a meta-analysis which increases the power of each separate study.

In our project comparing a cognitive-behavioral approach to the treatment of adults in groups to various control conditions, we carried out four studies, which had a common target of evaluation (Tallant et al., in press; Tolman and Rose, 1985; Subramanian and Rose, 1988; and Whitney and Rose, 1989). Several more are now being carried out. Even prior to actual publication, the first four studies have received sufficient attention to be considered by various agencies for inclusion in their ongoing programs.

### Defining the Method in Terms of Both
### Data Collection and Intervention Strategies

What distinguishes a program to enhance utilization of a practice method from one which aims at enhancing utilization of research? In the latter program, the method itself is defined in terms of both evaluation, data collection, and intervention tools. If the practitioner is merely carrying out the treatment strategies, it should be made clear that he or she is not making ample use of the method's potential.

In our agency (The Interpersonal Skill Training and Research Project) integration of measurement strategies is required whether or not a given treatment approach is part of a research project. This includes a post-session questionnaire to be filled in by the clients and the group therapist, as well as pre-post testing with inventories and behavioral checklists. It also includes data on attendance, drop outs, population characteristics, rate of homework completion, and participation data. Prescriptions are defined as how to use this information as part of the approach. In this way the researcher conveys to the practitioners that the measurement is an integral part of treatment.

Data requirements are not foreign to agencies. Most require information on the activities performed, the frequency of attendance, and drop outs from the program. Some require summaries of what went on in conferences or meetings.

In addition to promulgation of the method, there are many advantages to an approach that integrates both intervention and data collection. Such a data system not only provides rich information to the practitioner to improve his or her own practice, but it improves the overall quality of service to the community according to the testimony of the staffs we have worked with. Finally, the use of data integrated into the method enhances the reputation of the agency and increases the probability of obtaining increased or new sources of funding.

By using both the intervention and measurement strategies as a combined package, the practitioner is provided with an opportunity for self-correcting feedback through the collection and use of data. If practitioners utilize the method in its entirety they will also use the post-session questionnaire which provides them with session-by-session perception of the group by its members. Furthermore, the pre-post tests are also described in detail in the manual. Although it is clear that most users prefer a program that contains a clear set of clinical parameters only, we estimate from our correspondence that at least a small percentage of users make use of the measures to evaluate their own practice and to compare their findings with ours. In order to facilitate this feedback to us, we have recently begun to send a small questionnaire to all persons who request our treatment manual. We have also sent a similar questionnaire to former students and workshop participants. The questionnaire asks whether the measures were included in their use of the treatment package and their findings if any. How this works remains to be seen as this study is still in progress. If we are successful, not only are group workers utilizing a program with an empirical foundation, but they have the possibility of adding to and enriching that foundation.

In my opinion it should eventually become common practice for the tools to evaluate a program to be part of every treatment package. When the treatment is taught to students and/or the practitioner, they should be instructed in a package in which measurement and treatment strategies are integrated. Presently, in most packages research or evaluation is something tacked on if one has the time – and that seldom happens. The measurement should be seen as an inherent part of the package, and those who make use of only the clinical components of the package are not making use of its full potential. For the practitioner to add on two attitudinal or behavioral inventories and a roleplay test and to utilize a post-session questionnaire at the end of every session extends the cost of the group about three to six hours of staff time. It costs the members the equivalent of one session. Until practice scholars advocate the universal application of modest evaluation instruments in all clinical treatment, few will pay the cost.

### Training Practitioners in the Use of Data and Intervention Strategies

Once an agency is interested in the given approach, a training program for practitioners in a given agency is necessary to ensure that the data collection and use are indeed integrated and used consistently. Even if the practitioners are familiar with the intervention strategies, staffs are rarely familiar with the ways in which data can be used.

Case examples of how the data can be utilized should be included in the training package just as one includes examples of how one uses a given intervention strategy. For example, if one has found that in administering stress training with groups in a family service agency with women who are victims of violence and the pre-post measures for that one group are not comparable to established norms, one has the basis for reconsidering the package itself for that population or the skills of the group worker in using such a package. If more immediate feedback is necessary, and if the post-session evaluation indicates low satisfaction and little cohesion among the members (as determined by a post-session questionnaire), the group worker can adjust his or her intervention strategies to deal with these issues.

### Promoting Utilization Through Workshops and Courses

A broader strategy than in-service training to gain utilization of the research findings by a wide range of practitioners is to publicize the approach and its research foundation through one- to three-day workshops. Workshops have the advantage of providing training to a broad sample of the professional community. Because of the experience of many of the participants, such an intensive experience is likely to influence their practice. Once again the link of the method to its empirical foundation is essential to point out not only the value of the clinical method, but its foundation in experimental research and its use of data to improve the quality of practice. My colleagues and I have given numerous workshops in cognitive-behavioral group work throughout the U.S., Canada, and Europe. According to our correspondence, this has been the result of most of our workshops with a small percentage but large number of workshop participants. These workshops, leader guides, and books all interact and publicize the other. In a sense this multi-faceted approach to utilization increases dramatically the number of people utilizing the approach and evaluating the findings.

If one is affiliated with a college or university, the researcher has sufficient time to teach courses on the data-based group work approach to students who would be likely to use them. As an instructor it is possible to encourage and oversee whether the integration of data collection methods and intervention strategies are carried out. Of greater impact are similar courses in extension for practitioners who have ready access to groups. They are the ones who have the greatest need and often the greatest enthusiasm for the approach although many prefer not to address the data collection component.

### Developing Practitioner Handbooks

Since most practitioners require a great deal of direction when trying out a new method, it is extremely helpful to convert the measurement and interventive directives to the practitioner into a practitioner's handbook, to publicize these handbooks, and to make them readily available to the prospective audience. Furthermore, the handbooks become an excellent tool in training. As a result of our experiments we published in-house three manuals (Rose et al., 1982; Rose and Subramanian, 1987; and Rose, Tolman, and Hanusa, 1985) which we have advertised in a newsletter and distributed as part of the activities of a group therapy interest group.

In addition to handbooks or leader guides, method textbooks with as much of the research foundation that is available serve as well the purpose of utilization. Even in a didactic article there is insufficient space to elaborate on the details of the approach. The manuals too are limited because they avoid a clear discussion of the general principles. To this end we have written a practice textbook (Rose, 1989) for professional group practitioners and students. This is probably the most time consuming of the utilization strategies and can lead the researcher away from his or her research activity.

Both manuals and the theoretical textbook contain a description of the measurements used and how and when they are to be administered. The textbooks contain the logic of the measurement and how the findings can be used. One of the limitations of our manuals, like many others, is that they fail to go into sufficient detail about how to use the measurement instruments.

## Making Results and Description of the Program Readily Available

Research results of the studies should be published, preferably in journals readily accessible to the population who might use the information, in order to make the empirical foundation of the approach publicly available. The predominantly research or theoretical sociological or psychological journals seldom find their way to the libraries of social agencies and practitioners. Each of the research articles of our group projects were published primarily but not exclusively in social work journals (*Social Work, Journal of Social Service Research, Social Work Research and Abstracts,* and *Research in Social Group Work*, an edited selection of research articles).

Since, as we already pointed out, practitioners are notorious for not reading research reports, it is usually necessary to publish a clinical article in the more well-read practice journals of the field. Such an article gives the researcher an opportunity to amplify the intervention methods used. However, if the goal is research utilization, the data collection methods and outcomes of the research cannot be ignored. Such clinical articles also permit some advocacy of the approach. Following each of our experiments or of a set of related experiments, a clinical article has been or is now being written which indeed emphasizes the data and interventive attributes of the approach but also contains some abbreviated information about methods and results. One article (Tolman and Rose, 1985) appearing before the research articles provided the theoretical background for the experiments and the emphasis on data collection as part of the approach.

## Investing Resources for the Promotion
## of Utilization

As one may observe from the above discussion, resources must be invested in activities that promote research utilization, not only the research itself. These costs may take the form of time and/or money (although some of these activities may pay for themselves). Time must be taken from the research to write and publish and distribute the manuals, to present one's programs to agencies, to provide workshops and other demonstrations, and so forth. But without such an investment, it is our experience that very little happens to influence the practice community in making use of an empirical approach in a way that includes the use of its measurement strategies.

## CONCLUDING COMMENTS

In this chapter I initially reviewed the state of research utilization in group work which is slowly growing but not impressive. I have suggested that those who do research should incorporate a utilization plan into their research. I have discussed the principles involved in development of such a program and the difficulties in its implementation.

Is the program for utilization of the practice method to be distinguished from utilization of the research that provides the foundation of the approach? They are obviously closely linked. In spite of all our efforts, I am aware that many are using the intervention strategies associated with the method with little regard for its empirical foundation and data collection techniques. In fact, the users may have been recruited by effective public information programs rather than the research and the belief in the potential of data for improving one's practice. This is the danger of such an all out approach to encourage practitioners to use the results of one's research. The major protection of the consumer remains his or her ability to distinguish good from bad research and the ability of the researchers to link unequivocally the intervention and measurement strategies for effective and humane treatment.

## REFERENCES

Anderson, J. D. (1986). Integrating research and practice in social work with groups. *Social Work with Groups, 9*(3), 111-122.

Bell, W. J., Charping, J. W. and Strecker, J. B. (1989). Client perceptions of the effectiveness of divorce adjustment groups. *Journal of Social Service Research, 13*(2), 9-32.

Cartwright, D., and Zarder, A. (1968). *Group dynamics: Research and theory* (3rd ed.). New York: Harper and Row.

Feldman, R. A. (1986). Group work knowledge and research: A two-decade comparison. *Social Work with Groups, 9*(3), 7-14.

Haley, W. E., Lane Brown, S., and Levine, E.G., (1986). Experimental evaluation of the effectiveness of group intervention of dementia caregivers. *The Gerontologist, 27*, 376-382.

Lieberman, M. A., and Borman, L. D. (1979). *Self-help groups for coping with crisis*. San Francisco: Jossey-Bass.

Lieberman, M., Yalom, I., and Miles, M. (1973). Encounter groups: first facts. New York: Basic Books, Inc.

Lovett, S., and Gallagher, D. (1988). Psychoeducational interventions for family caregivers: Preliminary efficacy data. *Behavior Therapy, 19*, 321-330.

Rose, S. D. (1989). *Working with adults in groups: Integrating cognitive and small group approaches*. San Francisco: Jossey-Bass.

Rose, S. D., Hanusa, D., Tolman, R. M. and Hall, J. A. (1982). *Group leader's guide to assertiveness training*. Crownsville, MD: Crownsville Medical Center.

Rose, S. D., Siemons, J., and O'Bryan, K. (1979). The use of groups in therapy by members of AABT. *Behavior Therapist, 2*, 23-24.

Rose, S. D., and Subramanian, K. (1987). *Group leaders guide for pain management training in groups*. Madison, WI: University of Wisconsin, School of Social Work.

Rose, S. D., Tolman, R. M., and Hanusa, D. (1985). *Group leader's guide to stress management*. Interpersonal Skills Training Project, Madison, WI: University of Wisconsin, School of Social Work.

Rose, S. D., Tolman, R., Tallant, S., and Subramanian, K. (1986). A multi-method group approach: Program development research. *Social Work with Groups, 9*, 71-88.

Smith, M., Glass, G., and Miller, T. (1980). *The benefits of psychotherapy*. Baltimore, MD: Johns Hopkins Press.

Subramanian, K., and Rose, S. D. (1988). Group training for the management of chronic pain in interpersonal situations. *Health and Social Work, 21*(3), 29-30.

Tallant, S., Rose, S. D., and Tolman R. (in press). Recent support for stress management training in groups, *Behavior Modification*.

Tolman, R. M., and Rose, S. D. (1985). Coping with stress, A multimodal approach. *Social Work, 30*, 151-159.

Toro, P. A., Reischl, T. M., Zimmerman, M. A., Rappaport, J., Seidman, E., Luke, D. A., and Roberts, L. J. (1988). Professionals in mutual help groups: Impact on social climate and members' behavior. *Journal of Consulting and Clinical Psychology, 56*(4), 631-632.

Toseland, R., Rossiter, C., and Labrecque, M. (1988). *The effectiveness of peer-led and professionally-led groups for caregivers*. Unpublished manuscript, School of Social Work, SUNY-Albany.

Vinter, R. (1974). The essential components of social group work practice. In P. Glasser, R. Sarri, and R. Vinter (Eds.). *Individual Change Through Small Groups*. New York: The Free Press, 9-33.

Whitney, D., and Rose, S. D. (1989). The effect of process and structural content on outcome in stress management groups. *Social Service Research, 3*, 120-128.

# Research Utilization
# in Social Work Practice
# of Family Treatment

Hamilton I. McCubbin
Marilyn A. McCubbin

In social work practice, the bridging of family research and theory building has generally been lacking (Meyer, 1984; McCubbin, Olson and Zimmerman, 1985). Although some effort has been made in this regard during the past two decades, it has primarily been because of a single scholar-therapist having adopted and utilized all three orientations with a family systems orientation in mind and generally not because of any cooperative efforts by several individuals specializing in theory, research, and practice. Unfortunately this lack of integration of theory, research, and practice has delayed the development of each of these domains and curtailed the development of much needed research questions, propositions, hypotheses, measures, and theory building which would have fostered and accelerated such integrative efforts. However, it is important to call attention to the notable advances that family research in treating relationships has made to advance our understanding of and appreciation for the complex but important dynamics of family life. It is the purpose of this chapter to identify and highlight those emerging domains of family research which are of particular relevance to social work practice, and in so doing underscore the critical importance of research utilization in the field of social work as the profession takes a leadership role in integrating a family systems orientation into social casework, groupwork, and family-based child welfare services and programs. If we only consider the proliferation of family-based placement prevention services (Halpern, 1986; Bribitzer and Verdieck, 1988; Heying, 1985) since the enactment of the

Adoption Assistance and Child Welfare Act of 1980 (P.L. 96-272), we can recognize the magnitude of the challenge to master and integrate family research from all disciplines, namely social work, family science, nursing, family medicine, family sociology, and psychology, and attest to the importance of research utilization in family-based service agencies.

In recent reviews of family research in the area of family intervention and therapy (Olson, 1980; McCubbin, Olson and Zimmerman, 1985), family scientists noted that the exploration and refinement of existing ideas have characterized the two most recent decades of research rather than the introduction of dramatically new theoretical approaches. The most recent family intervention literature has been devoted to either: (1) the integration and refinement of previous models (i.e., Hills family stress framework (1949); Minuchins's (1974) synthesis of family development, family systems, and structural-functionalism); (2) simplified descriptions of previous theoretical work (i.e., cookbooks or working guides of family therapy and textbooks of family therapy); or (3) extensions of existing theoretical frameworks to specific problems like chemical addiction (Stanton, 1979; Steinglass, 1976) and aging (Herr and Weakland, 1979).

Out of these 20 years of research we note the emergence of five major developments in family research of particular relevance to family-based social work practice:

1. the continuous testing of the effectiveness of family systems-oriented interventions;
2. the re-emergence of family stress theory and the concomitant identification of critical family processes as targets for intervention;
3. the advancement of family typologies for classification and intervention:
4. the theory building and research emphasis upon family strengths and capabilities as critical targets for intervention; and
5. the continuous development, testing, and refinement of family assessment measures for research, clinical assessment, and program evaluation.

In briefly reviewing these major developments, we can reaffirm the importance of research utilization in family-based social work practice and intervention.

## TESTING THE EFFECTIVENESS
## OF FAMILY-BASED INTERVENTIONS

During the last two decades of family research, the empirical outcome literature has improved in both quantity and quality. This progress is clearly documented by the several comprehensive reviews already available (e.g., Gurman, 1973, 1975; Beck, 1976; Jacobson and Martin, 1976; Wells et al., 1976; Gurman and Kniskern, 1978a, 1978b; Jacobson, 1978; Wells and Denzen, 1978; Jacobson and Margolin, 1979).

The trend in the family research appears to be toward specifying which mode of family-based intervention is most effective for which group of families presenting which sorts of problems (Olson et al., 1980). This is a more effective approach to therapeutic outcome studies. As Frank (1979:312) has suggested:

> Instead of continuing to pursue the therapeutic relatively unrewarding enterprise of statistically comparing the effectiveness of different therapies, we should focus on particular forms of therapy that seem to work exceptionally well with a few patients and seek to define the characteristics of both the therapy and the patients that lead to this happy result.

An alternative to focusing on presenting symptoms is to focus on the type of family system. Olson et al. (1980) have emphasized the importance of system diagnosis prior to intervention. A given "symptom" may serve multiple functions in a relationship system. Therefore, the "system diagnosis" and presenting complaint may not uniformly covary. For instance, Killorin and Olson (1980) describe the course of therapy with four alcoholic families, each of whom operated at different (through extreme) levels of family cohesion and adaptability. There are other recent projects where the type of system is diagnosed prior to treatment, specific treatment programs are planned, and outcome is assessed for a narrowly defined treatment group (e.g., Alexander and Barton, 1976; Minuchin et al., 1978; Stanton et al., 1979; Steinglass, 1979a, 1979b).

Table 1 provides a summary of relationship-oriented treatment strategies which have yielded some degree of documented effectiveness. Unfortunately, we do not have sufficient manuscript space to provide a detailed review of the current literature on outcome research.

However, Table 2 may be used as a brief summary of improvement rates for four family therapy approaches by "identified patient." Details of these studies can be obtained from Gurman and Kniskern's (1978b) relatively recent review. Overall, it appears that marital and family therapy improvement rates are superior to those reported for individual therapies.

The following implications for practice are supported by the empirically based family research and overlap with the recommendations Gurman and Kniskern (1978b) make for training marriage and family therapists:

1. Conjoint marital therapy appears more useful than individual therapy for improving marital relationships.
2. Family therapy appears as effective as individual therapy for a wide range of presenting problems. It is not possible to specify the best type of family treatment.
3. No one "school" of marital or family therapy has been demonstrated to be effective with a wide range of presenting problems.
4. Therapist relationship skills are important regardless of the conceptual orientation or "school" of the family therapist.

### Family Stress Research: Emerging Targets for Social Work Intervention

Since the classic studies by Burgess (1926), Angell (1936), Cavan and Ranck (1938), and Koos (1946), and particularly Reuben Hill's (1949) research and theory building efforts based on observations of family responses to war-induced separation and reunion, we have witnessed a major shift in family research. Specifically, the last two decades of family stress research raised the exciting possibility of not only explaining and predicting dysfunctional family behavior in

TABLE 1. Relationship-oriented Treatment Strategies Yielding Some Degree of Documented Effectiveness by Presenting Problem

| Presenting problem | Behavioral exchange contracting | Conjoint couples group therapy | Behavioral family therapy | Conjoint interactional family therapy | Structural family therapy | Strategic family therapy | Zuk's triadic approach | Multiple family therapy | Drug therapy plus marital therapy | Family crisis intervention[c] |
|---|---|---|---|---|---|---|---|---|---|---|
| Alcoholism | x | x | | | | | | | | |
| Drug abuse | | | | | x | x | | x | | |
| Juvenile status offense | | | x[a] | x[b] | x | | | | | |
| Adolescent psychopathology | | | | x | | | x | | | |
| Childhood conduct problems | | | x | | | | | | | |
| School and work phobias | | | | | | | | x | | x |
| Psychosomatic symptoms | | | | | | x | | | | |
| Adult depression | | | | | | | | | x | |
| Marital distress | x | | | | | | | | | |

[a]Limited primarily to outcome studies reported 1970-79.
[b]Though labeled behavioral, the Alexander group at Utah actually used a mix of behavioral and communication approaches in conjoint family sessions.
[c]Langsley et al.

TABLE 2. Summary of Improvement Rates for Marital and Family Therapy

| | Number of Studies | Number of patients | Improved | Outcome(%) | |
| | | | | No change | Worse |
|---|---|---|---|---|---|
| *Marital therapy* | | | | | |
| Conjoint | 8 | 261 | 70[a] | 24 | 1 |
| Conjoint group | 15 | 397 | 66 | 30 | 4 |
| Concurrent and collaborative | 6 | 464 | 63 | 35 | 2 |
| Individual | 7 | 406 | 48 | 45 | 7 |
| Total | 36 | 1,528 | 61 | 35 | 4 |
| *Family therapy* | | | | | |
| Child as identified patient | 10 | 370 | 68 | 32 | 0 |
| Adolescent as identified patient | 9 | 217 | 75 | 25 | 0 |
| Adult as identified patient | 11 | 475 | 65 | 33 | 2 |
| Mixed identified patient | 8 | 467 | 81 | 17 | 2 |
| Total | 38 | 1,529 | 73 | 26 | 1 |

[a]Five percent unknown.

*Source:*Abstracted with permission from A.S. Gurman and D.P. Kniskern, "Research on marital and family therapy: Progress, perspective, and prospect,"in *Handbook of Psychotherapy and Behavior Change*, by Garfield and Bergin (1978).

response to stress, but understanding how family members interact with and support each other, what strengths and capabilities families call upon to adjust and adapt, the specific roles and transactions the community plays and enacts in family coping and adaption, and suggesting ways to improve the resiliency in families. Concomitantly, we have witnessed the emergency of prevention-oriented family action studies designed to strengthen families as well as promote the physical and psychological well-being of its members.

Family scholars have struggled with the design of research and the development of theories aimed toward uncovering why some families are better able to negotiate their way through transitions and tragedies and to cope with and even thrive on life's hardships, whereas other families, faced with similar if not identical stressors or family transitions, give up or are easily exhausted. Family stress theory has been advanced and adapted to guide this line of scientific inquiry and family system interventions. The importance of family stress theory to the study of normative family transitions and adaptation to major life changes and illnesses is based on the central roles that family type and family strengths and capabilities play in understanding and explaining family behavior. Family stress theory highlights the complex but meaningful role which certain family typologies such as the Balanced family type (Lavee et al., 1985; McCubbin et al., 1988; Olson et al., 1983), and Resilient, Regenerative, or Rhythmic family types (McCubbin et al., 1987) play in buffering the impact of stressful life events and in facilitating family adaptation following a crisis situation. In contrast to family therapy frameworks which tend to underscore the deficiencies and dysfunctional aspects of family systems, family stress theory sharpens its focus on and targets the strengths and resistance resources families have as part of their innate abilities to endure hardships. Social work has chosen to emphasize the importance of crisis theory and family strengths as part of its overall strategy of family-based interventions (Halpern, 1986; Whittaker and Garbarino, 1983).

Family stress research and theory building has been based on ten fundamental assumptions about the ecological nature of family life and intervention in family systems:

1. Families face hardships and changes as a natural and predictable aspect of family life over the life cycle.
2. Families develop basic strengths and capabilities designed to foster the growth and development of family members and the family unit and to protect the family from major disruptions in the face of family transitions and changes.
3. Families also face crises that force the family unit to change its traditional mode of functioning and adapt to the situation.
4. Families develop basic and unique strengths and capabilities designed to protect the family from unexpected or nonnormative stressors and strains and to foster the family's adaptation following a family crisis or major transition and change.
5. Families benefit from and contribute to the network of rela-

tionships and resources in the community, particularly during periods of family stress and crisis.

6. Family functioning is often characterized as predictable with shaped patterns of interpersonal behavior, which in turn are molded and maintained by intergenerational factors, situational pressures that have evolved over time, the personalities of the family members, and the normative and nonnormative events that punctuate family life throughout the life cycle.

7. Family interventions can be enhanced and families supported by both a diagnostic and an evaluation process which takes the strengths, resources and capabilities in the family system as well as the deficiencies of the family system into consideration.

8. Family functioning can be enhanced by interventions that target both the vulnerabilities and dysfunctional patterns of the family unit.

9. Family functioning can be enhanced by interventions that target both the family's interpersonal capabilities and strengths which, if addressed, can serve as a catalyst for other family-system, wellness-promoting properties.

10. Families develop and maintain internal resistance and adaptive resources, which vary in their strength and resiliency over the family life cycle but which can be influenced and enhanced to function more effectively. These resources can play a critical role in fostering successful family adjustments and adaptations even after the family unit has deteriorated to the point of exhibiting major difficulties and symptoms of dysfunction.

Family stress research may be described as attempting to describe families at two related but discernible phases in their response to life changes and catastrophes. The *adjustment phase* focuses first on those family types, and strengths and capabilities that explain why some families are better suited than others to adjust to minor changes. The *adaptation phase* focuses on what family types, strengths, and capabilities are needed, called upon, or created to manage a major transition and change calling for family reorganization and systemic change. Two major propositions (McCubbin and

McCubbin, 1989) have emerged from family stress and crisis research which may also serve to guide clinical and social work intervention:

### Proposition I: The Adjustment Phase:

*The level of family adjustment and/or the family's transition into a crisis situation (X) (and into the adaptation phase or exhaustion)* in response to a stressor event or transition is determined by: *A* (the stressor event or transition and its level of severity) — interacting with the *V* (the family's vulnerability determined in part by the concurrent pileup of demands, stressors, transitions, and strains and by the pressures associated with family's life-cycle stage) — interacting with T (the family's typology, i.e., regenerative, resilient, rhythmic, balanced, etc.) — interacting with *B* (the family's resistance resources) — interacting with *C* (the appraisal the family makes of the event — interacting with *PSC* (the family's problem-solving and coping repertoire and capabilities).

### Proposition II: The Family Adaptation Phase:

*The level of family adaptation (XX) and/or the family's transition back into a crisis situation (or exhaustion)* in response to a crisis situation is determined by: *AA,* the pileup of demands on or in the family system created by the crisis situation, life-cycle changes, and unresolved strains — interacting with *R,* the family's level of regenerativity determined in part by the concurrent pileup of demands (stressors, transitions, and strains) — interacting with *T*, the family's typology (resilient, rhythmic, balanced, etc.) — interacting with *BB,* the family's strengths (the family's adaptive strengths, capabilities, and resources) — interacting with *CC,* the family's appraisal of the situation (the meaning the family attaches to the total situation) and *CCC*, the family's schema (i.e., world view and sense of coherence which shapes the family's situational appraisal and meaning) — interacting with *BBB,* the support from friends and the community (social support) — interacting with *PSC,* the family's problem solving and coping responses to the total family situation.

These propositions about resilience in family units bring several dimensions of family functioning to center stage — family processes, family typologies, and family strengths and capabilities — and thus may be viewed as critical dimensions for social work intervention, planning, and programming.

## ISOLATING CRITICAL FAMILY PROCESSES

Although it is useful to describe and evaluate various approaches to family intervention, a critical step has been made to begin integrating concepts and principles and develop theoretical models. Understandably, family processes involve interactions within the family unit and through transactions outside of the family system. Four major processes have been documented in the research literature with great regularity and may be viewed as vital to family-based social work intervention: cohesion, adaptability, communication, and social support.

One recent attempt to develop an integrative model of the family was made by Olson, Russell, and Sprenkle in their Circumplex Model (Olson et al., 1979, 1980). In developing the Circumplex Model, three dimensions emerged from the conceptual clustering of concepts from six social science fields, including family therapy. The three dimensions were cohesion, adaptability, and communication. Evidence for the salience of these three dimensions is the fact that numerous theorists and therapists have independently selected concepts related to these dimensions as critical to their work (Table 3). (See Fisher and Sprenkle, 1978 and Sprenkle and Fisher, 1980 for empirical evidence of the importance of these three dimensions.)

The theme of cohesion is highly developed in Minuchin's work (1974; Minuchin et al., 1975, 1978). He writes that the human experience of identity has two elements: a sense of belonging and a sense of separateness. A family's structure may range from the one extreme of the "enmeshed" family to the other extreme of the "disengaged" family. In the former, the quality of connectedness among members is characterized by "tight interlocking" and extraordinary resonance among members. The enmeshed family responds to any variation from the accustomed with excessive speed

TABLE 3. Theoretical Models of Family Systems Utilizing Concepts Related to Cohesion and Adaptability and Communication Dimensions

| Cohesion | Adaptability | Communication | References |
|---|---|---|---|
| Affiliation | Interdependence | | Benjamin (1974 and 1977) |
| Affective Involvement | Behavior Control Problem Solving Roles | Communication Affective Responsiveness | Epstein, Bishop, and Levin (1978) |
| | Capacity to Change Power | | French and Guidera (1974) |
| Affect Dimension | Power Dimension | | Kantor and Lehr (1974) |
| Affection-Hostility | Dominance-Submission | | Leary (1957) and Constantine (1977) |
| Closeness Autonomy Coalitions | Power Negotiation | Affect | Lewis et al. (1976) and Beavers (1977) |
| Expressive Role | Instrumental Role | | Parsons and Bales (1955) |

and intensity. In sharp contrast, individuals in disengaged families seem oblivious to the effects of their actions on each other. "Actions of its members do not lead to vivid repercussions . . . the overall impression is one of an atomistic field; family members have long moments in which they move as in isolated orbits, unrelated to each other" (Minuchin et al., 1967:354).

Minuchin also devotes considerable attention to family adaptation. He stresses the importance of the family's capacity to change in the face of external or internal pressures, i.e., those related to developmental changes such as the addition or loss of members or changes in life-cycle stages. Minuchin notes that many families in treatment are simply going through transitions and need help adapting to them. "The label of pathology would be reserved for families who, in the face of stress, increase the rigidity of their transactional patterns and boundaries, and avoid or resist any exploration of alternatives" (Minuchin, 1974:60).

Family communication has been stressed by most family theorists from Ackerman to those associated with the "Palo Alto" communications group (Watzlawick et al., 1967, 1974; Satir, 1972). Also, many practitioners have begun to isolate the specific components of effective marital and family communication (Miller et al., 1975) and have created skill development workshops to facilitate family communication (Miller et al., 1976; Guerney, 1977).

Family research has contributed to the emergence of a relative sense of consensus among family therapists about the salience of the cohesion, adaptability, and communication dimensions. How these dimensions are operationalized, hypothesized to relate to each other, and utilized in therapy are still areas requiring considerable investigation.

Although social support is discussed as a separate topic in the social work literature (see, for example, Whittaker and Garbarino, 1983), it deserves brief mention here as an integral part of family system processes and family-based research. The role of the social network and the potential support it offers to alleviate or mediate the effects of stress have emerged as a major domain of family research in the past two decades. In general, both theory building and empirical studies have focused on three major lines of inquiry. First, what is social support? Investigations of this type have attempted to define and categorize types of support, such as emotional and financial. Second, what kinds of social networks offer support to the family or individuals within the family in times of stress? Investigations of this sort have looked at kin, friends, neighbors, social service institutions and special self-help groups, noting differences in the kind of support they offer, their accessibility to families, and the degree to which they are utilized by families. Third, in what ways and for which types of stressor events is social support a mediator of family stress?

The concept of social support has been defined in a myriad of ways, making it difficult to synthesize any core definition. The most widely referenced definition has been advanced by Cobb (1976). Cobb views social support as information exchanged at the interpersonal level which provides (1) emotional support, leading the individual to believe he or she is cared for and loved; (2) esteem support, leading the individual to believe he or she is esteemed and valued; and (3) network support, leading an individual to believe he or she belongs to a network of communication involving mutual obligation and mutual understanding. Granovetter (1973) has referred to social support as information disseminated with regard to problem solving and new social contacts for help. Other investigators have categorized social support as typical of service agencies such as churches and the Red Cross who offer material aid and tangible services in the form of babysitting, financial aid, temporary housing, etc., in times of emergency.

The major social support networks studied were neighborhoods, family and kinship, and mutual self-help groups. It should be noted, however, that while this review finds that these networks generally do provide a great deal of support which is positive in its effect in reducing stress, the question of accessibility of such networks is not discussed. Both the availability of such networks and the ability of such networks to provide support have been found to vary greatly. Many have noted that the elderly are particularly likely to have low social network involvement due to lack of money, loss of family and friends, and lack of transportation (Lee, 1979), although this finding has been questioned (Lowenthal and Robinson, 1976). Lower-class families have been found to give support in the form of services, in contrast to middle-class families who are more likely to provide money, valuable gifts, or loans (Troll, 1971; Lee, 1979).

*Neighborhoods.* Litwak and Szelenyi (1969), in their study of Hungarian housewives in Detroit, found that neighbors and friends provide an important source of assistance for short-term problems such as one day illnesses or needing a babysitter. A number of studies have detailed the creation of a range of significant social support groups for the elderly and latch-key children, for the mentally ill in rural communities (Patterson, 1971), and for widows of war (Zunin, 1974).

*Family and kinship network.* Caplan (1976) has described the following supportive characteristics of the family and kin systems when they are functioning effectively as modulators of stress: (1) collectors and disseminators of information about the world; (2) a feedback guidance system; (3) sources of ideology; (4) guides and mediators in problem-solving; (5) sources of practical service and concrete aid; (6) a haven for rest and recuperation; (7) a reference and control group; (8) a source and validator of identity; and

(9) a contributor to emotional mastery. Ethnic and minority families have made extensive use of extended family support (Lopata, 1978; Lin et al., 1979).

*Intergeneration supports* do not disappear as children leave home and establish families of their own. As Troll (1971) and Sussman (1976) have concluded from their review of research, most older persons maintain close, viable, and satisfying relationships with their adult children. In addition, most older and younger family members report satisfaction with the frequency and quality of intergenerational family relationships. This pattern of frequent and satisfying interaction among generations of adult family members living in independent households has been referred to by Hill (1970) as a modified extended family system. Hill's (1970) landmark study of family development among three generations, i.e., grandparents, parents, and young married children, revealed that: (1) the grandparent generation received the most assistance and was viewed as dependent; (2) the parental generation contributed the most assistance and held a patron-like status; and (3) the young married children provided and received moderate assistance and were viewed as reciprocators. The important point is that all three generations — older, middle, and younger — were involved in patterns of support and resource exchange which increased their viability and protected them against the harmful effects of stress.

*Mutual self-help groups* have been defined as associations of individuals or family units who share the same problem, predicament, or situation and band together for the purpose of mutual aid (Katz, 1970; Lieberman et al., 1979) Mutual help groups, in addition to being supportive of their members are also action oriented, often focusing on changing attitudes and policies which affect their problem situations. One of the more vivid examples of the 1970s was the coalition of families of American prisoners of war and men unaccounted for in Vietnam. Through this mutual aid group, families influenced the U.S. Congress and developed policies which ultimately supported them all, ensured their financial stability, and offered their children safeguards for a guaranteed college education (McCubbin, 1979).

Research on the mediating influence of social support for specific stressor events has emphasized the role of social support in protecting against the effects of stressors and thereby contributing to a family's resiliency. Research has also emphasized the importance of social support in promoting recovery from stress or crisis experienced in the family as a result of life changes, thereby contributing to the family's adaptive power. Research has revealed the influence of social support as a protective factor against complications of pregnancy and childbirth (Nuckolls et al., 1972) and in promoting medical compliance (Baekland and Lundwall, 1975). Investigations have indicated that social support makes individuals and family units less vulnerable to crisis when they experience stressors such as job terminations or difficult work environments (Gore, 1978), illnesses due to asthma (deAraujo et al., 1973) or leukemia (Kaplan et al., 1973), and natural disasters such as floods (Erickson, 1976) or tornadoes (Drabeck et al., 1975). The role of social support in promoting the family's recovery from crisis has been indicated in the case of psychiatric illnesses (Caplan, 1976); death (Parkes, 1972); divorce (Colletta, 1979); and multiproblem families (Burns and Friedman, 1976).

## DEVELOPMENTS IN FAMILY TYPOLOGIES

The use of typologies of couples and families constitutes a major breakthrough for family research because they help to bridge the gap between research, theory, and practice (McCubbin, 1988; McCubbin, Thompson, Pirner, and McCubbin, 1987; Olson, 1980). Typologies, whether developed empirically or intuitively (theoretically and clinically), offer numerous conceptual and methodological advantages over traditional variable analysis.

Conceptually, they bridge research and practice by focusing on actual couples and families, rather than on variables. Classifying a family system as a "rigidly enmeshed" type provides considerable information about the family, since the typology incorporates and summarizes a cluster of variables uniquely related to each type. Typologies enable a researcher or therapist to: (1) classify and describe couples and families on a number of variables; (2) summarize numerous characteristics of all the cases of a particular type; (3) establish criteria which determine whether a couple or family fits within a particular type; and (4) distinguish and describe differences between types. Methodologically, typologies enable an investigator to: (1) pool statistical variance across a number of variables uniquely related to each type; (2) empirically discover more stable and meaningful relationships between variables and types; and (3) translate the findings directly to couples and families rather than to variables.

In the last few years there has been increasing interest among family action researchers in identifying types of martial and family systems. For example, Cuber and Haroff (1955) developed one of the first inductively derived typologies of marriages based on interviews with high status couples. A typography of husbands' and wives' personality traits was derived from condensed interview reports with 200 couples (Ryder, 1970a, 1970b). Kanton and Lehr (1975) developed a typology of families based on the concepts of open, closed, and random systems. Constantine (1977) extended the four-player model into a more comprehensive and unified typology. A descriptive analysis of dysfunctional, mid-range, and healthy families was developed by Lewis et al. (1976), while Wertheim (1975) developed a typology based on three aspects of the morphogenesis-morphostasis dimension which described eight types of family systems related to the empirical types of families described by Reiss (1971). Most major typologies, however, have been developed intuitively and have suffered from one or more of the following problems: (1) criteria for classifying are not clearly specified; (2) procedures for assigning couples to types are subjective and ambiguous with unknown reliability; and (3) types are not exhaustive or mutually exclusive (Miller and Olson, 1978).

The empirical approach to developing typologies of marital and family systems is becoming more popular because of recent developments in computer programs on cluster and small-space analyses. Some of the first attempts to empirically develop "couples types" were done by Goodrich et al. (1968) and Ryder (1970b), using profile analysis to describe newlywed couples. Shostrum and Kavanaugh (1971) used a self-report instrument to develop types of couples based on their scores on the dimensions of anger-love and strength-weakness, and Moos and Moos (1976) developed a typology of families based on their Family Environment Scale. Similarly, using the Ravich Interpersonal Game-Test, Ravich and Wyden (1974) described eight types of marital interaction patterns. Olson and his colleagues have been working for several years on developing two different approaches to couple and family typologies, one empirical and the other theoretical. The empirical approach has focused on typologies of couples and families based on their verbal interaction patterns (Miller and Olson, 1978) generated by the Inventory of Marital Conflicts (Olson and Ryder, 1970) and other related inventories. The theoretical typology is the Circumplex Model of Marital and Family Systems developed by Olson et al. (1979).

Family stress research (McCubbin & McCubbin, 1989; McCubbin, Thompson, Pirner, and McCubbin, 1988) and family systems research (Olson et al., 1983) brings family typologies to center stage as one of the major influential variables involved in the family processes of resistance, adjustment, accommodation, and adaptation. Family typologies are defined as a set of basic attributes about the family system which characterize and explain how a family system typically appraises, operates, and/or behaves. These predictable and discernible patterns of family life, which are reinforced by rules and norms and guided by family values and goals, play an important role in explaining family behavior in the face of stressful life events and transitions. Once identified and measured, these characteristics of family life may be used to classify each family unit. Once families are classified or placed within a typology, it is possible to use the typology to make predictions about a family unit, its capabilities, responses, and outcomes in the face of stressful life events and/or crisis situations (Olson et al., 1983; McCubbin, Thompson, Pirner, and McCubbin, 1988). Thus, family typologies play a vital role in family stress research and clinical intervention. To bring the research and measurement-based constructs of family typologies to center stage for analysis and discussion as to their clinical relevance and possible utilization, we turn out attention to the concept of resilient families.

Family research emphasizes the importance of established patterns or typologies of family functioning which, if understood, can serve well the therapist, crisis manager, and educator helping families move from being a Fragile family unit (i.e., Low on Bonding and Flexibility) to being Resilient (i.e., High on Bonding and Flexibility). Current research (McCubbin, Thompson, Pirner, and Mc-Cubbin, 1988) provides initial evidence that these family types — Resilient, Rhythmic, and Regenerative — may be at the hub of family functioning; if touched and improved upon, the family unit would then be in a better position to manage its own recovery and adaptation to stressful and crisis situations.

## DEVELOPMENTS IN MARITAL AND FAMILY STRENGTHS

Family strengths and capabilities became the focus of a panel study of families before, during, and following a long-term (nine months) separation, with the military member at sea (McCubbin and Patterson, 1981). By interviewing families before the separation, during the initial phases of the nine-month wait, and after the families reunited ten months later, investigators could begin to examine what family factors appeared to make a difference between families who adapted well to the separation and those who struggled. Briefly, the data presented from this study rendered support to the stated hypothesis that families struggle with the pileup of several stressors and strains, and not just the initial stressor of family separation. Furthermore, families which attended to the needs of family members were better able to cope with and adapt to the situation. Specifically, the investigators observed that families who made an effort to enhance the self-esteem and self-reliance of its members and develop and maintain social supports from friends, relatives, and community programs were better able to endure the hardships of a nine-month separation and were also more self-reliant and better prepared for the separation. In other words, family members had personal strengths such as self-reliance and they developed the coping skills and strengths before the family even experienced the stressor event. These families prepared for the separation by actually obtaining a power of attorney and tying up all loose ends (e.g., car, home, finances, etc.) ahead of time. (See McCubbin et al., 1980; McCubbin and Patterson, 1981; Patterson and Mc-Cubbin, 1983.)

Research on family strengths conducted with nonmilitary families is also informative and need to be referenced in the context of this review. Pollack (1953) identified the following family strengths as keys to family adaptation: altruism (giving to others); a balance of independence, positive outlook, flexibility and compromise; the ability to foster growth of members; and supportive relationships.

In a pilot investigation, Otto (1963) called attention to the importance of: (1) concern for family unity, loyalty, and interfamily cooperation; (2) utilizing consciously fostered ways to develop strong emotional ties; (3) mutual respect for individual members; (4) flexibility in performing family roles; (5) ability to grow through children; (6) effective communication; (7) sensitive listening; (8) meeting spiritual needs of family; (9) ability to maintain relationships outside the family; (10) ability to seek help when appropriate; (11) ability to maintain relationships outside the family; (12) love and understanding; (13) spirituality commitment; and (14) active participation in the community.

Stinnett and his associates have made a substantial contribution to research on family strengths through their internationally recognized annual conferences and the resulting four volumes of writings on family strengths. Focusing attention on two classic investigations (Stinnett and Sauer, 1977; and Stinnett, 1981) underscores some of the salient family strengths they identify: (1) ability to deal with crisis in a positive manner: (2) spending time together; (3) love; (4) appreciation and commitment; (5) respect for individuality; (6) good communication patterns; and (7) high degree of religious orientation.

Through a survey of family professionals in the field of family counseling and family life education, Dolores Curran (1983) identified what she refers to as "Traits of a Healthy Family." Specifically, Curran identified 15 traits: (1) the healthy family communicates and listens; (2) the healthy family affirms and supports one another; (3) the healthy family teaches respect for others; (4) the healthy family develops a sense of trust; (5) the healthy family has a sense of play and humor; (6) the healthy family has a balance of interaction among members; (7) the healthy family teaches a sense of right and wrong; (8) the healthy family has a strong sense of family in which rituals and traditions abound; (9) the healthy family has a balance of interaction among members; (10) the healthy family has a shared religious core; (11) the healthy family respects the privacy of one another; (12) the healthy family values service to others; (13) the healthy family fosters table time and conversation; (14) the healthy family shares leisure time; and (15) the healthy family admits to and seeks help with problems.

A national survey of 1,000 families (Olson et al., 1983) involved in the Healthy Families at the Family Stress and Coping projects at the University of Minnesota and the University of Wisconsin, respectively, attempted to identify those family strengths which appeared to foster family "balance" over the family life cycle. The results of this survey which takes a family life cycle perspective of family strengths merit a brief summary:

*Families without Children* underscored the importance of: (a) Family Pride; (b) Family Accord; (c) Conflict Resolution; (d) Personality; (e) Conventionality; (f) Family and Friends; (g) Family Satisfaction; and (h) Marital Satisfaction.

*Families with Young Children*, that is with preschool and school-age children, emphasized the importance of: (a) Marital Communication; (b) Financial Management; (c) Conflict Resolution; (d) Family Satisfaction; (e) Resolution of Personality Differences (f) Marital Satisfaction; (g) Family and Friends; and (h) Quality of Life.

*Families with Adolescent Members* were the most stressed and therefore required a wider and broader range of family strengths in order to achieve a balance in family functioning. These families pointed to the importance of: (a) Family Pride; (b) Family Accord; (c) Conflict Resolution; (d) Resolution of Personality Issues; (e) Sexuality; (f) Commitment to Children; (g) Family and Friends; (h) Financial Management; (i) Religious Orientation; (j) Congregational Activities; (k) Spiritual Support; (l) Reframing; (m) Family Satisfaction: (n) Marital Satisfaction; (o) Quality of Life; (p) Parent-Adolescent Communication; and (q) Marital Communication.

*Families in Empty Nest Stage and Retirement Stage* struggled with financial strains, illness, losses, marital strains, work-family strains (retirement) and intrafamily strains. Their critical family strengths were: (a) Communication; (b) Resolution of Personality Issues; and (c) Health Practices. At each stage of the life cycle, family adaptation to normative transitions and stressful life events appeared to be facilitated by family strength, personal resources of family members, and community support.

*Family Resiliency and Coping.* The picture of family adaptation to change depicts the family as a reactor to stress and as a manager of resources within the family system. The active processes of family adaptation involving coping strategies within the family as well as in transactions with the community have received limited attention in both research and theory building (McCubbin, 1979).

However, there is a mounting belief among researchers and family clinical workers that understanding how families cope with stress is just as important as understanding the frequency and severity of life changes and transitions themselves (Coelho, Hamburg, and Adams, 1974; Moos, 1977). This is partially the result of accumulating empirical evidence linking coping to successful individual adjustment. More importantly, the present interest in family coping signals an important shift in our priorities in the study of family behavior under stress.

Traditionally, family stress and the demand for adaptation has been viewed as a deleterious situation to be contrasted with the smooth operation of the family unit. Predictably, the Traditional approach to the study of family stress has been to document the numerous psychological, interpersonal, and social aberrations in the family's response to stressors and related hardships. Most investigations appear to be shifting away from this dysfunctional emphasis to an interest in accounting for why some families are better able to endure hardships over the life span. This recent emphasis, which views stress as prevalent but not necessarily problematic, has let to an increasing interest in coping.

Coping research as part of family research has drawn from cognitive psychological theories (Hann, 1977), as well as from sociological theories (Mechanic, 1974; Antonovsky, 1979; Pearlin and Schooler, 1978). Cognitive coping strategies refer to the ways in which individual family members alter their subjective perceptions of stressful situations. This perspective focuses on the individual family member and his or her psychological states and subjective experiences as the dominant factors determining coping behavior. External influences and situations are taken into account through their impact on internal motivational and emotional states. The family member responds to the stress in a passive but reactive posture. Sociological theories of coping have emphasized a wide variety of actions directed at either changing stressful conditions or alleviating distress by manipulating the social environment.

Four basic hypotheses have been suggested in the limited number of family-oriented coping studies conducted in the 1970s. Coping behaviors will: (1) decrease the presence of vulnerability factors (e.g., emotional instability of a family member is a vulnerability factor which may need attention in the face of stressors) (Pearlin and Schooler, 1978; Boss et al., 1979), (2) strengthen or maintain those family resources (e.g., family cohesiveness, organization, and adaptability which serve to protect the family from harm or disruption (Adams, 1975), (3) reduce or eliminate stressor events and their specific hardships, and (4) involve the process of actively influencing the environment by doing something to change the social circumstances (McCubbin et al., 1976; Pearlin and Schooler, 1978).

These investigations have revealed that the family strategy of coping is not created in a single instant, but is progressively modified over time. Because the family is a system, coping behavior involves the simultaneous management of various dimensions of family life (McCubbin et al., 1980): (1) maintaining satisfactory internal conditions for communication and family organization, (2) promoting member independence and self-esteem, (3) maintaining family bonds of coherence and unity, (4) maintaining and developing social supports in transactions with the community, and (5) maintaining some effort to control the impact of the stressor and the amount of change in the family unit. Coping then becomes a process of achieving a balance in the family system which facilitates organization and unity and promotes individual growth and development.

One promising trend in family research has been the increasing interest in developing and evaluating marital and family enrichment programs. Reviews of the historical development of the marital enrichment movement have been completed by L'Abate (1974), Mace and Mace (1976), and Otto (1963). Most marital and family therapists have been so preoccupied with treating problematic relationships that they have failed to develop or use more preventative approaches. Although a general goal of enrichment programs has been prevention through the attempt to improve the quality of the marital and family relationship, there have been two basically different types of enrichment programs.

While both types of enrichment approaches have primarily focused on couples rather than families, one approach has focused on structured communication skill building programs, and the other (often called "marriage encounter") has been composed of more loosely focused programs. Although marriage encounter programs were developed in the last two decades, they have gained increasing acceptance as churches have begun sponsorship. The Catholic Church developed one of the earliest versions (Bosco, 1972; Koch and Koch, 1976), and now most church denominations have developed some type of marriage encounter program. David and Vera Mace (1976) have been leading advocates of marriage enrichment. They have developed an Association for Couples for Marital Enrichment (ACME) which offers weekend retreats and other programs. Communication skill building programs have been more systematically developed and researched than marriage encounter programs and represent a significant advance in the field. Miller and associates (1976) have developed a Couples Communication Program (CCP) and recently completed a program for families entitled "Understanding Us." Guerney (1977) and colleagues have developed a Conjugal Relationship Enhancement (CRE) program (Rappaport, 1976) and a program for Parent-Adolescent Relationship Development (PARD). L'Abate (1974, 1977) and associates have developed and evaluated a variety of programs for marital and family enrichment.

In a recent review of marital enrichment programs, Gurman and Kniskern (1978b) concluded that one must be cautious about the overzealous claims about the impact of these programs — especially the marriage encounters. They reviewed 29 studies of marital and premarital enrichment programs and found only six had an untreated control group. Although these studies generally demonstrated positive change, the results should be tempered by the serious methodological limitations.

Another promising preventative approach is the development of premarital programs and tools for preparing couples for marriage. There is growing evidence that traditional lecture programs for premarital couples most often offered by churches are not very effective (Druckman et al., 1979; Norem et al., 1980). A recent Canadian study by Bader and associates (Microys and Bader, 1977) demonstrated that experiential programs are helpful to premarital couples. Another recent study (Druckman et al., 1979) found that a structured premarital instrument called PREPARE was more useful than traditional education programs.

## DEVELOPMENTS IN FAMILY SYSTEM ASSESSMENT

Although a variety of diagnostic tools have been developed which could be used by marital and family therapists (Cromwell and Fournier, 1976), the statement made by Olson (1970:512) in an earlier review of the field still applies: "Most therapists seem to make their diagnostic evaluations in rather unsystematic and subjective ways using unspecified criteria that they have found helpful in their clinical practice." However, for the field to advance it is important to learn what types of therapeutic intervention work best with specific presenting symptoms or family systems. As Broderick (1976:xv) stated: "It is a simpleminded but often overlooked concept that couples are different and require differential diagnostic procedures leading to different treatment procedures."

There are a variety of reasons why most martial and family-oriented social workers do not currently use standardized diagnostic tools for their clinical assessment. First, most practitioners have not clearly identified the conceptual dimensions they consider important for diagnostic assessment. Second, there is a lack of concern with systematic diagnosis since it has often had little relationship to the therapeutic approach or intervention used. Third, most marital and family assessment tools do not assess clinically relevant concepts, are not designed for use in clinical or social work settings, and do not adequately capture the complexity of marital and family systems that the social workers feel is important.

There are, however, some recent attempts to base the treatment program on the diagnostic assessment. These bridging projects are different because they can be accomplished only when the conceptual, clinical, and empirical domains are integrated. Six examples of projects where this integrated approach has been attempted are the McMaster Model of Therapy by Epstein and colleagues (Epstein et al., 1978; Santa-Barbara et al., 1977), the Circumplex Model by Olson and colleagues (Olson et al., 1979, 1980); the Timberlawn project by Lewis and colleagues (Lewis et al., 1976; Beavers, 1977); the Social Ecology project at the Veterans Administration Medical Center in Palo Alto (Moos, 1974; Fuhr, Moos, and Dishotsky, 1981); the Family Stress, Coping and Health project (McCubbin and Thompson, 1987; McCubbin and McCubbin, 1989); and the Boysville project (Grasso and Epstein, 1988; Grasso, Epstein, and Tripodi, 1989; McCubbin, Kapp, and Thompson, 1988). All six projects have developed clinical indicators for diagnosis and research-based procedures for assessing family systems and their properties, as well as individual members and their functioning. These assessment tools enable the investigators to do clinical diagnosis before treatment, progress during treatment and post-evaluation at the end of treatment.

There are also attempts to develop more clinically relevant and useful diagnostic tools for couples and families. In this regard, Cromwell and colleagues are continuing to describe the value of "systemic diagnosis" (Cromwell and Keeney, 1979) which integrates systems theory and a multi-level (individual, interpersonal, and total system), multi-trait, and multi-method assessment. This comprehensive approach is very ambitious but reflects the type of systematic assessment that has been lacking in the field to date.

Few therapeutic models integrate the clinical assessment and the therapeutic approach. However, this type of integration could be accelerated it family therapists and family researchers worked together in a more collaborative manner. Numerous benefits could be accrued by both therapists and researchers it they formed a more cooperative relationship (Olson et al., 1980). Promising new directions for family research include the development of integrative models that bridge research, theory, and practice. Theoretical and empirical typologies are being developed which facilitate the bridging process and ultimately the value of family research (Grasso and Epstein, 1988).

Research on families will continue to move forward with the concerted efforts by social, behavioral and health scientists to advance theory-building, measurement, and intervention. While we have witnessed a proliferation of theory building efforts, some of which are creative and innovative, and other limited but interesting recapitulations of extant conceptualizations, we have only begun to advance the development of family-system–level measures which are needed for hypothesis testing, for assessment, to guide interventions, and to guide evaluations. Given the understandable limitations of time and space it is not possible to review the relevant research-based, family-oriented assessment measures for clinical practices. However, a review of systematic analysis of these instruments, particularly self-report measures in the areas of child research (McCubbin and McCubbin, 1988), family medicine research (McCubbin et al., 1989), and family stress research (McCubbin and Thompson, 1987) would shed light on the complexity of the family assessment issue and the importance of assessment to clinical work and program evaluation. A brief overview of a select number of major family assessment measures related to stress theory, family types, and family strengths and capabilities are summarized in Table 4 to again highlight the advances in theory and research and to underscore their extant importance and future relevance for clinical practice and evaluation.

Interventions can be enhanced by systematic assessments. While the clinician may feel more comfortable and skilled with assessments by interview, current studies (see Olson et al., 1983; McCubbin and Thompson, 1987) suggest the emerging value of family-system–level assessments, particularly in the use of self-report measures, as part of therapy, health care intervention, crisis intervention, and family life education. A multi-dimensional strategy for family assessment, which draws from social work practice, is suggested in this chapter.

### Challenge for Ongoing Dialogue in Social Work Practice: Foundation for Research Utilization

Family-oriented social work research has been an integral and valued part of the emerging field of family research. Motivated by the social work profession's commitment to family preservation and

TABLE 4. Family Measures Related to Family Stress Research

| Components of the Stress Typology Model for Families | Family Measure | Major Variable |
|---|---|---|
| Family Demands | FILE -Family Inventory of Life Events & Changes | **Pile Up**<br>Intra-family Strains<br>Marital Strains<br>Pregnancy Strains<br>Finance & Business Strains<br>Work-Family Strains<br>Illness Strains<br>Losses<br>Transitions<br>Legal Strains |
| Family Vulnerability | **FILE - Family Inventory of Life Events & Changes** | **Pile Up**<br>Intra-family Strains<br>Marital Strains<br>Pregnancy Strains<br>Finance & Business Strains<br>Work-Family Strains<br>Illness Strains<br>Losses<br>Transitions<br>Legal Strains |
| | **FS - Family Stressors** | **Pile Up**<br>Changes<br>Transistions<br>Losses |
| | **FST - Family Strains** | **Pile Up**<br>Intra-family Conflicts<br>Relative Conflicts |
| | **FCS - Family Changes and Strains** | **Pile Up**<br>Major Life Changes and Strains |
| | **AFILE-Adolescent- Family Inventory of Life Events & Changes** | **Pile Up**<br>Transitions<br>Sexuality<br>Losses<br>Responsibilities & Strains<br>Substance Use<br>Legal Strains |

TABLE 4 (continued)

| | | |
|---|---|---|
| | **YAFILES-Young Adult-Family Inventory of Life Events & Changes** | **Pile Up**<br>Transitions<br>Sexuality<br>Losses<br>Responsibilities &<br>    Strains<br>Substance Use<br>Legal Strains |
| | **FAPGAR**- Family APGAR | Adaptation, Partner<br>ship, Growth, Affec-<br>tion, and<br>Resolve |
| **Family Typologies** | **FACES I** - Family Adapt-ability and Cohesion | **Balanced Type**<br>Cohesion and<br>Evaluation Scales<br>Adaptability |
| | **FACES IIa** | **Resilient Type**<br>Bonding and<br>Flexibility |
| | **FACES III** - Family Adapt-ability and Cohesion Evaluation Scales | **Balanced Type**<br>Cohesion and<br>Adaptability |
| | **FHI - Family Hardiness Index** | **Regenerative Type**<br>Control, Confidence,<br>Challenge, Co-<br>oriented<br>Commitment |
| | **FTRI- Family Time and Routines** | **Rhythmic Type**<br>Family Time Together<br>and Family Routines<br>Together<br>Child's Play<br>Parent's Togetherness<br>Meals Together<br>Parent-Child/<br>Adolescent<br>    Togetherness<br>Family Time Together<br>Relatives Together<br>Kids/Adolescent<br>Chores<br>Family Organization |

|  | **SRI - Self Reliance Index** | **Self Reliance Type**<br>Autonomy<br>Decision-Making<br>Assertiveness |
|---|---|---|
| **Family Resources** | **FIRM- Family Inventory of Resources for Management** | **Family Strengths** of **Esteem and** Communication, Mastery Extended Family Social Support, Financial Well-being and Health, and Resource Strains |
|  | **FES-** Family Environment Scales | Expressiveness, Conflict, Independence, Cohesion, Achievement Orientation, Intellectual-Cultural Orientation, Active-Recreational Orientation, Moral, Organization, and Control |
|  | **FTS - Family Traditions Scale** | **Family Traditions** |
|  | **FCELBI - Family Celebration Index** | **Family Celebrations** Unique Celebrations Intra-Family Celebrations |
| **Family Coping and Problem Solving** | **CHIP- Coping Health Inventory for Parents** | **Parental Coping** Family Integration, Cooperation, Optimism Social Support, and Understanding of Medical Situation |
|  | **FCOPES- Family Crisis Oriented Personal Evaluation Scales** | **Family System Coping** Reframing Passive Appraisal Acquiring Social Support Seeking Spiritual Support Mobilizing to Acquire Help |

TABLE 4 (continued)

| | |
|---|---|
| **FCI - Family Coping Inventory** ( for Single Parents & Separated Parents) | **Spouse Coping** Maintaining Family Integrity Developing Inter - personal relationships Tensions Maintaining an Optimistic Definition of the Situation Developing Self Reliance & Self Esteem Believing in the Value of Spouse's Profession |
| **A COPE- Adolescent Coping Orientation for Problem Experiences** | **Adolescent Coping** Ventilating Feelings Family Problem Solving Seeking Spiritual Support Engaging in demanding Activity Investing in Close Friendships Developing Self Reliance Avoiding Problems Being Humorous Seeking Diversions Developing Social Support Seeking Professional Support Reading, Television, Music |
| **YACOPE -Young Adult Coping Orientation for Problem Experiences** | **Young Adult Coping** Avoidance Low Activity Level Family Problem- Solving Ventilation Self Reliance and Positive Appraisal High Activity Level Humor Emotional Connections Spiritual Support |

|  | DECS- Dual Employed Coping Scales | **Family Problem-Solving & Coping** Maintaining Family Procurement of Support Modifying Roles and Standards Maintaining a Positive Perspective Reducing Tension |
|---|---|---|
| **Social and Community Support** | **SSIndex - Social Support Index** | **Family Social Support** Emotional, Esteem and Community Support |
|  | **SSI** -Social Support Inventory | **Social Support** Emotional Support Esteem Support Network Support Appraisal Support Altruistic Support |
|  | **YASSInventory Young Adult Social Support Inventory** | **Young Adult Social Support** Parents & Sibling Spiritual Faith Special Persons Church/Synagogue groups High School friends Professionals Relatives Co-workers College friends College faculty, Counselors, Administrators Reading, Television, Music |
| **Family Schema and Coherence** | **FIC-Family Index of Coherence** | **Family Coherence** Order, Trust, Competence |
|  | **FSOC-** Family Sense of Coherence, | **Family Coherence** Comprehensibility Manageability Meaningfulness |

TABLE 4 (continued)

| Family Adjustment and Adaptation | | |
|---|---|---|
| | FAD- Family Assessment Device | Family Functioning Problem-Solving, Communication, Roles Affective Responsiveness Affective Involvement Behavioral Control General Functioning |
| | FAM- Family Assessment Measure | Family Functioning Affective Involvement Control Role Performance Task Accomplishment Communication |
| | FDI - Family Distress Index | Family Discord Emotional Distress Substance Abuse Violence Sexual Difficulties Separation/Divorce |
| | FWB - Family Member Well-being | Family Member Well-being Psychological Strains Emotional Strains |
| | FAC - Family Adaptation Checklist | Family Difficulties Marital Strains Financial Strains Legal Conflict |

homebuilders' programs, the inspiration of family life educators' interest in strengthening families, the clinicians' desire to improve on the quality of family life for struggling and dysfunctional families, and the policy makers' commitment to structure an environment to better suit and support a major social institution, the family, family scholars and scientists have seized opportunities to conduct meaningful action research. Their scientific effort has and will continue to impact on professionals as well as the families they serve. In many respects, family research has flourished through its collaborative efforts with educators, therapists, corporations, and governments. Through these collaborative ventures, five major research challenges have been addressed in the aforementioned investigations and continue to present themselves as future challenges for family research in social work settings:

*Challenge 1: to further our understanding of family strengths and capabilities in order to guide programs and social work practice.* The development of children and families will be enhanced by family action investigations which attempt to identify the critical aspects of family life which promote the well-being of family members and the family unit.

*Challenge 2: to seek greater understanding of families over the life cycle and to use such knowledge of normality to guide programs and social work practice.* The needs of children and other family members will vary by family stages of individual and family development. The well-being of children and families will be enhanced by family action investigations which attempt to identify the critical aspects of family life at each stage of development, which promotes family member and family unit well-being.

*Challenge 3: to seek greater understanding of specific types of family and their resiliency and to use such knowledge to advance programs and social work practice.* The degree to which children' needs are met and the family unit is able to develop and endure over time will depend on the type of family interaction and functioning each family creates and maintains; family typologies vary and some typologies are more effective than others. The well-being of children and families will be enhanced by family action investigations which attempt to identify family typologies and which determine the efficacy of the various types, and under what conditions.

*Challenge 4: to create, foster, and implement national, state, and agency-based policies which support families.* The degree to which children's needs are met and the family unit is able to develop and endure overtime and in the face of normative and non-normative stressors and transitions will depend on the nature of and impact of social policies and programs emanating from agencies, businesses, corporations, and the state and federal governments. The well-being of children and families will be enhanced by family action investigations which attempt to identify policies which promote or undermine children and families and which attempt to advance policies designed to strengthen children and families.

*Challenge 5: to evaluate the efficacy of family programs and to use the knowledge to improve program and social work services.* The degree to which children's and families' needs are met, particularly in those situations where they are supported by programs tailored to meet their needs, will be determined by the efficacy of these programs. Therefore, the well-being of children and families would be enhanced by family action investigations designed to assess the efficacy of child and family programs.

*Challenge 6: to take a more active posture in developing a more systematic effort to foster the integration of knowledge gained from family research into programs and social work practice.* The degree to which children and family needs are met, particularly in those situations where they are supported by programs designed to meet their needs, will be determined by the rapidity with which family-based research findings are integrated into the service offered and the level of interpersonal and case planning skills of the practitioners on the front line of the social service delivery system.

The past two decades of family research have been fruitful. Through collaborative research between social and behavioral scientists and government agencies, service agencies, and corporations, we have all benefited. The scientists have been able to advance the development of theories, particularly in the areas of family impact analysis, treating relationships, and family stress, coping, and strengths. Research methods have evolved and been tested through these collaborative investigations. For example, the recent Department of the Army family investigation involving both husbands and wives as respondents confirmed (86% return rate on questionnaires from both military members and their spouses) the value of including spouses in future military surveys. Consequently the collaborating agencies have gained meaningful information about areas in which their programs could be enhanced, new targets for intervention (prevention and treatment), and what new and relevant programs and policies can and should be developed to better meet the needs of families.

Obviously, family research has flourished in the past and this growth pattern is likely to continue, even in the face of reduced funding. Family research has the potential of moving forward undaunted by overzealous government scientists and agencies. Families have pressured the government and corporations (McCubbin and Thompson, 1989) to move ahead with such research because they believe that family research data are needed to guide government and corporate policies, programs, clinical interventions, and family-based social work services. In the face of this pressure, we can be assured that family-oriented social work research will survive and even thrive. The total arena of family research has and will continue to make meaningful contributions to both the professional literature and to programs and services designed to serve families. But the ultimate success of family research will only be determined by the degree to which the knowledge gained through research will be utilized in the future by social work practitioners and family therapists and educators in shaping their own services, programs, and social policies.

The application of stress theory to both assessment and intervention is based on the belief that planful and focused analyses of family behavior will serve as a better guide to practitioners involved in influencing and shaping family functioning. Under the watchful eye of the family theorist, family practitioners of all disciplines — social work, psychology, family science, the health sciences, and particularly nursing — have benefited from the conceptualization and systematic measurement of the complex properties of family life. We have come to believe that family crisis intervention and therapy will be enhanced by knowledge about how families behave under a wide range of stressful situations and in response to crises across stages of the family life cycle.

In the context of family stress research, we are confronted by the realization that families negotiate change and stressful life events with an innate, planful, systematic, and in some situations a surprising "knee jerk" reaction to fight to remain stable and resistant to systemic changes in the family's instituted patterns of behavior. On the other hand, in crisis situations, the family system must also change systemically to survive; by design families are called upon to expand and contract, to incorporate and to launch, and to achieve stability while introducing instability in order to evolve and develop.

This line of scientific inquiry, commonly referred to as situational and developmental stress research, has attempted to understand and explain this dynamic process of resisting change and adapting to change by isolating those individual, family unit, and community properties that interact and shape the course of family behavior over time and in response to a wide range of circumstances.

Findings from family research to date encourage the social work family practitioner, crisis counselor, health educator, and family life educator responsible for families under stress to recognize and appreciate the natural healing qualities of family life which, if understood, could become targets for intervention. Such interventions, however, would be different from the penetrating probes and strategic manipulations of the family therapist, at least in the beginning. In crisis situations, the emphasis would be on family problem-solving strategies to release the blocks to the family's own natural healing abilities and on family enhancement strategies to promote this natural process of family resiliency.

The practitioner would be the catalyst for system response and change by dwelling on the current issues affecting family life—the pressures, the pileup of stressors and strains, the normative transitions that disturb and disrupt the family's coping repertoire, and the family's innate abilities to find supports, to cope, and to adapt. The social worker would accentuate what is happening in the family, here and now, and encourage families to initiate strategies that can help the family to better manage the current situation with ease and effectiveness. Sometimes hurdle help to overcome the immediate pressure may be all that is needed. Practical advice and concrete suggestions would be a part of the practitioner's and educator's repertoire of intervention strategies complemented, naturally, by efforts to foster the family's self-discovery of the truth and its own unique patterns of coping with the situation.

We have quite a way to go before we can fully appreciate and demonstrate the contribution of family stress theory to therapy, crisis intervention, health care intervention, and family life education. We remain convinced, however, that families are durable and resilient interpersonal and social systems. They have enduring qualities of bonding, flexibility, hardness, coherence, and underlying patterns or types (such as resilient or rhythmic) which are legitimate targets for catalytic change. Family stress research encourages us to examine a host of strategies that can be employed in support of families under stress. Penetrating family therapy and its emphasis on structural change is but one among many alternatives available to the social work practitioner involved in supporting families under stress. We can be guided by systematic interventions but should not become slaves to empirical data. We can become diagnosticians without being dependent on our heuristic classifications. We can become educators, facilitators, and catalytic agents as part of our becoming therapists and change agents. Family stress research can steer and temper our approach to families and offer us tools to guide our probes and the depth of our interventions. In this regard, stress research has already made a difference in our work with families, but the degree to which this line of research is utilized or is even applicable to high risk populations served by the social work profession remains to be confirmed.

## REFERENCES

Adams, B. (1975). *The family: A sociological interpretation* (2nd ed.). Chicago: Rand McNally.

Alexander, J., and Barton, C. (1976). Behavioral systems therapy with delinquent families. In D. Olson (Ed.), *Treating relationships*. Lake Mills, IA: Graphic Publishing Company, pp. 167-88.

Angell, R. (1936). *The family encounters the Depression*. New York: Scribner.

Antonovsky, A. (1979). *Health, stress and coping*. San Francisco: Jossey-Bass.

Baekland, F., and Lundwall, L. (1975). Dropping out of treatment: A critical review. *Psychological Bulletin, 82,* 738-83.

Beavers, W. (1977). *Psychotherapy and growth: A family systems perspective*. New York: Brunner/Mazel.

Beck, D. (1976). Research findings on the outcomes of marital counseling. In D.

Olson (Ed.), *Treating relationships*. Lake Mills, IA: Graphic Publishing Company, pp. 433-73.

Benjamin, L. (1974). Structural analysis of social behavior. *Psychology Review*, 81, 392-425.

Benjamin, L. (1977). Structural analysis of a family in therapy. *Journal of Counseling and Clinical Psychology*, 45, 391-406.

Bosco, A. (1972). *Marriage encounter: The re-discovery of love*. St. Meinrad, IN: Abbey Press.

Boss, P. McCubbin, H., and Lester, G. (1979). The corporate executive wife's coping patterns in response to routine husband-father absence. *Family Process*, 18, 79-86.

Bribitzer, M., and Verdieck, M. J. (1988). Home-based, family-centered intervention: Evaluation of foster care prevention programs. *Child Welfare*, 117, 3, 255-66.

Broderick, C. Forward. (1976). In D. Olson (Ed.), *Treating relationships*. Lake Mills, IA: Graphic Publishing company, pp. xv-xvii.

Burgess, E. (1926). The family as a unity of interacting personalities. *The Family*, 7, 3-9.

Burns, K., and Friedman, S. (1976). In support of families under stress: A community based approach. *The Family Coordinator*, 25, 41-46.

Caplan, G. (1976). The family as a support system. In G. Caplan and M. Killilea (Eds.), *Support systems and mutual help*. New York: Grune & Stratton, pp. 19-36.

Cavan, R., and Ranck, K. (1938). *The family and the Depression*. Chicago: University of Chicago Press.

Cobb, S. (1976). Social support as a moderator of life stress. *Psychosomatic Medicine*, 38, 300-14.

Coelho, G., Hamburg, D., and Adams, J. (1974). *Coping and adaptation*. New York: Basic Books.

Colletta, N. (1979). Support systems after divorce: Incidence and impact. *Journal of Marriage and the Family*, 41, 837-46.

Constantine, L. (1977). A verified system theory of human process. Paper presented at Department of Family Social Science, University of Minnesota.

Cromwell, R., and Fournier, D. (1976). Diagnosing and evaluation in marital and family counseling. In D. Olson (Ed.), *Treating relationships*. Lake Mills, IA: Graphic Publishing Company, pp. 499-516.

Cromwell, R., and Keeney, B. (1979). Diagnosing marital and family systems: A training model. *Family Coordinator*, 28, 101-8.

Cuber, J., and Haroff, P. (1955). *The significant Americans: A study of sexual behavior among the affluent*. New York: Appleton-Century Crofts.

Curran, D. (1983). *Traits of a healthy family*. Minneapolis: Winston.

deAraujo, G., Van Arsdel, P. P., Holmes, T., and Dudley, D. L. (December 1973). Life change, coping ability and chronic intrinsic asthma. *Journal of Psychosomatic Research*, 17, 359-63.

Drabeck, T., Key, W., Erickson, P., and Crowe, J. (1975). The impact of disaster on kin relationships. *Journal of Marriage and Family*, 37, 481-94.

Druckman, J., Fournier, D., Robinson, B., and Olson, D. (1979). Effectiveness of five types of pre-marital preparation programs. Final Report for Education for Marriage Conference, Grand Rapids, MI.

Epstein, N., Bishop, D., and Levin, S. (1978). The McMaster model of family functioning. *Journal of Marriage and Family Counseling*, 40, 19-31.

Erikson, K. (1976). *Everything in its path: Destruction of the community in the Buffalo Creek flood.* New York: Simon & Schuster.

Fisher, B., and Sprenkle, D. (1978). Therapists' perceptions of healthy family functions. *International Journal of Family Counseling*, 6, 9-18.

Frank, J. (1979). The present status of outcome studies. *Journal of Counseling and Clinical Psychology*, 47, 310-16.

French, A. P., and Guidera, B. J. (1974). The family as a system in four dimensions: A theoretical model. Paper presented at American Academy of Child Psychiatry, San Francisco.

Fuhr, R., Moos, R., and Dishotsky, N. (1981). The use of family assessment and feed-back in on-going family therapy. *American Journal of Family Therapy*, 9, 24-36.

Goodrich, D., Ryder, R., and Rausch, H. (1968). Patterns of newlywed marriage. *Journal of Marriage and the Family*, 30, 383-89.

Gore, S. (1978). The effect of social support in moderating the health consequences of unemployment. *Journal of Health and Social Behavior*, 19, 157-65.

Granovetter, M. (1973). The strength of weak ties. *American Journal of Sociology*, 78, 1360-80.

Grasso, A. Epstein, I. (1988). Management by measurements: Organizational dilemmas and opportunities. *Computers in Human Services*, 4, 89-100.

Grasso, A., Epstein, I., and Tripodi, T. (1989). Agency-based research utilization in a residential childcare setting. *Administration in Social Work*, 12, 61-80.

Guerney, B. (1977). *Relationship enhancement.* San Francisco: Jossey-Bass.

Gurman, A. (1973). The effects and effectiveness of marital therapy: A review of outcome research. *Family Process*, 12, 145-70.

Gurman, A. (1975). The effects and effectiveness of marital therapy. In A. Gurman and D. Rice (Eds.), *Couples in conflict.* New York: Jason-Aronson, pp. 383-406.

Gurman, A., and Kniskern, D. (1978a). Deterioration in marital and family therapy: Empirical clinical and conceptual issues. *Family Process*, 17, 3-20.

Gurman, A., and Kniskern, D. (1978b). Research on marital and family therapy: Progress, perspective, and prospect. In S. Garfield and A. Bergin (Eds.), *Handbook of psychotherapy and behavior change.* New York: Wiley, pp. 817-901.

Halpern, R. (1986). Home-based early intervention: dimensions of current practice. *Child Welfare*, 115, 4, 387-98.

Hann, N. (1977). *Coping and defending: Processes of self-environment organization*. New York: Academic Press.

Herr, J., and Weakland, J. (1979). *Counseling elders and their families*. New York: Springer-Verlag.

Heying, K. (1985). Family-based, in-home services for the severely emotionally disturbed child. *Child Welfare*, 114, 5, 519-27.

Hill, R. (1949). *Families under stress*. New York: Harper & Row.

Hill, R. (1970). *Family development in three generations*. Cambridge, MA: Schenkman.

Jacobson, N. S. (1978). Specific and non-specific factors in the effectiveness of a behavioral approach to marital discord. *Journal of Consulting and Clinical Psychology*, 46, 442-52.

Jacobson, N., and Margolin, G. (1979). *Marital therapy: Strategies based on social learning and behavior exchange principles*. New York: Brunner/Mazel.

Jacobson, N., and Martin, B. (1976). Behavioral marriage therapy: Current status. *Psychological Bulletin*, 83, 540-56.

Kanton, D., and Lehr, W. (1975). *Inside the family*. San Francisco: Jossey-Bass.

Kaplan, D., Smith, A., Grobstein, R., and Fischman, R. (1973). Family mediation of stress. *Social Work*, 18, 60-9.

Katz, A. (1970). Self-help organizations and volunteer participation in social welfare. *Social Work*, 15, 51-60.

Killorin, E., and Olson, D. (1980). Clinical application of the Circumplex Model to chemically dependent families. Unpublished manuscript, Family Social Science. St. Paul, University of Minnesota.

Koch, J., and Koch, L. (1976). The urgent drive to make good marriages better. *Psychology Today*, 10, 33-35.

Koos, E. (1946). *Families in trouble*. New York: Kings Crown Press.

L'Abate, L. (1974). Family enrichment programs. *Journal of Family Counseling*, 2, 32-44.

L'Abate, L. (1977). *Enrichment: Structured intervention with couples, families, and groups*. Washington, DC: University Press of America.

Lavee, Y., McCubbin, H., and Patterson, J. (1985). The Double ABCX model of family stress and adaptation: An empirical test by analysis of structural equations with latent variables. *Journal of Marriage and the Family*, 47(4), pp. 811-25.

Leary, T. (1957). *Interpersonal diagnosis of personality*. New York: Ronald.

Lee, G. (1979). Effects of social networks on the family. In W. Burr, R. Hill, R. Nye, and I. Reiss (Eds.), *Contemporary theories about the family* (Vol. 1). New York: Free Press, pp. 27-56.

Lewis, J., Beavers, W., Gussett, J., and Phillips, V. (1976). *No single thread: Psychological health in family systems*. New York: Brunner/Mazel.

Lieberman, M., Borman, L., and associates. (1979). *Self-help groups for coping with crisis*. San Francisco: Jossey-Bass.

Lin, N., Ensel, W., Simeone, R., and Kuo, W. (1979). Social support, stressful life events and illness: A model and an empirical test. *Journal of Health and Social Behavior*, 20, 108-19.

Litwak, E., and Szelenyi, I. (1969). Primary group structures and their functions: Kin, neighbors, and friends. *American Sociological Review*, 34, 465-81.

Lopata, H. (1978). Contributions of extended families to the support systems of metropolitan area widows: Limitations of modified kin network. *Journal of Marriage and the Family*, 40, 355-66.

Lowenthal, M., and Robinson, B. (1976). Social networks and isolation. In R. Binstock and E. Shanas (Eds.), *Handbook of aging and the social sciences*. New York: Van Nostrand Reinhold.

Mace, D., and Mace, V. (1976). Marriage enrichment: A preventive group approach in couples. In D. Olson (Ed.), *Treating relationships*. Lake Mills, IA: Graphic Publishing Company.

McCubbin, H. (1979). Integrating coping behavior in family stress theory. *Journal of Marriage and the Family*, 41, 237-44.

McCubbin, H., Boss, P., Wilson, L., and Lester, G. (1980). Developing family invulnerability to stress: Coping patterns and strategies wives employ. In J. Trost (Ed.), *The family and change*. Sweden: International Library Publishing.

McCubbin, H., Dahl, B., and Hunter, E. (1976). Research on the military family: A review. In H. McCubbin, B. Dahl, and E. Hunter (Eds.), *Families in the military system*. Beverly Hills, CA: Sage, pp. 291-319.

McCubbin, H., Joy, C., Cauble, A., Comeau, J., Patterson, J., and Needle, R. (1980). Family stress, coping and social support: A decade in review. *Journal of Marriage and the Family*, 42, 855-71.

McCubbin, H., Kapp, S., and Thompson, A. (1988). Systematic monitoring of family system functioning, young adult coping and residential treatment. Unpublished manuscript. Boysville, MI.

McCubbin, H., McCubbin, M., Thompson, A., and Huang, S. (1989). Family assessment and self-report instruments in family medicine research. In C. N. Ramsey, Jr. (Ed.), *Family systems in medicine*. New York: The Guilford Press, pp. 181-214.

McCubbin, H., Olson, D., and Zimmerman, S. (1985). Family dynamics: Strengthening families through action in research. In R. Rappaport (Ed.). *Children, youth, and families: The action-research relationship*. New York: Cambridge, pp. 126-65.

McCubbin, H., and Patterson, J. (1981). Broadening the scope of family strengths: An emphasis on family coping and social support. In N. Stinnett, J. DeFrain, K. King, P. Knaub, and G. Rowe (Eds.), *Family strengths*. Vol. 3: Roots of well-being. Lincoln: University of Nebraska Press.

McCubbin, H., Thompson, A., Pirner, P., and McCubbin, M. (1988). *Family types and family strengths: A life-span and ecological perspective*. Edina, MN: Burgess International.

McCubbin, H., and Thompson, A. (1987). *Family assessment inventories for research and practice*. Madison: University of Wisconsin.

McCubbin, H., and Thompson, A. (1989). *Balancing work and family life on*

*Wall Street: Stockbrokers and families coping with economic instability.* Ednia, MN: Burgess International.

McCubbin, M. (1988). Family stress, resources and family types: Chronic illness in children. *Family Relations*, 37, 203-10.

McCubbin, M., and McCubbin, H. (1988). Family systems assessment. In P. Karoly (Ed.), *Handbook of child health assessment*. New York: John Wiley, p. 227-61.

McCubbin, M., and McCubbin, H. (1989). Theoretical orientations for family stress and coping. C. Figley (Ed.), *Treating Stress in Families*. New York: Brunner/Mazel, p. 3-43.

Mechanic, D. (1974). Social structure and personal adaptation: Some neglected dimensions. In G. Coelho, D. Hamburg, and J. Adams (Eds.), *Coping and adaptation*. New York: Basic Books, pp. 32-44.

Meyer, C. H. (1984). Integrating research and practice. *Social Work*, 29, 323.

Microys, G., and Bader, E. (1977). Do pre-marriage programs really help? Unpublished manuscript, University of Toronto.

Miller, B., and Olson, D. (1978). Typology of marital interaction and contextual characteristics: Cluster analysis of the IMC. Unpublished manuscript, Family Social Science. St. Paul, University of Minnesota.

Miller, S., Corrales, R., and Wackman, D. (1975). Recent progress in understanding and facilitating marital communication. *The Family Coordinator*, 24, 143-52.

Miller, S., Nunnally, W., and Wackman, D. (1976). Minnesota couples communication program (MCCP): Premarital and marital groups. In D. Olson (Ed.), *Treating relationships*. Lake Mills, IA: Graphic Publishing Company.

Minuchin, S. (1974). *Families and family therapy*. Cambridge, MA: Harvard University Press.

Minuchin, S., Baker, L., Rosman, B., Liebman, R., Milman, L., and Todd, T. (1975). A conceptual model of psychosomatic illness in children. *Archives of General Psychiatry*, 32, 1031-38.

Minuchin, S., Montalvo, B., Guerney, B., Jr., Rosman, B., and Schumer, F. (1967). *Families of the slums: An exploration of their structure and treatment*. New York: Basic Books.

Minuchin, S., Rosman, B., and Baker, L. (1978). *Psychosomatic families: Anorexia nervosa in context*. Cambridge, Massachusetts: Harvard University Press.

Moos, R. (1974). Family environment scale preliminary manual. Palo Alto, CA: Consulting Psychologist Press.

Moos, R. (1977). *Coping with physical illness*. New York: Plenum.

Moos, R., and Moos, B. (1976). Typology of family social environments. *Family Process*, 15, 357-71.

Norem, R. H., Schaefer, M., Springer, J., and Olson, D. H. (1980). Effective premarital education: Outcome study and follow-up evaluation. Unpublished manuscript, St. Paul, University of Minnesota, Family Social Science.

Nuckolls, K., Cassel, J., and Kaplan, B. May (1972). Psychosocial assets, life crisis and the prognosis of pregnancy. *American Journal of Epidemiology*, 95, 431-41.

Olson, D. (1980). Effective premarital education: Outcome study and follow-up evaluation. Unpublished manuscript, St. Paul, University of Minnesota.

Olson, D. (Ed.). (1970). Marital and family therapy: Integrative review and critique. *Journal of Marriage and the Family*, 32, 501-38.

Olson, D., McCubbin, H., Barnes, H., Carsen, A., Muxen, M., and Wilson, M. (1983). *Families: What makes them work*. Beverly Hills, CA: Sage.

Olson, D., Russell, C., and Sprenkle, D. (1980). Circumplex model of marital and family systems. II: Empirical studies and clinical intervention. In J. Vincent (Ed.), *Advances in family intervention, assessment and theory* (Vol. 1). Greenwich, CT: JAI Press, pp. 129-76.

Olson, D., and Ryder, R. (1970). Inventory of marital conflicts: An experimental interaction procedure. *Journal of Marriage and the Family*, 32, 433-88.

Olson, D., Sprenkle, D., and Russell, C. (1979). Circumplex model of marital and family systems: I. Cohesion and adaptability dimensions, family types, and clinical applications. *Family Process*, 18, 2-28.

Otto, H. (1963). Criteria for assessing family strength. *Family Process*, 2(2), 329-37.

Parkes, C. (1972). *Bereavement: Studies of grief in adult life*. New York: International Universities Press.

Parsons, T., and Bales, R. F. (1955). *Family socialization and interaction process*. New York: Free Press.

Patterson, S. E. (1971). Twenty older natural helpers: Their characteristics and patterns of helping. *Public Welfare*, 29, 400-03.

Patterson, J., and McCubbin, H. (1983). The impact of family life events and changes on the health of a chronically ill child. *Family Relations*, 32, 255-64.

Pearlin, L., and Schooler, C. (1978). The structure of coping. *Journal of Health and Social Behavior*, 19, 2-21.

Pollak, O. (1953). Design of a model of health family relationships as a basis for evaluative research. *Social Services Review*, 31, 369-76.

Rappaport, A. F. (1976). Conjugal relationship enhancement program. In D. Olson (Ed.), *Treating relationships*. Lake Mills, IA: Graphic Publishing Company.

Ravich, R., and Wyden, B. (1974). *Predictable pairing*. New York: Wyden Publishing.

Reiss, D. (1971). Varieties of consensual experience: I. A theory for relating family interaction to individual thinking. *Family Process*, 10, 1-27.

Ryder, R. (1970a). A topography of early marriage. *Family Process*, 9, 385-402.

Ryder, R. (1970b). Dimensions of early marriage. *Family Process*, 9, 51-68.

Santa-Barbara, J., Woodward, C. A., Levin, S., Streiner, D., Goodman, J. T., and Epstein, N. B. (1977). Interrelationships among outcome measures in the McMaster family therapy outcome study. *Goal Attainment Review*, 3, 47-58.

Satir, V. (1972). *Peoplemaking*. Palo Alto, California: Science and Behavior Books.

Shostrum, E., and Kavanaugh, J. (1971). *Between man and woman*. Los Angeles: Nash Publishing.

Sprenkle, D., and Fisher, B. (1980). Goals of family therapy: An empirical assessment. *Journal of Marriage and Family Therapy*, 6(12), 132-36.

Stanton, M. (1979). Family treatment approaches to drug abuse problems: A review. *Family Process*, 18, 251-80.

Stanton, M., Todd, T., Steier, F., Van Deusen, J., Marder, L., Rosoff, R., Seaman, S., and Skibinski, I. (1979). Family characteristics and family therapy of heroin addicts: Final report 1974-1978. Report prepared for the Psychosocial Branch, Division of Research, National Institute on Drug Abuse, Department of HEW. Washington, DC: Government Printing Office.

Steinglass, P. (1976). Experimenting with family treatment approaches to alcoholism 1950-1975: A review. *Family Process*, 15, 97-123.

Steinglass, P. (1979a). The alcoholic family in the interaction laboratory. *Journal of Nervous and Mental Disease*, 167, 428-36.

Steinglass, P. (1979b). An experimental treatment program for alcoholic couples. *Journal of Studies on Alcohol*, 40, 159-82.

Stinnett, N. (1981). In search of strong families. In N. Stinnett, B. Chesser, and J. DeFrain (Eds.), *Building family strengths: Blueprints for action*. Lincoln: University of Nebraska Press.

Stinnett, N., and Sauer, K. (1977). Relationship characteristics of strong families. *Family Perspectives*, 11(4), 3-11.

Sussman, M. (1976). The family life of older people. In R. Binstock and E. Shanas (Eds.), *Handbook on aging and the social sciences*. New York: Van Nostrand Reinhold, pp. 218-43.

Troll, L. (May 1971). The family of later life: A decade review. *Journal of Marriage and the Family*, 33, 263-90.

Watzlawick, P., Beavin, J., and Jackson, D. (1967). *Pragmatics of human communication*. New York: Norton.

Watzlawick, P., Weakland, J., and Fisch, R. (1974). *Change: Principles of problem formation and problem resolution*. New York: Norton.

Wells, R., and Denzen, A. (1978). The results of family therapy revisited: The non-behavioral methods. *Family Process*, 17, 251-74.

Wells, R. A., Dilkes, T., and Burckhardt, T. (1976). The results of family therapy: A critical review of the literature. In D. Olson (Ed.), *Treating relationships*. Lake Mills, IA: Graphic Publishing Company, pp. 499-516.

Wertheim, E. (1975). The science typology of family systems. II. Further theoretical and practical considerations. *Family Process*, 14, 285-308.

Whittaker, J, and Garbarino, J. (1983). *Social support networks: Informal helping in the human services*. New York: Aldine.

Zunin, L. (1974). A program for the Vietnam widow: Operation second life. In H. McCubbin, B. Dahl, P. Metres, Jr., E. Hunter, and J. Plag (Eds.), *Family separation and reunion*. Washington, DC: Government Printing Office, pp. 218-24.

# INTRODUCTION TO SECTION III

# Research Utilization in Administration and Community Organization

## Harold Weissman

The chapters in this section deal with three problems: What is the supply of available research? What do community organizers, administrators, and policy makers want in the way of research? How can supply and demand for research be brought into some congruence?

In the discussion which followed the presentation of these papers, Harold Lewis made the point that administrators are reasonable rather than rational. Administrators cannot simply maximize any one choice no matter what the data seems to indicate, because decisions made in one sphere of organizational life impact on other spheres. What is rational action in terms of maximizing one goal may be quite irrational in terms of that action's effect on another equally important goal.

Nevertheless, it is understandable that researchers would seek to have the knowledge and information they generate utilized by policy makers and administrators. The rationalists among the conference participants argued for a research utilization model of study, design, and development. In this model theory and research guide practice. Developmental research is conceived as consisting of those methods by which the social technology of human service is analyzed, designed, created, and evaluated. The phases of developmental research are viewed as the early and essential phases that come before the subsequent phases of utilization, which are diffusion and adoption. The full sequence of these phases—analysis, development, evaluation, diffusion, and adoption—with their constituent steps and conditions, is called developmental research and utilization (DR & U) (Thomas, 1984, p. 23).

In their comments others argued that such an approach is far removed from the reality of the working concerns or modus operandi of administrators, policy makers, and community organizers. They argued that DR & U or Social R&D assumes an orderly environment that is controllable; goals that are fixed, definable, and nonconflictual; financing that is available on an as-need basis; and an ability to produce innovations far beyond the capacity possible with present levels of knowledge.

> Engineering technologies, powerful and elegant when judged from a narrowly technical perspective, turn out to have unintended and unpredicted side effects that degrade the environment, generate risk, or create excessive demands on scarce resources . . . [a researcher] may discover that his client is unwilling to listen to his attempts to describe the situation's uniqueness and uncertainty, . . . He will be caught, then, in a thicket of conflicting requirements: a wish to keep his job, a feeling of professional pride in his ability to give usable advice, and a keen sense of his obligation to keep his claims to certainty within the bounds of his actual understanding. (Schön, 1987, p. 6)

Social workers operating at any level—policy, administrator, program—are troubled by indeterminate zones of practice where there is uncertainty, uniqueness, and value conflict. Developmental research cannot be the primary means for addressing such concerns because of the limitations noted above. Schön argues that professionals do not simply operate as rational problem solvers; rather, they are skilled improvisors, selectively managing large amounts of information, spinning out long lines of invention and inference, examining several ways of looking at a situation at once, holding an ongoing reflective conversation as they take action (Schön, 1987, pp. 26-27).

Mizrahi in her chapter details a number of supply and demand issues which affect the utilization of research in community practice and which bear on the above dispute. She points out that the way one conceptualizes and defines a problem determines how one analyzes and researches it. The community researcher has to be able to reconcile different definitions of the problem and make creative use of multiple sources of data to reflect the complexities involved in attempting to address them. She also draws attention to the enabling and disabling effects of ideology on research utilization as well as to the potential effects of the information explosion generated by the use of computers. She notes areas in community practice where supply does not keep pace with demand and concludes with a community practice research agenda for the 1990s.

In their chapter, Hasenfeld and Patti directly challenge the technocratic view that social welfare administrators can or even should be primarily guided by social science theory and research. The paper presents the results of a number of empirical studies which document what activities occupy the time of social welfare managers and the types of information and knowledge these activities demand. They conclude that administrators seldom have sufficient time or control over time for the kind of primary search processes that are thought to be necessary in the DR & U model to inform professional practice.

They detail four different types of research relevant to administration and suggest three different forms of utilization. The chapter concludes with a detailed statement of how research can be made relevant to the needs of administrators in terms of specific actions both researchers and administrators can take. As such, the article is quite sanguine about the possibilities of adjusting supply and demand for research about administrative concerns.

The last article in this chapter, by Rehr, is in effect a case study of how a sophisticated hospital social work director used research as an administrative tool. She describes how research studies on the services offered by her department played a crucial role in the hospital's decision to expand the social work department, how it protected the department from cutbacks, how research helped to improve practice through staff involvement in research, and above all how research helped to anticipate trends in service delivery and made possible the development of techniques and procedures which often served as a model for practice around the country.

If anything, these three chapters document the specific needs for research in these three areas of practice. They strongly argue that research is an important tool for supporting practice, yet not a superordinate one given the nature of the domains. And finally, they imply that sophisticated policy makers, administrators, and community organizers can use research as a very powerful tool to attain programmatic ends—with the caveat that they, rather than the researchers, must determine the ends.

## REFERENCES

Schön, Donald. *Educating the Reflective Practitioner,* San Francisco: Jossey-Bass, 1987.
Thomas, Edwin. *Designing Interventions for the Helping Professions,* Sage Publications, 1984.

# The Future of Research Utilization in Community Practice

Terry Mizrahi

The development of research utilization in community practice has been complex and uneven. Community practice — which generally includes organizing, development, planning, class advocacy, and social change — has had wide and shifting parameters. Beyond changing boundaries and definitions, other reasons for the lack of a unified body of applied research in community practice include: ambivalence about how much as well as what type of system/structural change is desirable and possible; differences about how change occurs; ambiguity about the derivation of the roots and sources of theory and practice; resistance from the community practitioners who see research as inimical to or diverting social action; and reaction to the political and economic conditions which affect educational and professional opportunities for community practice. Moreover, it is difficult to predict or control outcomes of community interventions because of the interconnectedness and uncertainty of conditions, ideology, goals, strategies, and resources. As a result of this difficult history, the models of practice-research utilization as well as the scope and content of the field are least developed within social work.

This chapter will discuss the state of community practice research utilization and present some of the major theoretical, methodological, and technological considerations for enhancing the development and application of research in the field. It will present some of the continuing as well as new directions for utilizing research in community work along the problem-solving continuum: the problem formulation and analysis phase, the implementation phase, and the evaluation (effectiveness and outcome) phase. Finally, it will discuss the roles of schools of social work in conducting, teaching and facilitating practice-research models, and identify a community practice-research agenda embedded in the tradition of social work.

Research utilization involves three related roles for the community practitioner: research consumer (the use of information obtained from other sources including findings from already conducted research and data already collected by outside agencies); research creator (the use of information gathered and analyzed directly by or for the practitioner); and research communicator (the presentation, dissemination, and publication of information to various constituencies). Little is systematically known about how research is consumed, created, and communicated in community practice.

## *ASSUMPTIONS*

Given the general goals of community practice as improving the conditions and quality of life through collective problem-solving, a primary assumption is that the gathering and use of information should be viewed in an action research framework where one is simultaneously trying to understand the situation while changing it (Karger and Reitnor, 1983; Schein, 1987; Epstein and Tripodi, 1978; Rubin and Rubin, 1986). It is also assumed that it is not possible to be objective as in value-free and neutral. The researcher (as well as the research itself), whether employing qualitative or quantitative approaches, has implicit or explicit ideology, assumptions, or hypotheses. It is further assumed that it is not possible to be unobtrusive, regardless of the methods used. Community meetings cannot be observed using one-way mirrors. The community practitioner when in the research mode, and the researcher engaged in community research, affect and are affected by the research transaction. At best, by utilizing the social work concepts of self-awareness and conscious use of self, the worker can anticipate and articulate these dilemmas and minimize their impact on the process and outcome of the research. It is not assumed, however, that the above means that all research is biased and therefore unreliable or invalid, but rather it must be recognized that data collection and interpretation do not occur apart from the people and their environments. It is additionally assumed that there is an obligation on behalf of those collecting and utilizing information to inform and involve the relevant participants in data process, interpretation, and application. Utilizing the concepts of empowerment and exchange, this means sharing information in appropriate and relevant ways, mediating the ideal with the pragmatic, and giving back something to the community as a trade-off for taking something. Finally, it is assumed that many community practitioners already engage in systematic information gathering and interpretation without necessarily conceptualizing that function as research.

## THE STATUS OF COMMUNITY PRACTICE RESEARCH

While the number of new and expanded texts for students and practitioners in community practice — exclusively for, or including, social workers — has increased in the 1980s (Burghardt, 1982a and 1982b; Staples, 1984; Rubin and Rubin, 1986; Cox et al., 1987; York, 1982; Brager, Specht, and Torczyner, 1987; Taylor and Roberts, 1985; Bicklin, 1983; Ecklein, 1984), only some of them devote a chapter or section to information gathering and research. Rarely do they explicitly incorporate or integrate findings or research-based concepts; Rubin and Rubin (1986) is a rare exception. A few articles in *Encyclopedia of Social Work* highlight the major themes in the broad field (Burghardt, 1987; Gilbert and Specht, 1987; Spergel, 1987; Rothman, 1987), but only a few of them identify research trends or needs. Moreover, the number of research-based articles relating to community practice appearing in *Social Work Research and Abstracts* remains small. The status and projections of research in community work remain largely unchanged since Thomas (1980) discussed the scene in Great Britain (which was also relevant to the United States) some time ago.

During the 1980s it appeared that the leadership and investment in maintaining and promoting a research-based community practice agenda had diminished. When Epstein and Tripodi (1978) discussed incorporating research into macro-level practice, they focused primarily on administration and agency service. Management and program evaluation have come a long way since then — the clarity of and supports for these areas are evident. Although there are knowledge, skill, and resources common to all macro areas (Austin, 1986; Jansson, 1987), and this should include research, community practice must remain a distinct method if social work is to contribute to this vital field.

## PROBLEM FORMULATION AND ANALYSIS PHASE

### Problem Definition

The way in which one conceptualizes and defines a phenomenon will affect how one analyzes, intervenes, and evaluates it. Generally put, a value-based or ideological lens usually interacts with, if not precedes, action and problem-solving. For the community researchers (the term I will use to mean both the community-based researcher and the research/fact-finding community practitioner), perspectives on constructs such as social structure, social problems, community, and even human development, while not in the every day conversation or even consciousness of most people involved in social change, very much shape the goals and strategies selected.

One of the first steps in systematic inquiry is to clarify the definition of the problem by posing questions: Who is defining it? What are alternative ways of defining it (Thayer, 1977)? For whom is it a problem/issue and why? Also important are other questions: How does change occur, and more specifically, who can affect or change the situation? How can groups influence both the definition and solution to the problem? The community researcher ideally begins the research process by assessing or reassessing his/her own and others' answers to these fundamental questions. Questions here include: What do we know already? What do we want to know? Why do we want to know? Neither the researcher nor the organizations involved in social change are neutral or free agents; unstated assumptions and desired outcomes of all parties need articulation and clarification (Jones and Harris, 1987), if not reconciliation.

Problem definition has had direct impact on major action research efforts (see Katan and Spiro, 1987; Warren, 1988; McGrath, 1983). It affects the kind of research undertaken, the methodologies employed, and how findings are interpreted and utilized. For example, the terms "community" and "neighborhood" have differing, and at times conflicting, meanings that shape the information gathering and interpretation phases (see discussions by Rothman [1987a], Lyon [1987], Warren and Lyon [1988], for the relationships among understanding, studying and changing the community; see Mc-Knight and Kretzman [1984] and Gilroth [1985] on how differing views on neighborhoods affect perspectives on the viability of organizing at that level; see Blau [1988] for an historical analysis of how ideology about the causes and cures of homelessness affected the way the problem was documented and data were interpreted).

The components of the problem-analysis phase that need systematic investigation include: (1) the geographic community (its institutions, people, resources, problems); (2) the needs and concerns of the people (whole or subpopulations of an identified geographic or functional community); (3) the resources, capacities, and commitment of institutions (formal and informal) to meet these needs; and (4) community and institutional power and decision making.

## *Traditional Tools and Techniques of Problem Documentation*

The methods to directly collect and analyze data for community practice have received the most attention. These tools are carefully explained in the literature (Siegel, Attkisson, and Carson, 1987; Collette, 1984; Neuber et al., 1980; Wilson and Mondros, 1982; Adler and Adler, 1987; Lyon, 1987; Schein, 1987). Less known, however, is how and whether community practitioners actually use them. Those closest to practice either omit or simplify them considerably in the materials they prepare for training (Thomas, 1980).

These techniques generally include the creation and use of existing social indicators; in-person, telephone, and mailed surveys; group data gathering processes such as focused group interviews, nominal group techniques, community forums, and public hearings; and observational techniques in natural or contrived settings conducted by members/insiders, participant observers, and outside observers. Each of these techniques has strengths and limitations in terms of ease and practicality of use, and the nature, quality, and quantity of data obtained.

Information gathering, informed by different theories, produces different types of information. For one example, there is a direct relationship between the theory of community power, the methodology used to study it, and the findings it produces (Lyon, 1987). For another, there is a linkage between concepts of need (Bradshaw, 1977) and different needs assessment strategies (York, 1982). In other words, there are different ways of knowing and different things to know.

The community researcher often will be in the position of having to reconcile different definitions of the problem and make creative use of multiple sources of data to reflect the complexities involved in attempting to address them. For example, consider how practice would be strengthened by utilizing only two of many documentation techniques — counting and observing — to analyze the problem of hunger. By documenting the increase in the number and location of soup kitchens and feed pantries over a five-year period, the community researcher concludes that the problem of hunger is becoming more pervasive. By spending time observing a soup kitchen in action (as Glasser [1989] did), the researcher discovers that, in addition to meeting a basic need, the food service also created a positive sense of community among the recipients. The use of these qualitative and quantitative data together informs practice in several ways: it demonstrates the magnitude of the problem; it documents the deficiencies in feeding programs (by also using waiting lists, turn-aways, provider-expressed ambivalence, etc.); and it humanizes the abstract concept of hunger; it points out the strengths, capacities and caring of givers and receivers of help, even in adverse situations. It also alerts the community researcher to another, less pathological interpretation of recipients' behavior if they resist changing their circumstances (e.g., leaving the program) when alternative programs or resources become available. An important link is made between micro and macro practice as the need is reaffirmed for service and advocacy strategies to be coordinated (Fabricant, 1986).

Here is another example of use of data in analyzing community problems and developing strategies for addressing them. A consumer health group concerned about utilization of a local hospital's emergency room obtained access to emergency room records and also spent time observing and interviewing there. They discovered that its use was related more to social conditions than to disease-related crises: accidents (automobile and home), assault (physical and sexual), bronchial conditions, alcohol and drug abuse, and dog bites. The community organization developed a series of short- and long-term strategies to address the various problems. They initiated a dog catching and education program involving neighborhood youth and animal protection agencies. They influenced the way the hospital collected data on accidents so that records included the causes and their sources and not merely the symptoms or results (e.g., a broken bone from (source), asphyxiation due to ingestion of poison, etc.). They also investigated and mapped the location of the automobile accidents. After pinpointing the locations, they sought to reintroduce two-way lanes through their neighborhood and to obtain a stop sign at the exit of certain parking lots. Additionally, since bronchial asthma is associated with poor nutrition, they launched a rooftop greenhouse program to grow and distribute vegetables (McKnight, 1978).

## New and Alternative Approaches to Problem Analysis

In recent years new and alternative paradigms for theory, research, and practice are influencing and involving community practice. The feminist, black nationalist, and ethnic/cultural perspectives have gained importance for many reasons: sensitivity and consciousness of these groups has increased; discontent has been vocalized among those who feel oppressed, disenfranchised, or misunderstood; and current interventions have had minimal impact on the depth and breadth of community problems and social conditions.

Collectively, this body of disparate work is providing cogent critiques of more traditional theory, methodology, and practice. At the same time, it is offering new, revised, and additional research-based approaches that may be more effective in working in those communities or with those populations. Conversely, these frameworks are contributing to more comprehensive understanding about and working with mainstream populations. A few of the many databased undertakings relevant to community practice are identified here to illustrate the impact these are beginning to have on the field.

The work of feminist scholars and researchers has begun to influence not only the knowledge about women, but knowledge about approaches to research, organizing, and social change (Brandwein, 1981; Weil, 1986; Davis, 1986 and 1987; Gottlieb and Bombyk, 1987; Maypole, 1987). For example, Mizrahi et al. (1989) have identified deficiencies and biases in organizing texts and are now surveying women organizers and materials used by women organizers to identify feminist organizing principles and practice-based theory. Other researchers are focusing on the organizing of poor women, women of color, and white, ethnic, working-class women. For example, a study of women's organizing revealed major differences by class (Naples and Gittell, 1982). Baver (1989) critiques the assumptions and approaches used to study Hispanic women in politics. She suggests that a broader definition which includes community organizing as political work produces a picture of greater political participation.

The black nationalist perspective is also permeating the content and methods of research. For example, while the role of the black church in organizing, planning, and advocacy has been discussed, recent studies are both deepening knowledge and challenging long held beliefs (Green and Wilson, 1989; Cox, 1984). The complex issues facing black women, their organizations, and organizers are being studied using both a feminist and nationalist lens (Smith and Stewart, 1983; Gilkes, 1983). Moreover, the culturally homogeneous, implicit, white Euro-American perspective for defining and solving problems is being exposed for both its bias and incompleteness (Rees, 1987; Rivera, 1987; Woodrum and Reid, 1987; Marti-Costa and Serrano-Garcia, 1987). At the same time, the results of such research endeavors are producing better tools for assessing and involving various ethnic communities (Heskin and Heffner, 1987; Humm-Delgado and Delgado, 1986). A more refined and complete description of rural communities is now appearing, in part because of recent farm and environmental crises (Herick, 1986; Fitchin, 1987). These are serving to dispel myths about rural life and produce a more realistic research-based organizing agenda.

## Use of Information Technology
## in Problem Definition and Analysis

Information technology, and the computer in particular, are revolutionizing society, significantly altering the delivery of human services, and of late, coming into use in community practice. As with any tool, computer technology can be used to empower or oppress, and community researchers are beginning to understand its power, problems, and potential. On a macro level, the impact of computers on a democratic society have great significance for community researchers (Barber, 1984; Perrolle, 1987; Danziger et al., 1982). At the service level, it is significantly altering agency life (Nurius, Hooyman, and Nicoll, 1988; Taylor, 1981; see also the journal *Computers in Human Services* for up-to-date accounts of social service applications and issues).

Grassroots and social change organizations have been slow to come on board because of resource deficiencies and/or an ideology that links computers with profit, exploitation, and social control. Many groups, however, are now beginning to make use of computers to do their work more efficiently and effectively. Beyond the traditional uses for office management, they are also being utilized for research-based data analysis and problem formulation to inform community practice. Among those functions are: to store, organize, analyze, and disseminate information on problem areas; to create databases on contributions, constituencies, contacts, and decision makers; to target political and social action campaigns; to share information by creating and using bulletin boards, local area networks, and teleconferencing (see McCullough, in press; Mizrahi et al., 1990; Rodberg, in press; Height and Rubins, 1983). A few examples: The New Jersey Self-Help Clearinghouse has created a database and other functions to tap, assist, develop, and facilitate the networking of hundreds of mutual aid groups across the state. In this way they are documenting and meeting needs, and through CompuServe (a national computer network) are hosting on-line conferencing (Madara, Kalafat, and Miller, 1989). A West Harlem community organization established an integrated computer system that enabled it to expand its housing management as well as planning capability, and the Clinton Housing Development Company created the Clinton Housing Inventory Program to monitor information on a neighborhood's residential properties, a vital aid in targeting tenant and housing organizing (Madeuno, 1986).

Beyond collecting and creating their own databases from their own sources, the computer is allowing groups to have easier access to and to store, analyze, and distribute data collected from government and other publicly available sources (Cordero, 1990; Spiegel, 1987). Integration of existing databases is one of the most exciting and challenging opportunities for community researchers. The concept of convergent analysis (Siegel, Attkisson, and Carson, 1987) is taking on new meaning as community researchers develop the software programs to integrate data from such sources as the U.S. Bureau of Census, the National Home Mortgage Disclosure Act, Police Departments, Health Departments, Boards of Elections, Departments of Housing, Real Estate, Taxes, the Environmental Protection Agency, among many other local, regional, state, and federal agencies.

At the same time, social change organizations have launched major social action, campaigns to require government to collect and disseminate information that can assist groups in organizing and planning more knowledgeably and effectively. Such organized action in the past has resulted in legislation and regulation mandating disclosure and access; two important examples are the federal and state Community Reinvestment Acts, and more recently, the Emergency Planning and Community Right-To-Know Act of 1986 building upon past Freedom of Information Acts (Goldman, in press).

For community researchers working on regional, state or national levels there are community information projects developed with, and by, universities and other large organizations that have financial and technical resources available to collect, house, disaggregate where necessary, analyze, produce, and disseminate public information. Many of these organizations are also doing their own data collection and analysis for the purpose of influencing public policy (see Wu and Korman, 1987; Woodrum and Reid, 1987; and Meyer, Share, and Radtke, 1986 for examples of the creative use of large-scale databases). Such programs include: the Infoshare Project of the Department of Urban Study at Queens College of the City University of New York, The Center for Law and Social Justice at Medgar Evers College of the City University of New York, and the Public Data Access, Inc. in New York City.

## PROGRAM IMPLEMENTATION PHASE

Research utilization at the implementation phase is much less developed than at the problem analysis phase, although all the methods, techniques, and technological tools used in the first phase can be adapted to track, monitor and assess ongoing practice. Several questions posed at this phase: Are the planned-for strategies and programs actually being undertaken? How are resources being used? Are the strategies and resources consistent with the goals and objectives?

At the implementation phase, research is concerned with what the community practitioner is doing and how she/he is doing it: the effort/input and process/throughput of community intervention. At this phase, it is generally strategies that are measured, not the goals themselves. The implementation (or action phase) includes activities such as monitoring involvement of consumers and other constituencies; assessing the type and usefulness of outreach techniques; assessing feedback and responsiveness of media, decision makers, funders, regulators; documenting survival and growth activity; and monitoring productivity of staff and volunteers.

Because so much of community practice involves informing, motivating, mobilizing, managing, and sustaining involvement of a variety of constituencies, tools and techniques to facilitate assessment of this activity are critical. Information technology is contributing to the way in which practitioners reach various constituencies. For example, in political campaigns, targeting software is allowing groups to reach and identify constituency using their own or already created lists such as registered voters, tenants, and property owners.

Another technique is the use of a time series analysis for the study of community group action. In one situation, this technique was used to ascertain that a campaign aimed at negatively affecting a bank's deposits by organizing a boycott worked (Stein and March, 1985). It could not be used, however, to evaluate outcome, that is, whether the ultimate goal to obtain a change in the bank's behavior was accomplished as a result of the strategy.

## Implementing Models of Community Practice

The implementation phase also includes knowing more about what is going on in community practice today, that is, doing and utilizing research to describe the scope, content, and auspice of community practice. Finally, it also means making research undertakings more relevant and applicable to the work of community practitioners.

We need to know more about how practitioners use data and what help they need to obtain, utilize, and disseminate information. In the only study identified about the relationship between data providers and community-based data users, it was found that very few community workers knew about existing data sources and even fewer used them, even when they were deemed relevant to their work (Spiegel, 1987).

While Rothman's three models of community organizing (1987) — locality development, social planning, and social action — are still the generally taught methods of community practice, ironically there are almost no systematic studies examining the extent to which these in fact ever reflected or now reflect community practice. Cnaan and Rothman (1986) identified only one previous study conducted in Israel before their study which operationalized Rothman's three models and applied them to community workers also in Israel. Clearly studies such as these are needed in this country. The field is ripe for examining both practice models and the locus of the social work trained community practitioner today. In other words, we need to know more about where they are and how they are functioning before we can strengthen their effectiveness through more comprehensive and targeted research utilization methods.

There is however, increasing recognition that the complexity, purpose, and scope of community practice needs additional conceptual and empirical analysis (Hyman, 1986). An additional or fourth model, "social change organization-building," seems needed to more accurately reflect community practice in the 1980s. This model encompasses and builds upon Burghardt's discussion of community-based social action (1987), Rothman's (1987) and Spergal's (1987) identification of citizen participation, social and interorganizational networking, and my own ongoing work on coalitions (Mizrahi and Rosenthal, 1988).

A body of research being done primarily by social workers has begun to describe and analyze organizations engaged in social change. These studies include some well-constructed, in-depth case studies (Harris, 1987; Lindgren, 1987; Roberts-Degenerro, 1986) and comparative studies of social change organization-building (see Mondros and Wilson [1989] on 42 social action organizations; Reisch [1986] on 70 advocacy organizations; and Mizrahi and Rosenthal [1988] on 40 social change coalitions). All these works have in common the fact that they are questioning the community practitioners and leaders in an attempt to describe more accurately the structure and dynamics of these organizations, and to begin to link these variables with evaluations of their effectiveness. Cumulatively, these should lead to research-based practice principles and more informed practice-based theory.

## THE EVALUATION PHASE OF COMMUNITY PRACTICE

### Research on Effectiveness and Outcome

As with all human service research, it is difficult to evaluate the effectiveness of interventions. The greater the number of variables involved, the more complex is the analysis with respect to accounting for and measuring the change, and the more uncertainty with respect to attributing cause and effect. Furthermore, beyond the question of what is being evaluated is the question of who is doing the assessment — the worker, the lay leadership, the membership or constituency, knowledgeable outsiders, professionals — and for what purpose? Different problems emerge when the evaluator is an outsider/consultant, in contrast to one who is an inside staff researcher (Epstein and Tripodi, 1978; Schein, 1987; Aaronson and Sherwood, 1967), or a community researcher engaged in action-analysis simultaneously (Farris and Ruckdeschel, 1981). Just as it is difficult to have total unanimity about the definitions of the problem, so too is it almost impossible to have a singular definition of success (Hunt, 1987). This is the phase of research utilization (as with all social work methods) that is the least developed. However, many of the perceptual and empirical techniques identified in the problem formulation and analysis phase also can be adapted to the effectiveness phase.

Nevertheless, it is essential to critically scrutinize what is being done, how, and why at all stages of the social change process, or at what Wilson and Mondros (1982) call the briefing action-debriefing phases. Community practitioners need tools and information to help their organizations analyze the results of their efforts and those of others (especially given the scarcity of resources available), and community practitioners need the means and the methods to examine their own and others' professional practice (self and peer review) in order to be efficient as well as effective.

Community researchers can make use of past analyses of social change organization-building efforts as well as studies that have attempted to link structure and process to outcome. Two major efforts worth scrutiny are the Alinsky models of neighborhood organizing (in geographic communities) and the organizing of welfare recipients (a functional community) (on Alinsky-style organization, see Fisk, 1973; Lancourt, 1979; Reitzes and Reitzes, 1982; Cruz, 1987; on welfare rights organizing, see Piven and Cloward, 1977; West, 1981). When viewed as a whole, these series of studies demonstrate that one cannot separate ideology, methodology, and outcome. There were clearly different definitions as well as measures and levels of success at different times and in different contexts.

Nevertheless, by reviewing findings from these research efforts, the competent practitioner will be in a better position to apply them to his/her own community or organization, and make more realistic assessments concerning the probable outcome of interventions.

A few, more limited, examples: Dear and Patti (1981) identified a series of practice strategies for those engaged in political advocacy based on a study of the factors influencing the passage of legislation. Refining concepts and examining components of effectiveness can lead to a better understanding of the relationship between the structure of leadership and successful outcomes (Biaggart and

Hamilton, 1987). The community researcher can learn more about the quality, quantity, representativeness, and effectiveness of neighborhood organizations by reviewing studies by Jones (1982); Jones and Tumelty (1986); and Ragab, Blum, and Murphy (1981). Hubbart's findings (1986) on community beliefs and community economic development help the practitioner understand that community-based development is neither a panacea nor a plot. There is a need to separate myth from reality, and to validate or challenge untested assumptions in order to build a more effective practice. In this way, community practice can define its objectives and strategies more realistically—without being overly idealistic or overly cynical.

## THE ROLE OF SCHOOLS OF SOCIAL WORK

The future development of community practice research depends to a great extent on the leadership and resource commitment of Schools of Social Work in partnership with the relevant social agencies and field-related practicum settings.

Research cannot be divorced from the arenas to which it will be applied, and instrument creation must reflect the realities of the everyday life of community practitioners.

1. Requirements can be instituted that all those students who do community profiles, community analysis, or community-based research (and ideally that should be all students) contribute their work to some social change organization in those communities. Alternately or additionally, schools can accumulate these documents and begin to serve as an information and resource center. The Education Center for Community Organizing at Hunter College School of Social Work (Mizrahi, 1987) and the Center for Community Education at Rutgers School of Social Work are two examples.
2. Social work schools can initiate or join consortia with other schools or departments within the university who have community practice-related components in their curricula. For example, the Hunter School of Social Work Community Organization and Planning faculty formed such a group with faculty from Urban

Affairs, Community Health Education, Sociology, and Social Research around a common commitment to train community-based practitioners and be of service to the community. One of its projects, now in process, is the production of a *Guide Book of Information Sources* for students as well as for community educators, organizers, and developers.

3. Schools and agencies need to make public data access a part of their research agenda. In promoting democratic information policies, schools, agencies, and social change organizations, can serve as intermediaries between large public or private bureaucracies and community-based groups. Government also must be encouraged to adapt affirmative action information policies as they did in Chicago (Kretzman, 1983). A "right to know" policy would make information accessible, affordable, and accountable to all citizens.

4. The formation in the early 1980s of the ACOSA (Association of Community Organization and Social Administration) is a promising direction for linking education, research, and practice. Since its inception, ACOSA Symposia have been held as adjuncts to the Annual Program Meetings of the Council on Social Work Education. Many of the papers presented there are research-based and have been published in relevant journals. In 1988 the organization was formalized, and has defined as one of its functions the need to strengthen theory and practice in community-based macro specialization. ACOSA could serve as the initiator as well as communicator of research-based practice models.

## COMMUNITY PRACTICE RESEARCH AGENDA FOR THE 1990s

There continues to be a need to conduct practice-related research and research utilization activities in the community practice end of the macro continuum (Epstein and Tripodi, 1978; Karger and Reitnor, 1983; Reisch and Wenocur, 1986; Thomas, 1980). The substantive areas of research that need priority and resources should include those that have the potential of contributing to a social work model of community practice. The body of expertise from other disciplines would continue to be adapted and integrated where applicable.

Community practice within social work has four special, if not unique, components that distinguish it from other planning and organizing disciplines. It is in these areas that social work-based research can make its special contribution to theory and practice.

First, it has a humanistic value base to answer the question (and paraphrasing Lyon [1987]): Planning for what? This usually includes the end values of social and economic justice, democracy and peace. We need to know more about the values in community practice (Rothman, 1987) and how these relate to goals, strategies and outcomes. Unclear or contradictory values which can emerge in community practice make the process of doing and the outcomes of research more problematic (Jones and Harris, 1987; see for example, Schwartz, 1979, for a discussion of the value conflicts inherent in the concept of neighborhood). Lauffer (1987) alludes to value issues as the limits of rationality.

Second, there is full acceptance of the fact that community practice is a sociopolitical as well as technical process (Gilbert and Specht, 1987). They and others stress the process skills essential in achieving social change goals. A need to refocus on, reexamine, and refine these interactional components is becoming increasingly articulated (Gilbert and Specht, 1987; Cnaan and Adar, 1987; Biaggart and Hamilton, 1987). These traditionally have included people-involving skills such as communication, group dynamics, leadership development, and negotiation. Additionally, social work emphasizes a commitment to the process and goal of empowerment. This means organizing and planning with and by, as well as on behalf of, an identified community or constituency. We need to know more about whether this is still being practiced and how better to balance process and goal.

Third is a recognition of the importance of the political/environmental context—the larger social system—in which community practice occurs. The premise here is that organizing and planning are political processes that involve the strategic use of power and conflict. More research is needed to document the process of change (Farris and Ruckdeschel, 1981); in particular to understand both the strategies of influence used in making change, and knowledge about the nature of and responses to resistance and opposition.

Fourth, social work community practice, like the profession as a whole, emphasizes self-awareness and the conscious use of self (Burghardt, 1982a). Inherent in professional development of the community worker is his/her relationships to colleagues, clients, sponsors, and decision-makers. (Transference and counter-transference have their analogs in macro practice!) There is very little information about the qualities, achieved and ascribed statuses, and worker styles as these relate to process and effectiveness. Overall we need to know more about each of these four components and how they combine to make for consummate community practice.

This chapter has presented both the complexity and creativity involved in collecting, analyzing, applying, and evaluating new and already collected data to strengthen community practice. In spite of past limitations, exciting prospects abound for deepening and broadening research utilization in this challenging but essential domain within social work.

## REFERENCES

Adler, P.A. and Adler, P. *Membership Roles in Field Research*. Newbury Park, CA: Sage, 1987.

Aaronson, S.M. and Sherwood, C.C. "Researcher–Practitioner: Problems in Social Action Research." *Social Work* 12(4); 89-96, October 1967.

Austin, M.J. "Community Organization and Social Administration: Partnership or Irrelevance," *Administration in Social Work* 10(3); 27-39, Fall 1986.

Barber, B. *Strong Democracy: Participating Politics for a New Age*. Berkeley: Off California Press, 1984.

Baver, S.L. "Political Participation of Puerto Rican Women: Mapping a Research Agenda." *Affilia: Journal of Women and Social Work* 4(1); 59-69, Spring 1989.

Biaggart, N.W. and Hamilton, G.G. "An Institutional Theory of Leadership." *Journal of Applied Behavioral Science* 24(4): 429-442, 1987.

Bicklin, D. *Community Organizing: Theory and Practice*. Englewood Cliffs, NJ: Prentice-Hall, 1983.

Blau, J. "On the Uses of Homelessness: A Literature Review." *Catalyst: A Socialist Journal of the Social Services* 6(2): 5-26, 1988.

Bradshaw, J. "The Concept of Social Need." In Gilbert, N. and Specht, H. *Planning for Social Welfare*. Englewood Cliffs, NJ: Prentice-Hall, 1977.

Brager, G., Specht, H., and Torczyner, J. *Community Organizing,* 2nd ed. New York: Columbia University Press, 1987.

Brandwein, R. "Toward Feminization of Community Organizing Practice." In Lauffer, A. and Newman, E., Eds. Community Organizing for the 1980s, Special Double Issue of *Social Development Issues* 5(2-3), Summer/Fall 1981.

Burghardt, S. "Community-based Social Action." *Encyclopedia of Social Work,* 18th ed. National Association of Social Work, 1987.

Burghardt, S. *The Other Side of Organizing: Resolving the Personal Dilemmas and Political Demands of Daily Practice.* Cambridge, MA: Schenkman, 1982a.

Burghardt, S. *Organizing for Community Action.* Beverly Hills, CA: Sage, 1982b.

Cnaan, R.A. and Adar, I. "An Integrative Model for Group Work in Community Organizing Practice." *Social Work With Groups* 10(3): 5-24, Fall 1987.

Cnaan, R.A. and Rothman, J. "Conceptualizing Community Intervention: An Empirical Test of 'Three Models' of Community Organizing." *Administration in Social Work* 10(3):41-55, 1986.

Collette, W. "Research for Organizing." In Staples, L., ed., *Roots to Power.* New York: Praeger, 1984.

Cordero, A. "Computers and Community Organizing: Issues and Examples from New York City." In Mizrahi, T. et al., eds. Computers of Social Change and Community Organizing – A Special Issue of *Computers in Human Services* (in press, 1990).

Cox, A.J., "Exploring the Black Clergy's Role in Effecting change in a Non-Urban Area of Southern Appalachia." *Human Services in the Rural Environment* 9(1): 24-27, 1984.

Cox, F., Erlich, J., Rothman, J., and Tropman, J.E., ed. *Strategies in Community Organizing,* 4th ed. Itasca, IL: F.E. Peacock, 1987.

Cruz, W. "The Nature of Alinsky Style Community Organizing in the Mexican American Community of Chicago: United Neighborhood Organization," Ph.D. Dissertation, October 1987.

Danziger, J.N. et al. *Computers and Politics: High Technology in the American Local Government.* New York: Columbia University Press, 1982.

Davis, L.V. "A Feminist Approach to Social Work Research." *Affilia* 1(1):37-47, Spring 1986.

Davis, L.V. "Views of Wife Abuse: Does It Make a Difference?" *Affilia* 2(2):53-66, Summer 1987.

Dear, R., and Patti, R. "Legislative Advocacy: Seven Effective Tactics." *Social Work* 25(4):289-296, July 1981.

Ecklein, J. *Community Organization,* 2nd ed. New York: John Wiley & Sons, 1984.

Epstein, I. and Tripodi, T. Incorporating Research into Macro Social Work Practice and Education." *Administration in Social Work* 2(3):295-305, Fall 1978.

Fabricant, M. "Creating Survival Services." *Administration in Social Work* 10(3), 71-84, Fall 1986.

Farris, B.E. and Ruckdeschel, R.A., "Phenomenological and Linguistic Turns in Social Thought: Impact on Community Organization Research and Practice," in Lauffer, A. and Newman, E., eds. Community Organizing for the 1980s, Special Double Issue of *Social Development Issues* 5(2-3):126-133, Summer/Fall 1981.

Fisk, J.H. *Black Power—White Control: The Struggle of the Woodlawn Organization in Chicago.* Princeton University Press, 1973.

Fitchin, J.M. "When Communities Collapse: Implications for Rural America." *Human Services in the Rural Environment* 10(4):48-57, Spring/Summer 1987.

Gilbert, N. and Specht, H. "Social Planning and Community Organization." *Encyclopedia of Social Work*, 18th ed. National Association of Social Workers, 1987:602-619.

Gilkes, C.T. "Going Up for the Oppressed: The Career Mobility of Black Women Community Workers." *Journal of Social Issues* 39(3):115-39, 1983.

Gilroth, R. "Organizing for Neighborhood Development." *Social Policy* 15(3):37-42, Winter 1985.

Glasser, I. *More Than Bread: Ethnography of a Soup Kitchen.* Tuscaloosa: University of Alabama Press, 1989.

Goldman, B. "Right to Know: Information for Participation." In Mizrahi, T. et al., Eds. Computers for Social Change and Community Organizing, A Special Issue of *Computers in Human Services* (in press).

Gottlieb, N. and Bombyk, M. *"Strategies for Strengthening Feminist Research."* *Affilia* 1(2) 23-35, Summer 1987.

Green, C. and Wilson, B. *Struggle for Black Empowerment in New York City: Beyond the Politics of Pigmentation.* NY: Praeger, 1989.

Harris, I.M., "Community Involvement in Desegregation: The Milwaukee Experience." In Cox, F., Erlich, J., Rothman, J., and Tropman, J.E., Eds. *Strategies of Community Organization*, 4th ed. Itasca, IL: Peacock, 1987:373-383.

Height, T. and Rubins, R. "How Community Groups Are Using Computers." *Journal of Communication* 109-117, Winter 1983.

Herick, J.M. "Farmers' Revolt! Contemporary Farmers' Protests in Historical Perspective: Implications for Social Work Practice." *Human Services in the Rural Environment* 10(1):6-11, Winter 1986.

Heskin, A.D. and Heffner, R.A. "Learning About Bilingual, Multicultural Organizing." *Journal of Applied Behavioral Science* 23(4):525-541, 1987.

Hubbart, I.M. "Community Beliefs and the Failure of Community Economic Development." *Social Service Review* 60(2):183-200, 1986.

Humm-Delgado, D.E. and Delgado, M. "Gaining Community Entree to Access Service Needs of Hispanics." *Social Casework* 67(2):80-89, 1986.

Hunt, S.M. "Evaluating A Community Development Project." *British Journal of Social Work* 17(6):662-667, December 1987.

Hyman, D. "On the Dialectics of Social Theory and Action: A Synthesis of Six Models of Community Engagement." *Journal of Sociology and Social Welfare* 13(2):265-286, June 1986.

Jansson, B.S. "From Sibling Rivalry to Pooled Knowledge and Shared Curriculum: Relations Among Community Organization, Administration, Planning and Policy Analysis." *Administration in Social Work* 11(2):5-18, Summer 1987.

Jones, D.J. "Are Local Organizations Local?" *Social Policy*, 13(2), Fall 1982.

Jones, D.J., and Tumelty, S.M. "Are There Really 10,000 Block Associations in New York City?" *Social Policy* 17(2); 52-53, Fall 1986.

Jones, E.R. and Harris, W.M. "A Conceptual Scheme for Analysis of the Social Planning Process." *Journal of the Community Development Society* 18(2), 18-41, 1987.

Karger, J.H. and Reitnor, M.A. "Community Organization for the 1980s: Toward Developing a New Skill Base Within a Political Framework." *Social Development Issues* 7(2):50-62, 1983.

Katan, J. and Spiro, S.E. "The Knowledge Base of Planned Change in Organizations and Communities." In Cox, F. et al., Eds. *Strategies of Community Organization*, 4th ed. Itasca, IL: Peacock, 1987:98-106.

Kretzman, J.P. The Politics of Information Reform in Chicago: An Experiment in Decentralization. Unpublished doctoral dissertation, 1983.

Lancourt, J. *Confront or Concede: The Alinsky Citizen-Action Organizations.* Lexington, MA: D.C. Heath, 1979.

Lauffer, A. "Social Planners and Social Planning in the United States." In Cox, F., Erlich, J., Rothman, J., and Tropman, J.E., Eds. *Strategies of Community Organization*, 4th ed. Itasca, IL: Peacock, 1987:311-325.

Lindgren, H.E. "The Informal-Intermittent Organization: A Vehicle for Successful Citizen Protest." *Journal of Applied Behavioral Science* 23(3):397-412, 1987.

Lyon, L. *The Community in Urban Society.* Chicago: Dorsey Press, 1987.

Madara, E.J., Kalafat, J., and Miller, B. "The Computerized Self-Help Clearinghouse: Using 'High Tech' to Promote 'High Touch' Supports Networks." *Computers in Human Services*, 1989.

Madeuno, A. "Computer Applications by Community-Based Groups to Development Projects." *Resources* 4(4), April, 1986. A publication of National Congress for Community Economic Development, Washington, DC.

Marti-Costa, S. and Serrano-Garcia, I. "Needs Assessment and Community Development: An Ideological Perspective." In Cox, F. et al., Eds. *Strategies of Community Organization*, 4th ed. Itasca, IL: Peacock, 1987:362-371.

Maypole, D.E. "Sexual Harassment at Work: A Review of Research and Theory." *Affilia* 2(1):24-38, Spring 1987.

McCullough, M. "Democratic Questions for the Computer Age." In Mizrahi, T. et al., Eds. Computers of Social Change and Community Organizing — A Special Issue of *Computers in Human Services* (in press).

McGrath, J.E. "Looking Ahead by Looking Backwards: Some Recurrent Themes About Social Change." *Journal of Social Issues* 39(4):225-239, Winter 1983.

McKnight, J. "Politicizing Health Care." In *Social Policy* 9(3):36-39, November/December 1978.

McKnight, J., and Kretzman, J. "Community Organizing in the 1980s: Toward a Post Alinsky Agenda." *Social Policy* 14(3):15-17, Winter 1984.

Meyer, F.A., Share, R.F., and Radtke, H.D. "A Systemic Approach for Identifying Planning Zones and Service Centers: A Nevada State Health Example," *Journal of Community Development Society* 17(1):16-30, 1986.

Mizrahi, T. "An Education Model for Meeting Community Organizing Needs of the Urban Community." Paper presented to APM of Council on Social Work Education, St. Louis, March 1987.

Mizrahi, T., Fasano, R., Downing, J., Friedland, P., McCullough, M., and Shapiro, J. Editors. Computers for Social Change and Community Organizing, special issues of *Computers in Human Services*. The Haworth Press (1990).

Mizrahi, T., and Rosenthal, B. "Building Effective Coalitions: Toward a Synthesis of Theory and Practice." Paper presented at Community Organizers and Social Administrations' Symposium, Council on Social Work Education, Atlanta, March 1988.

Mizrahi, T., Joseph, B., Lob, S., Peterson, J., McLaughlin, P., Sugarman, F., and Rosenthal, B. "Community Organizing from Women's Perspectives: Developing a Feminist Theory-Based Practice Model Through the Building of a Women Organizers' Network." Paper presented at COSA Symposium, APM-CSWE, Chicago, March 1989.

Mondros, J.B. and Wilson, S.M. "Structure as Strategy in Community Organizations." Paper presented at Community Organizing and Social Administration Symposium, Council of Social Work Education, Chicago, March 1989.

Naples, N. and Gittell, M. "Activist Women: Conflicting Ideologies." *Social Policy* 13(2):25-27, Summer 1982.

Neuber, K.A., Atkins, W.T., Jacobson, J.A., and Reuterman, N.A. Needs Assessment: A Model for Community Planning. Beverly Hills, CA: Sage, 1980.

Nurius, P., Hooyman, N., and Nicoll, A.E. "The Changing Face of Computer Utilization in Social Work Settings," *Journal of Social Work Education* 24(2):186-197, Spring/Summer 1988.

Perrolle, J. *Computers and Social Change: Information, Property and Power.* Belmont, CA: Wadsworth, 1987.

Piven, F.F. and Cloward, R. *Poor People's Movements: Why They Succeed, How They Fail.* New York: Pantheon Books, 1977.

Ragab, I.A., Blum, A., and Murphy, M.J. "Representation in Neighborhood Organizations." *Social Development Issues* 5(2-3):62-73, Summer/Fall 1981.

Rees, S. "The Culture-Bound State of Evaluation: Implication for Research and Practice." *British Journal of Social Work* 17(6):645-659, December 1987.

Reisch, M. "From Cause to Case and Back Again the Reemergence of Advocacy in Social Work." *Urban and Social Change Review*, 19:20-24, Winter/Summer 1986.

Reisch, M., and Wenocur, S. "The Future Community Organization in Social Work: Social Activism and the Politics of Profession Building." *Social Service Review* 60(1):70-93, March 1986.

Reitzes, D.C. and Reitzes, D.C. "Alinsky Reconsidered: A Reluctant Community Theorist." *Social Science Quarterly* 63(27):256-79, June 1982.

Rivera, J.A. "Self Help as Mutual Protection: The Development of Hispanic Benefit Societies." *Journal of Applied Behavioral Science*, 23(3):387-396, 1987.

Roberts-Degenerro, M. "Factors Contributing to Coalition Maintenance." *Journal of Sociology and Social Welfare* 13:248-264, 1986.

Rodberg, L., "Breaking From Big Brother: Computerizing Small Government Funded Organizations." In Mizrahi, T. et al., Eds. Computers of Social Change and Community Organizing, a special issue of *Computers in Human Services* (in press).

Rothman, J. "Community Research and Community Theory." *Encyclopedia of Social Work*, 18th ed. National Association of Social Work, 1987a.

Rothman, J., "Three Models of Community Organization Practice." In Cox, et al., Eds. *Strategies of Community Organizing Practice*, 4th ed. 1987.

Rubin, H.J. and Rubin, I. *Community Organizing and Development.* Columbus, OH: Merrill, 1986.

Schein, E.H. *The Clinical Perspective in Field Work–Qualitative Research.* Newbury Park, CA: Sage, 1987.

Schwartz, E. "Neighborhoodism: A Conflict in Values." *Social Policy* 9(5) 8-14, March/April 1979.

Siegel, L.M., Attkisson, C.C., and Carson, L.G., "Needs Identification and Program Planning in the Community Context." In Cox, F., et al., Eds. *Strategies of Community Organization*, 4th ed. Itasca, IL; Peacock, 1987:71-97.

Smith, A. and Stewart, A., Issue Editors. "Approaches to Studying and Research on Black Women's Lives." *Journal of Social Issues* 39(3):1983.

Spergel, I.A. "Community Development." *Encyclopedia of Social Work*, 18th ed. National Association of Social Work, 1987.

Spiegel, H.B.C. "New Tools for Neighborhood Development: A Look at Some Information Providers and Users." Graduate Program in Urban Affairs, Hunter College, April 1987.

Staples, L. *Roots to Power: A Manual for Grassroots Organizing.* New York: Praeger, 1984.

Stein, D.D. and March, M. "The Impact of a Community Action Group: An Illustration of the Potential of Time Series Analysis for the Study of Community Groups." *American Journal of Community Psychology* 13(1):13-30, 1985.

Taylor, J.B. *Using Microcomputers in Social Agencies.* Beverly Hills, CA; Sage, 1981.

Taylor, S.A. and Roberts, R.W. *Theory and Practice of Community Social Work.* NY: Columbia University Press, 1985.

Thayer, R. "Measuring Needs in the Social Services." In Gilbert, N. and Specht, H., Eds. *Planning for Social Welfare.* New York: Prentice-Hall, 1977.

Thomas, D.N. "Research and Community Work." *Community Development Journal* 15(1):30-41, January 1980.

Warren, R.L., "The Sociology of Knowledge and the Problems of the Inner Cities." In Warren and Lyon, Eds. *New Perspectives on the American Community*, 5th ed. Chicago: Dorsey, 1988:365-377.

Warren, R.L. and Lyon, L. *New Perspectives on the American Community*, 5th ed. Chicago: Dorsey Press, 1988.

Weil, M. "Women, Community and Organizing." *Feminist Visions for Social Work*. In N. Van Den Bergh and L. Cooper, Eds. Silver Spring, MD: NASW, 187-210, 1986.

West, G. *The National Welfare Rights Movement: The Social Protest of Poor Women*. New York: Praeger, 1981.

Wilson, S. and Mondros, J.B. "Program Assessment Strategies for Community Organization." *Social Development Issues* 6(3):25-39, Winter 1982.

Woodrum, E. and Reid, N. "Migration, Ethnic Community Organization and Prosperity Among Japanese Americans." *Arete* 12(1):1-46, Summer 1987.

Wu, S.Y. and Korman, M. "Socioeconomic Impacts of Divestment on Communities in New York State. *American Journal of Economics and Sociology* 46(3):261-72, July 1987.

York, R.O. *Human Service Planning: Concepts, Tools, and Methods*. Chapel Hill, NC: University of North Carolina Press, 1982.

# The Utilization of Research in Administrative Practice

Yeheskel Hasenfeld
Rino Patti

The grounding of social welfare administration in social science theory and research in general, and the utilization of research methods and findings in the management of human services, in particular, are considered axiomatic to the development of effective administrative practices. Glaser (1988:220-221) argues for a closer integration of research and management in order to institutionalize rationality in the organization. As he puts it, "If managers and researchers agree on agency goals and both accept research findings on facts, the ultimate in rationality is conceivable: policies and practices empirically and logically appropriate to maximizing goal achievement." Underlying this conception of administration is a rational model of decision-making. It suggests that administrators should have a clear and hierarchically ordered set of goals informed by social science research; engage in a comprehensive empirical study of the alternatives; study the potential costs and benefits of each alternative; select the most profitable alternative; and carefully evaluate the results. Nonetheless, the extent to which this normative model of administration is actually practiced or feasible is open to question. In this chapter we review the research on the behavior of executives, examine the forces that push for the use of research in administrative decisions, assess the empirical evidence on patterns of research utilization, and discuss the organizational conditions which are conducive to greater utilization of research in social welfare administration. We conclude with some thoughts about an appropriate model of administrative behavior and the role of research in it.

## MANAGEMENT ACTIVITIES
## AND INFORMATION UTILIZATION

In order to provide a context for understanding research utilization in management, it is useful to describe the salient characteristics of this type of work. Research describing the nature of managerial practice in human service organization is quite recent and
still sparse (Patti, 1977; Wolk, Way, and Bleeke, 1982; Cashman,
1978; Files, 1981; Schmid, Bar-Gal, and Hasenfeld, in press; Arguello, 1988; Ezell, Menefee, and Patti, 1989). Despite numerous
substantive and methodological limitations of this body of work, it
is possible to draw a broad and preliminary profile of managerial
activity in social welfare agencies.

The extant research in social welfare points to the conclusion that
management is characterized by diversity, brevity, and fragmenta-
tion. This finding is consistent with the ground-breaking research of
Mintzberg (1973), and several studies of managerial activity in
fields other than social welfare that followed (Kotter, 1982; Luthans
and Lockwood, 1984; Kurke and Aldrich, 1983). Although studies
have conceptualized managerial work in quite different ways, it is
apparent that executives are typically engaged in a wide array of
tasks, including but not limited to, acquiring and exchanging resources with organizations in the environment; assessing needs,
prospects, and threats both internal and external to the agency; planning for and directing the implementation of services and programs;
allocating resources and recruiting staff; and motivating, reinforcing, supervising, and evaluating subordinates.

The diversity of these tasks is accentuated by the fact that administrators tend to engage in contact with a wide variety of groups and
individuals whose needs and interests are often divergent. Schmid
and his colleagues (in press) found, for example, that executives of
community service agencies interacted with five major constituencies: agency staff, organizations in the environment, headquarters
representatives, consumers and volunteers. For example, on a given
day the executive of an agency is likely to engage several subordinates who have different programmatic and/or functional responsibilities, resource controllers such as legislators and funders who
may have varying expectations for agency performance, representa-

tives of other service organizations, clients, and so on. To some extent the information needs of administrators vary in each of these sets of relationships since the issues, problems, and goals dealt with in each case are likely to be different. It seems fair to conclude then that administrators will draw on a broad range of quite diverse types of information in order to transact business. No single type of information, e.g., program outcome data, community needs, or fiscal performance, is likely to provide the manager with all that he or she needs to know.

This complex activity configuration suggests a second characteristic of managerial work that may have implications for how research is utilized. In all of the studies examined, managers' time tended to be broadly distributed across many activities with relatively brief periods devoted to each. For example, Schmid, Bar-Gal, and Hasenfeld (in press) found that in an average work day of 10.2 hours, six of the eight activities with which directors were engaged consumed one or more hours. Similarly, Ezell, Menefee, and Patti (1989), using a classification scheme with 13 types of activity, found that ten required two or more hours a week. Studies by Files (1981), Patti (1977), and Arguello (1988) discovered similar patterns of time allocation for managers. Taken together, these findings describe a practice that tends to be fragmented, discontinued, and marked by multiple brief interactions. The still popular conception of administration as an orderly, sequential process characterized by systematic analysis and rational problem solving has little support in the empirical literature. Given this activity profile, it should not be surprising that administrators have little time to spend scanning literature for research pertaining to their organizations and distilling its implications. Rather, the administrator is more likely to select information that has immediate relevance to the tasks and decisions at hand and tends to rely on what is provided through verbal reports, contacts, or in summarized written form. Seldom is there sufficient time or control over time to allow for the kind of primary search processes that are thought to be necessary to inform professional practice.

While the time of top level administrators is broadly distributed, the evidence suggests that they tend to spend more time on internal tasks and issues than external ones. In all of the studies examined, management functions related to internal operations consumed a far greater amount of time than those which involved relations with the environment. This appears to be the case even with executives of social service agencies.

Moreover, among the internally oriented activities, those relating to interpersonal relations with staff tend to be more time consuming than those concerning planning for and evaluating the organizations' work. For example, Ezell, Menefee and Patti (1989) found that hospital social work directors averaged 12.6 hours per week in guiding and supervising subordinates (e.g., staffing, training and developing, motivating and reinforcing, managing conflict, and disciplining and correcting), but only 6.7 hours in planning, coordinating, monitoring, and controlling. Schmid, Bar-Gal, and Hasenfeld (in press) also found that administrators devoted an average of about 32% of their time supervising, staffing, and communicating, but only 17% of their time in planning. It seems that the social welfare administrator is more likely to be taken up with facilitating and supporting the performance of subordinates through face-to-face interactions than with the "rational" processes of analyzing the organization's problems, assessing alternatives, and deciding future courses of action. This being the case, it appears that managers in social service agencies are more likely to need and use information that pertains to the day to day operation of the organization and can be utilized for immediate problem solving, especially around staff performance, rather than that which informs longer term, strategic decision making.

## RESEARCH FOR ADMINISTRATIVE DECISIONS

Recognizing the broad diversity of activities and information administrators use, we need to define the concept of research within this context. We adopt the conception developed by Simon (1970) who distinguishes between programmed and heuristic decision-making processes. When the alternatives are fixed, research for management purposes involves an optimization process which includes a set of given alternatives of action (command variables), a set of environmental parameters which must be considered in the selection of the alternatives, and a utility function (desired ends) which may be supplemented by a number of constraints. "The optimization problem is to find an admissible set of values of the command variables, compatible with the constraints, that maximize the utility function for the given values of the environmental parameters" (Simon, 1970:135). Thus, the social science model of research utilization is more likely to occur in programmed decisions. When the alternatives are not given, research involves a means-end analysis which consists of setting goals, assessing differences between present situation and the goals, finding through various search procedures (which may range from controlled experiments to personal experiences) some tools or processes that are relevant to reducing the differences, and applying these tools and procedures. This is an iterative process until the over goal is attained or abandoned (Simon, 1977). In this process the function of research is to store information about states of the world and information about actions. "Ability to attain goals depends on building up associations, which may be simple or very complex, between particular changes in states of the world and particular actions that will (reliably or not) bring these changes about" (Simon, 1970:141). It is important to emphasize that in both forms of research, the rules of standard logic prevail. Since many managerial decisions are non-programmed, research utilization is more likely to be in a form of knowledge acquisition and learning, or in the form of monitoring actions taken. Much of our attention will be focused on utilization of research for heuristic decisions.

## TYPES OF RESEARCH AND UTILIZATION

Within this framework we distinguish between various forms of research and differentiate among patterns of utilization. Four different types of research are noted: (1) theory testing research: classic social science research directed at *explaining;* (2) applied research: directed at *predicting* social events or patterns such as demographic and economic trends, voting behavior, market analysis, or emergence of social needs; (3) action and intervention research: directed at improving the efficacy of practice technologies (e.g., social R&D, program evaluation); and (4) monitoring: use of research methods to collect and analyze empirical data to assess compliance with external and internal standards, regulations, and policies (e.g., need assessment, auditing, client tracking). We also distinguish between three forms of utilization (Beyer and Trice, 1982): (1) instrumental: use of research to make specific decisions; (2) conceptual: use of research to inform and enlighten the decision makers; and (3) symbolic: use of research to gain legitimacy. Clearly there are relationships between type of research and mode of utilization. On the basis of available research, to be reviewed below, we propose that administrators use mostly monitoring research and occasionally action research for instrumental purposes, while they use applied and action research for conceptual purposes. Theory testing research and applied research will typically be used for symbolic purposes (Figure 1). We should also point out that research can be used to avoid or delay making decisions, either by indicating the need for further research or by pointing to equivocal findings (Rothman, J., personal communication).

## THE IMPETUS TO USE RESEARCH

The impetus for and type of social science research used by social welfare administrators is influenced, in a significant way, by environmental forces — ideological and political, technological, and economic — that their agencies encounter. In the 1960s the rapid expansion of the welfare state resulted in the proliferation of social services which were justified on the basis of social science research, both basic and applied. Social science research on delinquency, pov-

FIGURE 1. Proposed Relationship Between Research and Utilization

| Type of Research | Utilization Instrumental | Conceptual | Symbolic |
|---|---|---|---|
| Theory testing | - | + | + |
| Applied | - | + | + |
| Action | + | ++ | + |
| Monitoring | ++ | + | - |

erty, discrimination, and education were used by policy-makers and administrators to initiate and legitimize new social programs (e.g., community action agencies), and research methodologies were adopted for the design of various demonstration projects (e.g., Head Start). In a paradoxical way, the oversimplified scientific views on the causes of poverty and inequality coupled with favorable public attitudes gave policy-makers and administrators ample ammunition to design very ambitious social programs which inevitably failed to meet the high expectations they generated. Moreover, the evaluation research that were commissioned to win political approval of the new programs failed to demonstrate their effectiveness, in no small measure, because of the inarticulate social science assumptions used to justify their mission and goals (Aaron, 1978). Program evaluation, a fledgling research methodology, was used by legislators and administrators to control the flow of fiscal resources from the federal government to local agencies. This is best exemplified in The Elementary and Secondary Education Act of 1965 which required local school districts to provide appropriate objective measures of education achievement (Cronbach et al., 1980).

The disenchantment with the Great Society programs in the 1970s and the change in the political climate resulted in increased requirements for administrative accountability and program evaluation by funding authorities. Indeed, evaluation was made a regular requirement for most publicly funded health, education, and welfare programs. In this sense, program evaluation was used as a mechanism to justify allocation of resources in an environment of scarcity. That is, much of the utilization of the program evaluation was conceptual and occasionally instrumental and symbolic. These developments were coupled with the increased technological sophistication of program evaluation including the use of experimental and quasi-experimental designs.

Indeed, technology has played a very important role not only in the impetus for program evaluation, but also in monitoring and auditing. The availability and increasing affordability of information technology have resulted in greater demands for information about the services, finances, and operations of human services. Agencies could no longer claim lack of capacity to generate and provide such information. Moreover, the development of data base information systems and the increased ease and sophistication of data manipulation have created potentials for linking various sources of data and have vastly expanded the capacity and reduced the cost of conducting research for management purposes (Rapp, 1984; Mutschler and Hasenfeld, 1986). Thus, the instrumental use of monitoring and auditing research has been made much more feasible and practical.

Finally, economic factors are also a significant force in shaping the use of research by social service administrators. The cutbacks in funding experienced by many social service agencies in the 1980s have produced a dual pressure on social service administrators. First, funding agencies have increased their demands for accountability. They are requiring greater empirical evidence of how resources are used, and often stipulate continued funding on the basis of efficiency and effectiveness measures. These are used as political weapons to allocate resources among programs. Second, administrators have had to devise cutback strategies that can be justified. Again, research in the forms of audits, need assessments, and evaluation are used to justify cuts and reallocation of resources and to neutralize countervailing pressures (Hasenfeld, 1984). Consequently, monitoring research has become a primary strategy in cutback management.

## USES OF RESEARCH BY ADMINISTRATORS

Contrary to conventional wisdom, administrators do use research albeit not in the content and form typically desired by social scientists. Social scientists tend to advocate a model of research utilization, especially for managerial decisions, which approximates the following steps (e.g., Boehm, 1982): (1) empirical validation of the nature of the problem; (2) review of previous research; (3) formulation of hypotheses or action guidelines; and (4) design of a study, preferably experimental, to test the hypotheses or the validity of the action guidelines; (5) analysis of the results; (6) implementation of managerial decisions on the basis of the results. The reality of organizational decision making suggests a different pattern of doing and using research. Both doing and using research in the organization is ''messy'' from a social scientist perspective because it is frequently subject to a number of constraints (Boehm, 1982; Weiss, 1980). These include: (1) limited time to undertake the research; (2) changes in importance of decision issues; (3) lack of adequate resources required for the research; (4) political considerations about the consequences of the research; and (5) organizational limitations that compromise the research design. Moreover, administrators are driven by the need to solve a problem in a manner acceptable within the political economy of their organization rather than conform to the research requirements or results.

Beyer and Trice (1982) reviewed 27 empirical studies on the use of research by policy makers and administrators. They found only two studies that reported considerable instrumental use of research. The first study (Alkin, Stecher and Geiger, 1982) found extensive use of evaluation research by local educational administrators to modify their programs; the second study (Caplan, 1975) reported that among a sample of federal government officials, 40% indicated using social science research, basis and applied, to make policy decisions. Rothman (1980), in a study of 12 administrators of British social service departments with a reputation of considerable use of research, also found that the administrators reported using research as an aid in planning, to correct false assumptions, and as a weapon to get certain objectives. More recently, McNeece, DiNitto, and Johnson (1983) reported of a study of 42 community mental health directors, 83% of whom reported doing evaluation studies. However, only 25% indicated that data on program effectiveness influenced decisions regarding program changes. Majchrzak and Blevins-Stepanich (1984) conducted a study of seven statewide social service agencies and 96 decision makers. They identified more than 150 unique decisions which were clustered into performance appraisal, establishing criteria for assessing effectiveness, program change, and resources requirements. The information used to make decisions was classified into four categories: quantity of service demand and delivery, quality and efficiency of service delivery, changed client behavior and client satisfaction, and changes in the community and community satisfaction. For most of the decisions, especially for establishing effectiveness criteria and for program change, the predominant information used was on quality and efficiency of the service delivery. The sources of the information on quality and efficiency were mostly archival agency data (e.g., agency client and management information systems) and evaluation and special audit studies. Thus, the decision makers did use mostly monitoring research for instrumental decisions.

Conceptual use of research is a common form of utilization by policy makers and administrators. This is not surprising because "conceptual use does not require immediate, direct application. Also, conceptual use is not so inhibited by the constraints of customary or prescribed repertoires of behaviors" (Beyer and Trice, 1982:596-600). Rich (1981) conducted a study of the use of survey research by several federal agencies. He defined instrumental use as impact of the information that can be documented, and found that within the first three months the survey was received the predominant use was instrumental, mostly because the survey dealt with "hot issues." In the long run, however, the use became mostly conceptual. Weiss (1980) conducted a study on the utilization of social science research by 150 mental health decision makers. In response to the questions: "Do you consciously use the results of social science research on your job?" and "In what ways do you use social science research on your job?" she obtained the following results:

| | |
|---|---|
| No, never | 11% |
| Not consciously | 22% |
| Yes, but did not describe any ways used | 10% |
| Yes, gave general uses | 50% |
| Yes, gave specific uses | 7% |

Weiss (1980:153-4) concluded that "the overall impression is that decision makers in mental health are remarkably receptive to social science research," mostly as general guidance for planning and for continuing education. The majority of her respondents (54%) obtained the research results from scientific and professional journals. Thus, much of the use of basic, applied, and action research seems to be conceptual rather than instrumental.

Finally, there is also evidence to suggest that decision makers often use research for symbolic and ritualistic purposes (Edelman, 1977). Policy makers and administrators alike often will cite research in order to buttress and legitimize their positions, and to justify their courses of action. In doing so, they use research results selectively, highlighting supportive results while ignoring challenging or negative findings.

There is a tendency to assume that the utilization of research is indispensable to good management. However, as Caplan (1980:5) points out, "there is a real danger in uncritically accepting utilization as desirable or in being oversold on its value." He goes on to quote Campbell who stated that, "the more any quantitative social indicator is used for social decision making, the more subject it will be to corrupting pressures and the more apt it will be to distort and corrupt the social processes it is intended to monitor." One can cite numerous instances in which latent biases in the underlying assumptions of the research and in its design produced results which blamed the victims, and yet served as guides to social programs. It must be underscored that numerous conditions can generate inaccurate findings (Cook, Levinson-Rose, and Pollard, 1980), such as the existing state of the art (e.g., cross-sectional rather than longitudinal research), biases in the underlying theory (e.g., the culture of poverty), inappropriate research design, biases in data collection, problems in replication, and biases in the interpretation of findings (e.g., the effects of negative income tax on work incentive and marriage). Especially troublesome is the tendency to assume that the research and its results are value-neutral and, therefore, exempt from a political dialogue where conflicting values compete for authority. Administrators can use research to "stack the cards" in favor of their own values and interests while buffering them from competing interests.

## ORGANIZATIONAL CONDITIONS AFFECTING RESEARCH UTILIZATION

Much of the explanation of the gap between research and utilization rests on the two-culture hypothesis (Rich, 1981) which posits that the culture of research and the culture of management are inherently incompatible. Shrivastava and Mitroff (1984) identified several cultural differences: (1) the researcher's emphasis on objective data versus the manager's stress on subjective experience; (2) the researcher's reliance on scientific theory versus the manager's confidence in intuition; and (3) the researcher's demand for empirical and observable data versus the manager's pragmatic orientation. More generally, the culture of management is directed toward problem solving under conditions of uncertainty and time pressure, while taking into account numerous interacting constraints and contingencies. The culture of research, on the other hand, is directed toward the generation of knowledge through prescribed research methodologies within a well-defined area, while holding constant as many extraneous conditions as possible.

Thus, much of the research on research utilization focuses on ways to reduce the potential incompatibility between the two cultures. Recognizing that the utilization of research involves a process of exchange, the central concern is to specify the conditions under which such exchange can take place and meet the needs of both parties. These can be classified into (1) the commodity to be exchanged, i.e., the research itself; (2) the attributes of the exchanging parties: the administrator and the researcher; (3) the incentives to engage in the exchange; (4) the process of the exchange, i.e., the linkages between the researcher and the administrator; and (5) the organizational context of the exchange.

## The Research Itself

Most studies indicate that the quality and credibility of the research are very important to its utilization. Decision makers are more likely to use research which they perceive to be of high quality and objectivity (Caplan, 1977; Rich, 1981; Rothman, 1980). Indeed, Weiss (1980:184-5) found that the criteria ranked highest by decision makers for using research were: "the recommendations were supported by the data," "understandably written," and "objective, unbiased." Burry and Alkin (1984) emphasized the importance of an appropriate methodology and rigor of the design from both the researcher's and the user's perspectives. Use of the research increases when it is presented in a manner that is understandable to the users and is timely (e.g., Rich, 1981; Rothman, 1980). Finally, use will increase when the research results are concrete and specific, and can provide guides for action.

## Researcher and User Attributes

Based on observations drawn from several empirical studies, Burry and Alkin (1984) concluded that the use of evaluation research increases when the researcher: (1) is personally committed to seeing the research put to use; (2) can establish credibility in terms of technical competence; (3) can assume a role appropriate to the setting; and (4) is willing to be cooperative and involved with the user. Similarly, the user must be: (1) committed and identified with the purposes of the research; (2) trained and have prior experience in using research; and (3) open to new ideas and change. Rothman (1980) reached similar conclusions in his study.

## Incentives for Research

Administrators are more likely to use research when it strengthens their political positions, reinforces their interests, and assists in mobilizing resources or buffers against attacks. Yin (1976) argues that successful utilization of R&D in organizations occurs only when it is linked to important organizational functions such as expansion, acquisition of resources, and development of new policies and programs. Undoubtedly, researchers whose rewards are contingent on the extent of the use of their work are much more likely to make efforts to increase the utility of their research. This is one of the advantages of having an in-house researcher (Rothman, 1980). In contrast, when the researcher's incentives are controlled by an organization, such as the academy, whose operative goals are incompatible with the agency's needs, the potential use of the research will greatly diminish.

## Links Between Researcher and Administrator

As a process of exchange of information, one cannot underestimate the importance of the communication channels and patterns that must be developed between the researcher and the user. A trusting and cooperative relationship is paramount to effective utilization (Rothman, 1980; Burry and Alkin, 1984). Participation of the users in the design of the research, the researcher's visibility and involvement in the organization, and the frequency of the interaction between the two parties are viewed as vital to use of research.

### Organizational Context

The organizational structure within which the research is embedded will be a significant determinant of its visibility, centrality, and ultimate utility. To the extent that the research is linked to or is anchored in units that are powerful in the organization, the more attention it will receive. Research acquires considerable power in the organization when it becomes indispensable to those units which (1) link the organization to external resources; (2) are central to the mission of the organization; and (3) are high in the hierarchy of authority. Similarly, research utilization increases when there is an organizational culture which reinforces learning, innovation, and boundary spanning activities. Finally, research utilization will increase when there is consensus about the domain of the organization and it is defined in clear and realistic terms (Wholey, 1981).

## IS THE EMPIRICALLY BASED ADMINISTRATOR THE APPROPRIATE MODEL?

Several conclusions can be derived from this review. First, administrative tasks are diverse, brief in duration, and focus more on internal rather than external tasks. Second, while administrators do rely on information and research, they confine instrumental use mostly to auditing and monitoring information. They are more likely to use action, and applied and basic research for conceptual and symbolic purposes. Third, there are many variables ranging from the nature of the research to the organizational context which influence the degree of utilization. What is patently clear is that the model of the empirically based administrator as espoused by management scientists is unrealistic. This is due partly to a faulty image of administrative decision makers as rational actors. As Sproull and Larkey (1979:95) put it, "constructing simplified representation of complicated decision situations or problems appears to be a universal characteristic of human behavior." Moreover, administrators simplify decision situations by using general or global assessments of the situation as a substitute for careful independent judgment about the attributes of the situation, even when adequate information exists. "More information is often the last thing the decision maker wants, needs or will use" (Sproull and Larkey, 1979:95).

Furthermore, the model of the empirically based administrator ignores the political and economic context of organizational behavior. The administrator functions in a political and economic environment in which mobilization and control of power and resources are important ingredients to the survival and success of the organization. Therefore, "the organization is concerned with much besides the logically best solution. Decisions are weighted not only against standards of effective performance, but also against considerations of organizational survival, growth, convenience, and reputation" (Weiss 1981:192). In such an environment, research use is one of an arsenal of tools administrators use to mobilize power and resources including political skills, connections to dominant interest groups, ability to forge coalitions, fund-raising acumen, and interpersonal skills.

Following Schon (1983), we propose that reflection-in-action is a more appropriate model of administrative behavior in which research utilization is only one of many ingredients in the decision-making process. In this process there is an application of tacit knowledge, prior learning and experiences, and intuition to the situation. When undertaking action the administrator reflects on his or her understanding of the situation, criticizing, restructuring, and incorporating the resultant knowledge into subsequent actions. Because the decisions are made within an organizational context, the administrator is bound by "repositories of cumulatively built-up knowledge: principles and maxims of practice, images of mission and identity, facts about the task environment, techniques of operation, stories of past experience which serve as exemplars for future action" (Schon, 1983:242). In this model, research is generally used not instrumentally, but for reflection. It becomes part of the repertoire of knowledge and experiences that the administrator may call upon in the process of making decisions. Research aids the reflective and, thus, the learning process to the extent that it enables the administrator to better understand the situation and the action. Moreover, administrators who have long-term objectives must undertake many intermediate steps, including research utilization, which cannot be shown to be directly linked to the final outcomes. Nonetheless, in this trial and error process research plays a significant role in enhancing the administrator's learning, in presenting new decision options, and in assessing prior decisions.

Reflection-in-action may, of course, be a highly biased and self-reifying process. Therefore, one of the key functions of research is to purge biases through the process of learning and understanding. Hence, the aim of research utilization should be less on direct use in decisions, which is unlikely to happen, and more on casting doubt on accepted administrative ideologies, increasing the administrator's repository of knowledge, and improving the capacity to assess decision outcomes. This can occur when the organization restructures itself to become a "self-learning" organization. In such an organization considerable resources are invested in its intelligence system both internally and externally, and in the provision of incentives and rewards to innovation, experimentation, and further training and education of its staff.

An example of such an investment is the development of the Boysville Management Information System (BOIS) whose purpose is to provide, on a regular basis, useful information to both administrators and direct service professionals. Consistent with our perspective, Grasso, Epstein, and Tripodi (1988) found that BOIS created a pro-research orientation among the staff, but that training and making the research more understandable and usable were especially important to increased utilization. Yet, the institutionalization of research in administrative practices is not merely a technological issue. It requires commitment from the executive leadership of the agency as well as structural transformations which integrate research into central organizational activities and reward its use.

## REFERENCES

Aaron, H. J. (1978). *Politics and the Professors: The Great Society in Perspective*. Washington, DC: The Brookings Institution.

Alkin, M., Stecher, B. M., and Geiger F. L. (1982). *Title I Evaluation: Utility and Factors Influencing Use*. Northridge, CA: Educational Evaluation Associates.

Arguello, D. (1988). "A comparative study of executives in New Mexico human service agencies." Unpublished doctoral dissertation, University of Washington, Seattle, WA.

Beyer, J. M., and Trice, H. M. (1982). "The Utilization Process: A Conceptual Framework and Synthesis of Empirical Findings." *Administrative Science Quarterly*, 27: 591-622.

Boehm, V. (1982). "Research in the 'Real World' — A Conceptual Model." In M. Hakel et al. (Eds.), *Making it Happen: Designing Research with Implementation in Mind*. Beverly Hills, CA: Sage, pp. 25-38.

Burry, J. and M. C. Alkin. (1984). *The Administrator's Role in Evaluation Research*. University of California, Los Angeles: Center for the Study of Evaluation.

Caplan, N. (1975). "The Use of Social Science Information by Federal Executives." In G. M. Lyons (Ed.), *Social Science and Public Policies*. Hanover, NH: Dartmouth College, Public Affairs Center, pp. 47-67.

Caplan, N. (1977). "A Minimal Set of Conditions Necessary for the Utilization of Social Science Knowledge on Policy Formulation at the National Level." In C. H. Weiss (Ed.), *Using Social Research on Public Policy-Making*. Lexington, MA: Lexington Books, pp. 183-197.

Caplan, N. (1980). "What Do We know About Knowledge Utilization?" In L. A. Braskamp and R. D. Brown (Eds.), *Utilization of Evaluative Information*. San Francisco: Jossey-Bass, pp. 1-10.

Cashman, B. (1978) "Training Social Work Administrators: The Activity Dilemma." *Administration in Social Work*, 2, 347-358.

Cook, T. D., Levinson-Rose, J., and Pollard W. E. (1980). "The Misutilization of Evaluation Research." *Knowledge: Creation, Diffusion, Utilization*, 1(4), 477-498.

Cronbach, L. J., et al. (1980). *Toward Reform of Program Evaluation*. San Francisco: Jossey-Bass.

Edelman, M. (1977). *Political Language*. New York: Academic Press.

Ezell, M., Menefee, D., and Patti, R. (1989). Managerial Leadership and Service Quality. *Administration in Social Work*.

Files, L. A. (1981). "The Human Services Management Task: A Time Allocation Study." *Public Administration Review*, 41, 686-692.

Glaser, D. (1988). *Evaluation Research and Decision Guidance for Correctional, Addiction Treatment, Mental Health, and Other People Changing Agencies*. New Brunswick, NJ: Transaction Books.

Grasso, A. J., Epstein, I., and Tripodi T. (1988). "Agency-based Research Utilization in a Residential Child Care Setting." *Administration in Social Work*, 12(4), 61-80.

Hasenfeld, Y. (1984). "The Changing Context of Human Services Administration." *Social Work*, 29:522-529.

Kotter, J. P. (1982). *The General Manager*. New York: Free Press.

Kurke, L. B., and Aldrich, H. E. (1983). "Mintzberg Was Right! A Replication and Extension of the Nature of Managerial Work." *Management Science*, 28, 975-984.

Luthans, F., and Lockwood, D. C. (1984). "Toward an Observation System for Measuring Leadership Behavior in Natural Settings." In J. G. Hunt, D. M. Hasking, C. A. Shreiseim, and R. Stewart (Eds.), *Leaders and Managers*. New York: Pergamon Press, pp.117-141.

Majchrzak, A., and M. E. Blevins-Stepanich. (1984). *Public Sector Organizational Decisionmaking: An Analysis of Information Use*. Working Paper No. 854. Krannert: Graduate School of Management, Purdue University.

McNeece, A. C., DiNitto, D. M., and Johnson P. J. (1983). "The Utility of Evaluation Research for Administrative Decision Making." *Administration in Social Work*, 7(3/4), 77-87.

Mintzberg, H. (1973). *The Nature of Managerial Work*. New York: Harper & Row.

Mutschler, E., and Hasenfeld, Y. (1986). "Integrated Information Systems for Social Work Practice." *Social Work*, 9, 67-79.

Patti, R. J. (1977). "Patterns of Managerial Activity in Social Welfare Agencies." *Administration in Social Work*, 1, 5-18.

Rapp, C. A. (1984). "Information, Performance, and the Human Service Managers for the 1980s: Beyond Housekeeping." *Administration in Social Work*, 8(2), 69-80.

Rich, R. F. (1981). *Social Science Information and Public Policy Making*. San Francisco: Jossey-Bass.

Rothman, J. (1980). *Using Research in Organizations*. Beverly Hills, CA: Sage.

Schmid, H., Bar-Gal, D., and Hasenfeld, Y. (in press). "Executive Behavior in Community Service Organizations." *Journal of Social Service Research*.

Schon, D. (1983). *The Reflective Practitioner: How Professionals Think in Action*. New York: Basic Books.

Shrivastava, P., and I. Mitroff. (1984). "Enhancing Organizational Research Utilization: The Role of Decision Makers' Assumptions." *Academy of Management Review*, 9(1), 18-26.

Simon, H.A. (1970). *The Sciences of the Artificial*. Cambridge, MA: MIT Press.

Simon, H. A. (1977). *The New Science of Management Decision*. Engelwood Cliffs, NJ: Prentice-Hall.

Sproull, L., and P. Larkey. (1979). "Managerial Behavior and Evaluator Effectiveness." In H. C. Schulberg and Jeanette M. Jerrell (Eds.), *The Evaluator and Management*. Beverly Hills, CA: Sage, pp. 89-104.

Weiss, C. H. (1980). *Social Science Research and Decision Making*. New York: Columbia University Press.

Weiss, C. H. (1981). "Use of Social Science Research in Organizations: The Constrained Repertoire Theory." In H. D. Stein (Ed.), *Organization and the Human Services*. Philadelphia: Temple University Press, pp. 180-204.

Wholey, J. S. (1981). Using Evaluation to Improve Program Performance. In R.

A. Levine et al. (Eds.), *Evaluation Research and Practice*. Beverly Hills, CA: Sage, pp. 92-106.

Wolk, J. L., Way, I. F. and Bleeke, M. A. (1982). "Human Service Management: The Art of Interpersonal Relationships." *Administration in Social Work*, 6, 1-10.

Yin, R. K. (1976). *R&D Utilization by Local Services: Problems and Proposals for Further Research*. Santa Monica, CA: Rand Co.

# Practice Uses of Accountability Systems in Health Care Settings: Social Work and Administrative Perspectives

Helen Rehr

This chapter describes an agency-based, research utilization program in a health care setting, and its underlying assumptions. More specifically, it draws on social work's perception and practice uses of a professional accountability system at The Mount Sinai Hospital in New York City. Our basic thesis is that broad-based, in-house studies of the delivery of care to our patients and their families is a necessary part of practice. In so saying, I agree with T. Franklin Williams' claim that, "research and care require each other; they interact with each other" (Williams, 1988, p. 579). More generally, the paper supports Ed Kilborne's opinion that for physicians and for social work practitioners as well, it is important that those "caring for the patients shall themselves engage in studies, since not infrequently careful observation of patients yields suggestions for lines of research which might be overlooked" (Kilborne, 1986, p. 47), and which can enhance practice.

It is important to assert the value of professional accountability via in-house studies — its significance for a staff and an administrator, for program enhancement within the institution, for health care colleagues, and finally its implication for our consumers and the field itself. In addition, I shall register the belief that social work academics have in general neglected a vital study arena and have failed to teach clinicians the need to be invested in the study of service delivery. It is also my belief that the language of research with its statistical determinants, important as it is to researchers, is an anathema to clinicians. Compounding the research write-up problem is its limited translation for clinical application. At this time we are still left with researchers talking to researchers, and clinicians learning from other clinicians with little access to meaningful research findings which could affect service delivery and quality performance. I will conclude with a few suggestions on how to reach clinicians and a description of a Mount Sinai model used with third-year medical students as a way to expose them to the relationship between practice and research.

## HISTORICAL OVERVIEW: ACCOUNTABILITY SYSTEMS IN HEALTH CARE

The 1965 amendments to Social Security mandated professional quality review for services under the federally reimbursed programs of Medicare, Medicaid, and Maternal and Child Health Care Services. Social workers in health care assumed the mandate included their services. As a result, a partnership between professional social workers and their administrators was created in an attempt to enhance the quality as well as the cost-effectiveness of social work services to their clientele.

Professional accountability is a concept not without its critics. It is still under attack and perceived as a sell-out of professionally determined service delivery to those in need. It is seen as a political ploy tied to cost-containment with the intent to cut back on the government-supported social services. Adding to the difficulty is the lack of clarity in perception of professional accountability by regulators, payers, providers, and consumers who bring their own definitions and expectations to quality assurance.

Professional accountability in the health care field has been sought for a long time. Florence Nightingale during the American Civil War assessed nursing care to casualties; Flexner in 1910 reviewed medical education in the context of its performance; in 1910 E.A. Codman reviewed hospital services, creating the term "end result" of care delivered as his tool of measurement (Rehr, 1979, p. 16). Since then, there have been a host of review committees in hospitals: mortality, pathology, and surgical reviews. The Professional Standard Review Organizations (PSRO) and End Stage Renal Disease (ESRD) organization set in 1972 by Congress were the means by which mandated audits were prescribed to deal with in-hospital problem identification and resolution. All of these were done by peer reviews within the institution determined by guide-lines set by the relevant professionals. By 1972 quality review and cost-containment were linked. In 1974 utilization review of in-hos-pital care was the mechanism set up to review, and set standards and criteria for admission. Also the Uniform Hospital Discharge Data System (UHDDS) was the beginning of what was to become a national data collection body (Rehr, 1979, p. 18).

It is important to recall that given the national fiscal crisis, the mandate for peer review and service audits was furthered because, by and large, the professionals and the institutions, while reviewing care, were *not* systematically implementing findings that dealt with institutional or colleague problems. Abuse, misuse, waste, and re-imbursement fraud in the marketplace brought on this rash of laws and regulations which were created "to promote effective and eco-nomical delivery of health services of proper quality for which pay-ment was made" (Rehr, 1979, p. 17).

The expectation of quality assurance and cost-containment was translated to mean maintenance of professional skills, keeping up with current knowledge, and sound utilization of care. It called for:

1. information: patient- and practitioner-relevant;
2. data: disease-specific, length of stay, procedures;
3. standard setting: for performance, services;
4. institutional and program evaluation;
5. professional performance assessment;

and ultimately cross-institutional comparisons.

As late as the end of the 1970, when information was collected within a medical institution it was perceived as the private purview of the reviewing body. By and large, institutions were not collect-ing data about patients served, services delivered, or/performance other than what was required for reimbursement. These were essen-tially visits, in-patient stays, and lab and other procedures. The technology for information collecting and dissemination was just coming into being. Institutions were slowly investing in systems that could be more extensive than billing and personnel processing. By the 1980s the expectations for data collection demanded by regulatory and paying agencies began to include such factors as demographics, admission and discharge dates, diagnoses, and facil-ities-services-manpower utilized, and translated to length of stay, out-patient and emergency visits, and occupancy-to-service ratios, the emphasis on costs to charges remained.

In regard to the review of professional performance, the preroga-tives of professional autonomy are still with us, but slowly shifting. The pressures from consumer groups and regulatory bodies have been more and more evident, resulting in recent public dissemina-tion of findings such as mortality rates in hospitals by the Health Care Financing Administration (HCFA). Rating systems dealing with quality and costs are wanted and sought by most purchasers of services, industry and consumers in particular. Rating systems on providers (doctors and hospitals) are currently in full discussion with emphasis on the appropriateness and necessity of services, as well as quality and cost-effectiveness (*Quality Review Bulletin*, Dec. 1982, p. 37). Similarly, CHAMPUS, which reimburses social work services for government employees, reviews them in the same context.

Social scientists and medical experts such as A. Donabedian (1973), R. Greene (1976), B. Starfield (1974), R. Brook and F. Appel (1973) had been working on ways to view quality of care since the 1960s. The machine technology was there, and quality, access, equity, and even the right to health, not just health care, were the social-health issues of that decade. With the advent of quality assurance in care as defined by Medicare and Medicaid, social workers in health care anticipated the need to undertake re-view of social work services, modeling on audits and peer review similar to what medicine was doing (Coulton, 1982). The new state and local regulations as well as the expectations set by the Joint Commission on Accreditation of Hospitals (JCAH) included social work services review in hospitals. These reviews were meaningful since at the state and local levels, it meant reimbursement rates would be set. At the JCAH level not only rates but quality determi-nants were made known, and nonaccreditation or suspended accred-itation could affect an institution in its medical education, house staff, professional, and even public perceptions. Accreditation was and is a highly sought commodity. Institutions responded to reviews set by guidelines of the JCAH, and state and local accrediting bodies. Social work in health care responding to accreditation reviews pioneered for the field-at-large by setting standards via the National Association of Social Workers and the Society for Hospital Social Work Directors. The two social work organizations worked together to establish reviewing methods, and to suggest studies to evaluate the quality of care delivered by social workers.

Avedis Donabedian (1973) set measures for quality assessment in the context of structure, process, and outcomes. These do not require definition for this audience other than to say that while much has been undertaken, developing a uniform and systematic means to deal with these concepts remains to be done even today (Zastowny and Lehman, 1988). Quality expectations did force the development of reviewing mechanisms to cover:

- professionally developed norms, criteria, and standards;
- a data retrieval system on patients, providers, and institutions;
- a utilization review system and periodic medical care evaluation studies;
- a peer review system based on established criteria;
- a means to correct identified deficiencies related to individual and organizational performance;
- continuing education as the corrective measure; and
- uniform information and data systems for regional and cross-institutional assessments (PSRO Program Manual, 1974, p. 1).

The intent was to set up a continuous, self-reviewing mechanism by those invested in the care (physicians and other health care professionals). The means to the review having been suggested, it left the major problems to be addressed: how to evaluate health and hospital care; how to define these in physical, psychological, or social functioning terms; what are the instrumentalities of care: a doctor, a team of health care professionals, selected procedures relevant to specific diseases; who is the actual client of services delivered: an individual, a family, a caseload, a population; and finally, what is the outcome of care. The last was the truly hard factor when we had to consider what it is, when to assess it, by what terms, and how and by whom the outcome should be judged (Rehr, 1979, p. 22).

## SOCIAL WORK ACCOUNTABILITY
## AT MOUNT SINAI HOSPITAL

Mount Sinai's Social Work Services Department moved very early in seeking professional accountability measures. The handwriting was on the wall: quality assurance was here to stay and social work had to come on board. In one sense the Medicare, Medicaid, and Maternal and Child Health legislation were a bonanza for hospitals. Reimbursement for services was based on a "reasonable cost plus" basis. The interpretation of "reasonable cost plus" was largely an in-house determination. While there has not been time to review our files for all the in-house studies we did in the 1960s and early 1970s in order to support the value of social services, I easily remember a particular early study. Anticipating the shift from multiple-bed ward care to semi-private services for Medicare patients, we studied the elderly in-patients, the numbers known to social workers, why they were known, and the services delivered. Within the institution our attending physicians generally believed that their private and semi-private patients were never in need of social services. We demonstrated to the contrary with heavy demand by the elderly irrespective of income level and were able to present the hospital administration with a documented rationale for increased services to the private and semi-private Medicare patients, and to those who would fill the beds in the renovated wards (Berkman and Rehr, 1967).

Almost a half-century ago Mary Jarrett (1946) did a study of Bellevue Hospital in-patients. In that study she arrived at a formula of those in need of social work services which was distributed along a high/mid and low ratio of 1/3, 1/3, and 1/3. For many years our own studies at Mount Sinai supported this notion, particularly when social work was serving predominantly the patients on the wards. That distribution no longer holds. Current studies geared to age, disease, multiple diagnoses, severity, length of stay, social supports, and functional limitations reveal that the distribution of social work services is targeted to these factors and not to bed utilization. In addition, Mount Sinai is now serving a sicker population than it did ten years ago. As a result social work services are in even greater demand today.

At Mount Sinai the Department of Social Work Services, convinced of the need to be informed and having had experience with outside research consultants attempting to interpret its work and practice, moved to invest itself in conceptualizing professional accountability for staff and administration. A basic tenet of this effort was that information and data were the property of the practitioners themselves, as well as of administrators. Together, they had to provide data on which judgments could be made in relation to practice and program. We had hopes for a uniform data system that could be arrived at for regional and national determinations (Rehr, 1979, pp. 48-57) and worked on the premise regionally (unsuccessfully) and nationally (now well established) (SHSWD, HSWIS Newsletter, #4, 1988).

At Mount Sinai we elected a social work approach to quality assessment rather than an interdisciplinary or team mechanism in the belief that it would force social work to develop its own method, criteria, process, and outcome measures. Once developed, social work could then be integrated with other disciplines (Lurie, 1978, p. 67). A number of components had to be defined and developed:

- an information system capable of reliable data retrieval;
- norms, standards, or criteria which have been difficult to determine because social work had values, but neither norms for performance (services) nor professionally accepted standards for the determination of "good" care (now being developed by the SHSWD with the assistance of the JCAH);
- structural components such as availability, accessibility, and guaranteed access; staffing patterns; adequate documentation of services delivered, et al.;
- process, performance, or the sequence of acts provided or to be provided which are functionally defined (service determinants have been projected by SHSWD); and
- outcome in the context of what happened to the individual or recipient unit of social services, recognizing the difficulty in

determining where one looks, how to measure it, and whether the service was the catalyst for the outcome (problem/s to service/s to outcome/s are in periodic review by the SHSWD and selected social work departmental studies).

Coulton (*Quality Review Bulletin*, 1982) translated quality assurance as involving a qualified staff in an acceptable program with defined structure and which delivers services in the context of "good" practice, capable of achieving desired results by patients/families, and which safeguards that those who need services do get them.

Because we believe that an uninformed social work department is powerless, and similarly, a social work staff will remain static without informational and practice assessment opportunities, we assumed that being informed was essential, particularly in multi-disciplinary settings in what some call "host" care systems (Jansson and Simmons, 1986). In institutions where many departments compete for support, information gives the department visibility and credibility in the organization, and the ability to command resources for defined purposes. It also helps a department to achieve comparable status to other departments in the institution, thus crediting a bio-psycho-social context of care, rather than medical predominance or that of a "host" care system.

An institutional administrator does not respond to an emotional appeal for service increments. S/he requires written documentation indicating the problem, objective data to support the need, alternative solutions with financial and value consequences, and a professional recommendation of what it will take to implement a change and how it will be evaluated. Responsible, documented need is required in program, labor, and cost terms, and not in social problem analyses terms. In our settings it has become more or less accepted that medical diagnosis alone without assessment of social, psychological, and environmental factors will not hold for treatment and care purposes. However, this concept continues to need demonstration. We have begun to face the fact that a service is only as good as its ultimate benefit to someone, both the client system and the members of the provider system.

Fairly quickly, we took a route with successive steps, all of which were functionally productive to staff, administrators, other health care providers, and the institution itself. We started with the staff and where they posed their first concerns. When social workers continued to report that referrals were reaching them very late in the patient's hospital stay, we did a study which confirmed referrals as late as the day before discharge (Berkman and Rehr, 1967 and 1972). There was open recognition that quality planning for patients' post-hospital care suffered from late referrals. The next step was to find the means to safeguard access to social work services as early as possible. Working with staff produced their variables for high social risk (Berkman and Rehr, 1973 and 1974) which have been subsequently refined (Rehr, *QRB*, 1986; Newsletter #4, HSWIS, 1988; Cunningham, 1982). Agreement was reached by staff and administration, following a study matching risk to case review, to introduce a casefinding screening device (Berkman, Rehr, and Rosenberg, 1980). Today high risk screening is also done preadmission at Mount Sinai (Reardon et al., 1988). Social work here and throughout hospitals in the country is in control of its own casefinding for patients hospitalized or to be hospitalized (*QRB*, 1982).

A concurrent major concern dealt with the credibility and value of services delivered. While this was a longtime professional goal of ours, it was catapulted into action by the Medicare legislation of 1966 which included a quality assurance expectation. As casefinding was to serve the guaranteed access component of quality assurance, we sought to review outcome. Given the state of the art of studies of outcome of care, we elected the consumer and provider satisfaction routes. Donabedian (1973), Starfield (1974), and Greene (1976) are some social scientists who have given credence to "satisfaction" as one outcome measure. We also considered that the "voice of the consumer" would have critical significance for hospital administration, health care colleagues, and the social work staff itself. The consumers' response to social work services had been documented by social workers over a period of time (Overton, 1960; Maluccio, 1979; Perlman, 1975). However, recently it appears to have been bypassed by social work researchers as a measure of outcome on the assumption that it is too soft a variable to be reliable.

We moved first to develop a social-health problem classification. Again with the staff, we approached it by a case content analysis and finalized a 29-problem classification for adult medical and surgical situations (Berkman and Rehr, 1972). The Berkman-Rehr problem classification has since been validated (Berkman, 1980) and updated. From problem classification we moved to problem contracting between the worker and the client system. It took a fiscal crisis at Mount Sinai to move from relationship-based, long-term services to problem-focused services with a goal structure set by client and worker. To achieve credibility with the hospital administration, we needed to find constituencies to support the Department's work. We asked the senior staff whether they could identify doctors who would commit themselves to social work support. The response was that if everyone was going to get hit financially doctors would want to protect themselves first. We then asked each to identify six clients who would attest to social work's helpfulness. We were told that a basic goal of social work intervention was for the client to conclude that all gains are self-achieved. In one of our studies, we had already found in early telephone follow-up that social work clients tended *not* to recall their experience with social workers as well as they did those with doctors and nurses (Berkman and Rehr, 1975). We then suggested an experiment where each social worker (20) would call any three clients (closed cases) to determine their recall of services received and their degree of satisfaction. We would meet again in six weeks.

As you might guess, we met with a very crestfallen bunch, none of whom had much positive to report. Before concluding that meeting, the conceptualization of contracting was discussed in full and it was agreed that we would draw on the Berkman-Rehr Problem Classification as an across-the-board measure attempting to structure a problem-to-contract approach. Drawing on the work of Reid and Epstein (1972) for task-oriented services and Maluccio and Marlow (1974) for contracting, we developed a measure of open mutual agreement between the client system and the worker regarding the problem to be dealt with. Having concretized the problem/s and implemented contracts of service, the client and the worker could each report perception of outcome and satisfaction (Berkman and Rehr, 1975) in relation to the agreed-upon problem contract.

Satisfaction with services, although difficult and subjective, is now being seen as a major measure by those in mental health in particular, (satisfaction is being studied for) its relationship to motivation and compliance — (and) especially (for how it is) related to the quality of care (Zastowny and Lehman, 1988). Social work, which had recognized the "voice of the consumer" as a component of care in the 1950s and 1960s, should regain its leadership in searching out this measure of service outcome. Clients' perception of care is critical to how care should be given. Provider satisfaction with delivery correlates highly with consumer satisfaction (Berkman and Rehr, 1975; Speedling et al., 1983) and could also serve as a valuable assessment of services.

To review, we developed with staff an information system; designed a social-health problem classification; built in a problem/contract-to-outcome concept so that we could determine "what happened" as perceived by the client system and the provider system, and correlated these. We developed a peer review system predicated on the belief that professional social workers could determine "good" from "bad" practice, and could set expectations and review for them. We also developed consumer (and provider) satisfaction instruments as quality assurance determinants not only for the Department but also for the hospital and its divisions (Speedling et al., 1983); engaged in program audits both within the Department and multi-departmentally; introduced in-house continuing education based on the findings of our studies and staff recommendations; conceptualized a self-directed, independent worker versus the ongoing worker-supervisor relationship; developed high social risk screening for social work services and casefinding to deal with guaranteed access; and engaged in a range of in-house departmental applied studies along with a number of interdisciplinary study partnerships. All this has served staff, administration, and institutional social work programs well. In the final analysis, drawing on present day technology, some outside research consultation, but essentially our own applied social work research center,* we are meeting the primary goal: to serve the client system and to enhance the quality

---

*Murray M. Rosenberg Applied Social Work Research Center, Mount Sinai Medical Center.

of care. In our opinion, the most powerful force which catapulted social work in health care to study its own services was the federal mandate for quality assurance and sound utilization of services.

## GENERATING STAFF SUPPORT

How do you invest a staff in joining an administrator in a partnership of study? An administrator can go in an executively determined unilateral power direction, or have the staff share in defining problems and in decision making. Fizdale (1974) said that the former method is dealing with "employees" who respond to orders, and the latter is dealing with "professionals" who must affect the quality of care they offer their clients — a major difference in administrative perception. Having experienced the executive-determined route and found almost immovable resistance and having learned at the same time that the staff's ideas and wishes for change were as clear as ours, it was not difficult to try to set an atmosphere that supported the belief that professional accountability resided in the professional with administrative support. Explanations for nonutilization of research findings by practitioners had been summarized by many researchers (Fanshel, 1980) and more recently by Grasso, Epstein and Tripodi (1988), with recognition that there is no single explanation. We drew on the mandate for professional accountability to activate the staff to assume responsibility for their practice. To do so, staff needed to be responsive to performance and service analysis.

If program and performance are to be in periodic review, workers need to feel stress, strain, curiosity, and even dissatisfaction, and an administrator needs to create the climate to let these feelings surface. Having said that, it follows that opportunities for open discussions and sharing questions, problems, frustrations, and ideas need to be made available. A partnership with shared power needs to be present. Shared decision making is a major tool to deal with resistance to change. This is coupled with the belief that a professional social worker has an investment in building his/her own continuous knowledge and in the enhancement of performance. Practitioners can make significant contributions and have done so. They transpose findings into action more readily then researchers. They know their settings and how to negotiate them, which can lead to sound application of change recommendations.

The following scheme worked well for us:

1. Diagnose the problem together; open communication.
2. Set objectives mutually.
3. Draw on a participatory approach involving open interactions and reaching group consensus.
4. Disseminate the maximum information available (not the least).
5. Invest all participants in the process.
6. Discuss findings for implications.
7. Discuss findings for recommendations, implementation of change, and role assignments.
8. Deal with resistances in the group and by the group.
9. Disseminate change recommendations and implement the training required.
10. Invest in a periodic review of the changes and continued open communication.

Internalization of change behavior is the most powerful gain for a staff member. A staff member needs to advocate for wanting something different, both within a professional, self-renewal context and in a departmental, structural context. Having a significant part in the study, owning it so to speak, leads to commitment to change and a stake in it. There are observations that workers make, as noted by Williams and Kilborne, which prompt questions that can be narrowed down to "one page" studies. If workers are invested in working on the problem, they see the potentialities of the findings for further study and for their ultimate use. Experimental and pilot projects by workers need to be welcomed with time allocated to do them, recognition and rewards should be forthcoming, publication and conference presentations should be encouraged.

The use of group investment in performance and program evaluations is itself a dynamic supportive process. It enhances knowledge and performance via the exchange and serves as the unit for continuing education as well as for periodic evaluation of changes. The staff in its own review of its investment in professional accountability measures indicates that their participation has helped them to deal with the real world of performance and service. They can answer such questions as, "what do I do?" "how do I do it?" "what did my client achieve?" "what did I achieve?" "what should I do differently?" and "what does the department need to do differently?" and they can report their responses to health care colleagues. The assumption herein is that competency and quality are sought by the serious professional, and since no fixed model of treatment for a bio-psycho-social diagnosis is yet available to us, we concentrate on "structure" and "outcome" as perceived by both the client system and the provider system, rather than the process per se (except via preceptor/supervisor). Comparison among cases is still not possible because of the highly idiosyncratic material of each case. Outcomes are not in a unilinear relationship to a worker's process, but similarities and differences can be observed in the aggregating of similar problems, specific diseases, social and/or physical limitations, age- or sex-related factors, class, and a range of other variables which can lend themselves to future epidemiological or bio-psycho-socially focused studies. Professional accountability measures offer workers a yardstick with which they can "measure and compare the benefits and risks" of their services (Laupacis, Sackett and Roberts, 1988). When asked about professional accountability, staff's primary comments were that they had become more self-disciplined, independent, self-directed, could evaluate the benefits of their services more readily (as to successful outcomes or not), and were in control of their own performance. Their investments had "moved the group to support structural approaches in assessing the work of the individual practitioner and in auditing the general delivery of care, and to regard their own investment in peer review and audit as components of professional accountability" (Rehr, 1979, p. 149).

On the administrative side, we have already indicated that speaking from an informed base removes vulnerability. A management information system which is functional, has a staff's backing, offers a quantification of services delivered to whom, by whom, and at what cost along with provider and consumer satisfaction measures, and supplies the opportunity to do applied studies, is invaluable. It is important to note that we have been discussing functional measures and applied studies. These are studies which have utility in the enhancement of service delivery and the quality of care and are invaluable, and cannot be successful without a partnership of staff and administration.

## *EDUCATIONAL IMPLICATIONS*

Our experience to date, however, leads us to the conclusion that present-day social work education does not produce the practitioner who can integrate a study attitude into the clinical enterprise. What seems to be still missing is the academic commitment to the value of applied studies — those with functional utility — although there are some beginning signs from those academics who look to the agency as the realistic and pragmatic focus for study (Grasso, Epstein, and Tripodi, 1988; Seidl (Fanshel), 1980; Mutschler, 1984). We encourage the development of the practitioner-scientist, for social work agencies. This type of researcher has been well received at Mount Sinai. But the paramount need is for clinical acumen which requires observational and questioning skills, pursuit of ideas, and new insights. Clinicians, who like T. F. Williams (1980), are curious about the "what" and the "why" of what they are doing and what happened as a result, have a curiosity that motivates them to explore further. Social workers who have learned that meaningful but simple documentation is critical for review of their cases, who look over their caseload periodically and raise questions, who can enjoy the opportunity to discuss failures and successes with peers, who are curious about alternative strategies, who have opportunities in which observational skills are enhanced and can have a "hands-on" study experience, will develop skills in user utilization of data.

If one is to draw on the medical model it could be a Case Review Committee, a multi-professional Audit Committee, a Peer Review Program, or a Journal Club — all opportunities which encourage reading and staying current in knowledge. There will be social work students who wish to go the route of the researcher, and they should be encouraged. However, what is most critical for the field is the clinician who can be a participant in studies and a consumer of research findings. S/he needs to have an interest in what s/he is doing in a system of personal services which must be responsive to need.

Again, a model in medical education that works for medical students' orientation to social-health research is the one designed by Deuschle and Dana and the Community Medicine faculty. In the third year each medical student is expected to engage in the study of a health problem which has social significance. There have been studies of drop-outs in adolescent clinics, medication compliance, emergency room use, and others. With the assistance of a faculty member over a month's time, the student is required to design a study (simple and do-able), do a literature search, collect information either via chart review or in-person interviews, analyze the data, interpret the findings, and make recommendations. S/he writes a report, makes a 20-minute presentation of the study to students, peers, and faculty, and leads a discussion of the findings. It teaches students to be consumers of research and respecters of the study process, and about the professional utility of applied studies along with the indispensable relationship between practice- and research, which require each other. These studies are intended to promote understanding of the relationship of the biological, social, and psychological factors in the definition and satisfaction of health problems. It also teaches presentation skills (Deuschle et al., 1972). Academics, both practice- and research-based, should seek opportunities in health care settings to work with the social work staff on professional accountability measures (Rehr and Rosenberg, 1977), and to open up opportunities for applied studies which have performance and program utility.

## FUTURE RESEARCH IMPLICATIONS

There are so many studies that we wish the Department could have claimed in the context of quality assurance. One in particular done by our then dean and a colleague demonstrated that savings in substituting ambulatory for in-patient care were evident only if the social costs were considered, and fewer services were given at home (Ancona-Berk and Chalmers, 1986). Although we had the data in social workers' records shortly after the Diagnosis-Related groups (DRGs) went into effect we did not get to this study, but are pleased it has been done. Social costs have not been introduced enough into the research arena (Fahs, 1988). Social workers are a natural for contributing to the significance of this factor, e.g., social supports input, productive time loss, quality of life, and functional status as an outcome of given studies. So many researchable questions remain for the future. Some of the professional accountability questions the Mount Sinai social workers are currently asking include the following:

- Are motivation and compliance related to satisfaction with care?
- What structure and provider environments facilitate sound and differentiated service delivery?
- Can we develop a classification of satisfaction dimensions for mental health services comparable to those developed for medical services?
- What are the vital dimensions in client-provider interaction?
- Who are and what makes for satisfied versus dissatisfied clients?
- Do targeted populations, e.g., disease-specific, age-specific, chronically ill patients, etc., require special services?
- Is there a relationship between "qualified" workers and outcome?
- How do we enhance peer review for concurrent quality assurance of services?
- Are services cost-effective, e.g., are volume, time involved, and outcomes efficiently related?
- Are "at home" services meeting needs of discharged patients?
- How do we view the relationship of multiple diagnoses, severity of illness, and social functioning limitations?
- Are the social work services reaching those in need; is there access to or rationing of health care services?
- Who stays in needed social work services; who drops out?
- How do we triage and differentiate problems, those at risk, and their service needs?
- How do we support services outside the institutional walls?

It is apparent that social work settings in health care are actively invested in quality assurance reviews. The NASW and the SHSWD have recently had a "clinical indicators" conference with the intent to develop standards and norms, and process and service modes relevant to outcomes (NASW and SHSWD, 1988). In addition the SHSWD has developed HSWIS (a management information system) which it hopes will be uniformly adopted by its members. There are now dozens of departments investing in management information systems and showing benefits therefrom in regard to control and planning systems (Nurius, Berger, and VanDerweele, 1988).

All of the work in health care settings to date has its beginnings in the recognition that professional accountability is lodged in the social worker and supported by an administrative partnership. What is paramount in those systems reported as successful is that the staff is seen as the mainstay and the guide to quality of care and the direction of needed services. Social-health policy deliberations may derive from in-house accountability studies and our social workers have testified, along with their health care colleagues, before subcommittees of Congress. This paper, however, has dealt with an approach to in-house performance and program assessments. Social work education needs to recognize the significance of professional accountability in social workers and to prepare them to make practice use of quality assurance research.

## REFERENCES

Ancona-Berk, V. A. and Chalmers, T. C. An analysis of the costs of ambulatory and in-patient care, *American Journal of Public Health*, Sept. 1986, 76(9), 1102-1104.

Berkman, B. Psychosocial problems and outcome: an external validity study, *Health and Social Work*, Aug. 1980, 5(3), 5-21.

Berkman, (Gordon) B. and Rehr, H. Aging ward patients and the hospital social work department, *Journal of American Geriatrics Society*, 1967, 15(12).

Berkman, B. and Rehr, H. Social needs of the hospitalized elderly: a classification, *Social Work*, July 1972(a), 17(4), 80-88.

Berkman, B. and Rehr, H. The Sick-role cycle and the timing of social work intervention, *Social Service Review*, December 1972(b), 46(4).

Berkman, B. and Rehr, H. Early social service casefinding for hospitalized patients: an experiment, *Social Service Review*, June 1973, 47(2), 256-265.

Berkman, B. and Rehr, H. The search for early indicators of need for social service intervention in the hospital, *Journal of the American Geriatrics Society*, Sept. 1974, 22(9), 416-421.

Berkman, B. and Rehr, H. Elderly patients and their families: factors relating to satisfaction with hospital social services, *The Gerontologist*, Dec. 1975, 15(16).

Berkman, B., Rehr, H., and Rosenberg, G. A social work department develops and tests a screening mechanism to identify high social risk situations, *Social Work in Health Care*, Summer 1980, 19(11).

Brook, R. and Appel, F. A. Quality of case assessment: choosing a method for peer review, *New England Journal of Medicine*, 1973, 288(25), 1323-1329.

Coulton, C. J. Approaches to quality assessment in social work, *Quality Review Bulletin*, Special Edition 1982.

Coulton, C. J. Quality assurance for social service programs: lessons from health care, *Social Work*, Sept. 1982, 397-402.

Cunningham, L. S. Early assessment for discharge planning: Adapting a high risk screening program, *Quarterly Review Bulletin*, Special Edition, Joint Commission on Accreditation of Hospitals, Spring 1982, 66-71.

Deuschle, K. W., Bosch, S. J., Banta, H. D., and Dana, B. The community medicine clerkship: a learner-centered program, *Journal of Medical Education*, Dec. 1972, 47.

Donabedian, A. *Aspects of medical care administration*, Cambridge, Harvard University Press, 1973, 58-207.

Fahs, Marianne C. Reconciling quality-social-health outcomes with cost-effectiveness, presented at the Doris Siegel Memorial Colloquium, New York City, 10/21/88.

Fanshel, D., ed. Future of social work research, Washington, DC, NASW, 1980. See in particular chapters by Fanshel, Briar, Reid, Seidl, Coulton.

Fizdale, R. *Social agency structure and accountability*, New Jersey, Burdick, 1974.

Grasso, A. J. and Epstein, J. Management by measurement: organization dilemmas and opportunities, *Administration in Social Work*, 1988, 11(3/4) 89-100.

Grasso, A. J., Epstein, I., and Tripodi, T. Agency-based research utilization in a residential child care setting, *Administration in Social Work*, 1988, 12(4), 61-80.

Greene, R. *Assessing quality in medical care*, Cambridge, Ballinger Publishing Co., 1976.

Jansson, B. S. and Simmons, J. The survival of social work units in host organizations, *Social Work*, 1986, 31, 339-343.

Jarrett, M. C. A method for determining the number of medical social workers needed for casework in a general hospital, Social Service Division, Bellevue Hospital, New York, 1946.

Kilborne, E. The emergence of the physician—basic scientist, *Daedalus*, Spring 1986, 15(2), 47.

Lurie, A. Social service conducts two quality assurance programs, *Hospitals*, Feb. 1978, 52.

Laupacis, A., Sackett, D. L., and Roberts, R. S. An assessment of clinically useful measures of the consequence of treatment, *New England Journal of Medicine*, June 30, 1988, 318(26).

Maluccio, A. N. and Marlow, W. The case for the contract, *Social Work*, Jan. 1974, 19(1).

Maluccio, A. N. *Learning from clients*, New York, Free Press, 1979.

Mutschler, E. Evaluating practice: A study of research utilization by practitioners. *Social Work*, 1984, 29, 332-337.

NASW Health and Mental Health Commission, The Society of Hospital Social Work Directors and the Joint Commission in Accreditation of Health Organizations joined in a first Quality Indicators Consensus Building Conference in Fall 1988 to identify and define indicators for appraising care.

Newsletter #4, 1988, Society for Hospital Social Work Directors, A.H.A., which discusses "A Computer Based Hospital Social Work Information System," HSWIS, 1988.

Nurius, P., Berger, C., VanDerweele, T. ASSIST: An alternative management information system for social services in health care, *Social Work in Health Care*, 1988, 13(4), 99-115.

Overton, A. Taking help from our clients, *Social Work*, April 1960, 5(2).

Perlman, R. *Consumers and social service*, New York, John Wiley, 1975.

*PSRO Program Manual*, USDHEW, Office of Professional Standards Review, U.S. Government Printing Office, March 15, 1974.

*Quality Review Bulletin*, Social work review: approaches to evaluation and analysis of patient care, Special Edition 1982. (This issue has 16 articles reflecting the range of quality assurance programs instituted by social work departments in hospitals.)

Reardon, G. T., Blumenfield, S., Weissman, A. L., and Rosenberg, G. Findings and implications from pre-admission screening of elderly patients waiting for elective surgery, *Social Work in Health Care*, 1988, 13(3).

Rehr, H. and Rosenberg, G. Today's education for today's health care social work practice, *Clinical Social Work Journal*, 1977, 5(4), 342-350.

Rehr, H. *Professional accountability for social work practice*, New York, Prodist, 1979.

Rehr, H. Editorial: Discharge planning: an on-going function of quality care, *Quality Review Bulletin*, Feb. 1986, 12(2).

Reid, W. J. and Epstein, I. *Task-centered casework*, New York, Columbia University Press, 1972.

Starfield, B. Measurement of outcome: a proposed scheme, *The Milbank Memorial Quarterly/Health and Society*, Winter 1974, 52(1), 39-50.

Speedling, E. J., Morrison, B., Rehr, H., and Rosenberg, G., Patient satisfaction surveys: closing the gap between provider and consumer, *Quality Review Bulletin*, August 1983, 9(8), 224-228.

Williams, T. F. 1987 Donald P. Kent Memorial Lecture, *The Gerontologist*, 1988, 28(5), 579.

Zastowny, T. R. and Lehman, A. F. Patient satisfaction with mental health services, *Quality Review Bulletin*, Sept. 1988, 284-289.

# INTRODUCTION TO SECTION IV

## Putting Research to Work in Agency Settings

James K. Whittaker

John Goodlad, distinguished researcher and professor of education at the University of Washington, noted in a recent faculty lecture that if colleges of education are to adequately meet the challenges of teacher training, they need to do many things differently. One critical recommendation Goodlad posed as an absolutely essential element in an overall reform strategy involved the creation of a link between the college of education and a few experimentally minded school districts, where teacher trainees could be exposed to several models of exemplary pedagogy and where the problems of curriculum design and classroom management would become the foci for a wide variety of faculty-student applied research efforts. The "R&D" component of this provocative recommendation harks back to a conception of mission-oriented research common to land grant higher education, particularly in agriculture and engineering. Thus, if the corn was blighted, one went to the university agricultural experiment station for analysis and problem-solving advice and recommendations. In a more recent example, if your contract was to build part of the heat shield for the space shuttle (as it was at the Boeing Company just a few years ago) and the tiles were falling off on re-entry, one went to the university's college of engineering and *that* problem became the focus for the appropriate graduate seminar in design and development.

That such examples are harder to identify in the human services was, in large measure, a reason for this conference. The relative scarcity of examples of what Bill Reid (1978) once wonderfully referred to as the social agency as "research machine," provided a particular stimulus to the provocative contributions by John Schuerman, Betty Blythe, David Fanshel, Elizabeth Mutschler, and Mel Raider, which make up this section on agency-based research utilization.

John Schuerman challenges us to think about the application of "average" findings to the individual case through the use of expert systems. He skillfully teases out the role of user needs, practice tasks, organizational variables, and available information technology in shaping the adoption and use of various expert systems. Betty Blythe urges us to more carefully examine the context of practitioner-based research and, in particular, the organizational requisites for the adoption and maintenance of such curricular innovations as the move toward integrating research and practice content through such things as empirically based practice. As the Council on Social Work Education has rather dramatically altered its accreditation standards for the teaching of research and practice content, Betty Blythe urges us to examine the effect of this shift in actual agency practice. She properly cautions against the simplistic acceptance of particular technologies, such as single system designs, as a sufficient answer to the problem of agency-based research and argues instead for a more variegated approach based on practice information needs at several levels.

As he has on so many previous occasions, David Fanshel argues the benefits of analyzing routinely gathered data as an aid to practice and administration. Building upon his landmark studies of status changes of children in foster care, Fanshel's present study of the Casey Family Program, a privately funded exemplary agency offering long-term subsidized foster care to troubled youth, breaks new ground in both design and analysis and offers intriguing opportunities for practice utilization. His time series analyses of youth in placement offer a unique life course perspective on adolescent development for a population of children who grow up in other than their biological families. The correlates of "successful" outcomes; the antecedents of "failed" placements; the intensity of various service packages; the complex interplay of youth, their biological and foster families, and case workers are all features of an impressive multi-variate analysis that both involves practitioners in the design and offers many tantalizing implications for practice. Over time, for example, could certain patterns of youth/family problems and placement histories help with the assessment of risk and acuity? Fanshel's study offers a fascinating "window" into the intake stream and service system of foster care which allows for continuing analysis and feedback and tracking. As his earlier work so clearly established, certain indicators such as parental visitation ought to be routinely monitored in the same manner as vital signs in a hospital as they are so integrally related to outcomes. In this impressive study, Fanshel has given us once again a template for agency-based research that is at once rigorous and utterly practical. It deserves replication.

Elizabeth Mutschler addresses the important question of how information technology influences human service agencies. She reminds us that all too often, the acquisition of hardware precedes sensible discussion of how it will be used and toward what informational needs. She reminds us as well how attitudes of both practitioners and administrators can have a powerful effect on both the form and substance of research utilization in a given agency. She offers a useful frame for thinking about the demand characteristics of various practice tasks and their informational needs. Finally, Mel Raider offers an interesting example of agency-based research designed to address the issue of familial involvement in the care and treatment of developmentally disabled family members.

Common to all the papers was an enduring commitment to pursue research in the agency context. All of these investigators are intimately familiar with the potential and liabilities of pursuing complex research questions in a constantly changing, often turbulent agency environment. Like their colleagues at the host agency, Boysville of Michigan, they passionately believe that that is precisely where social work research needs to be. Their excellent and stimulating studies presented here are proof positive of both the potential beneficial efforts of agency-based research and testimony to how much work remains to be done.

## REFERENCE

Reid, W.J. (1978) The social agency as a research machine. *Journal of Social Service Research* 2, 11-24.

# Expert Systems and Ordinary Research As Sources for Practice Guidance

John R. Schuerman

## *INTRODUCTION*

For the past two years, my colleagues and I at the Chapin Hall Center for Children at the University of Chicago and at the Juvenile Protective Association of Chicago have been engaged in an exploration of the development of expert consulting systems for child welfare decision making. An expert system is a computer program designed to give advice on decisions. These systems attempt to capture the knowledge and skill of human experts in a way that is usable by other workers. The program asks the user a series of questions about a case and then makes recommendations for action. Expert systems came out of the field of artificial intelligence and have been developed in a number of industrial, commercial, and medical applications. The most common type of expert system is based on large numbers of if-then rules.

Our project has involved work with staff of the Illinois Department of Children and Family Services and the Juvenile Protective Association. We conduct intensive interviews with experts in both agencies in an effort to understand how they arrive at decisions in child welfare cases. The decisions with which we are concerned are those that occur in cases of child abuse and neglect. We have focused on the decisions that must be made early in a case that has been reported for alleged child abuse: the decisions to indicate or

My colleagues in this work have included Steve Budde, Richard Calica, Penny Johnson, Edward Mullen, and Matthew Stagner. I am indebted to them for helpful comments on this paper. The research described in this paper has been supported by the Chicago Community Trust and the Arie and Ida Crown Memorial.

unfound a case, the assessment of risk, whether to take protective custody of the child, and what services should be provided to the child and family. The first objective of the work is to develop a computer program that can be used by relatively untrained and inexperienced child protective workers, those workers who must investigate allegations of abuse and neglect to determine their substance and recommend action.

Expert systems development tries to uncover and codify knowledge and make it available for practice decisions. Classic research, particularly evaluation and developmental research, attempts to do the same thing. In this chapter, expert systems and classic research as sources of guidance for practice activities are compared. In the following, "research" means "ordinary" research, particularly evaluative and developmental research as compared to expert systems development.

## WHEN SHOULD RESEARCH FINDINGS OR EXPERT SYSTEMS BE USED?

### Research

When can research findings be trusted as guides for practice activities? The answer to this question is usually sought by examining such things as external and internal validity and the quality of measurements. Two issues are considered here: generalizability and the applicability of aggregate findings to individual cases. To what group of individuals (or situations, etc.) do particular research findings apply? In the practice situation the question is whether such and such research findings can be applied to this case.

### Generalizability

Ideally, the generalizability of research is assured by developing a careful, operational specification of the population of interest and then sampling from that population using methods to insure that each member of the population has a known probability of being selected. With this procedure critical assumptions of inferential statistical techniques are met and the statistical procedures can be relied on to generate probabilistic statements about population characteristics.

We all know that this ideal is rarely met in real research. Populations are usually not precisely defined, often we do not randomly sample, and attrition from our nonprobabilistic samples almost always occurs in the form of nonresponse and subsequent drop-outs. As a result, the probabilities that come out of our statistical manipulations apply to some ill-understood subgroup of our original ill-defined population. In the face of these shortcomings the question is, to what group can we apply these findings, if any? To answer this question we appeal to reason. We try to figure out the extent to which the violations of accepted research practice affect the results. We develop a nonstatistical analysis making use of the characteristics of the sample and other facts to try to specify a group for which we believe the findings are likely to be true. The analysis invariably rests on one or more implicit or explicit assumptions about the relationship between the group studied and the population of interest, assumptions that are difficult to verify. In the end, it is left to the practitioner to determine whether the findings might apply to a case at hand.

## Applying Aggregate Findings to Individuals

A second problem in the application of research findings to specific cases arises from the fact that the results of an evaluation are expressed by statements such as "intervention $x$ is superior to intervention $y$ in situation $z$, $p$ percent of the time" or "intervention $x$ produces beneficial effects in $p$ percent of cases with $z$ characteristics." Usually an intervention is not universally superior or beneficial. Things do not always work out well even for the most resolutely empirical practitioner. Another way of saying this is that there invariably is variability in outcome. Thus, we do not know with certainty that the research findings will apply to a given situation.

At times it may be acceptable to simply "play the percentages," that is, it may be reasoned that although things may not work out in this case, we will use the technique that has the highest probability of success. This way of thinking works best when one is able to take a long view, when it is one's batting average at the end of the season that is most important. The approach is also reasonable when the costs of wrong decisions are not too high. However, when a child may die if you make the wrong decision about intervention it is harder to take the probabilistically long view, although even in this situation the hard-headed empiricist might insist that a cold expected benefit-cost calculation will produce the best decision. Obviously basing decisions on probabilities of success is also more acceptable the higher the probabilities of success are. If an intervention is almost 100% sure, we are far more likely to use it. Unfortunately, the evidence for most interventions is middling, often not much better than 50-50.[1]

These two problems, generalizability and the nonuniversality of findings, cause difficulties for the practitioner in determining whether or not to make use of research results in dealing with a particular case. When faced with a particular case, the practitioner may consider all of the available research but in the end must exercise at least some judgment as to whether the results might apply in this case. Research does not determine what is done but rather is used for guidance in making judgments about actions to be taken. It is hoped that the judgments will be "informed" by the research. But there will almost always remain aspects of the judgment that cannot appeal to research findings. Research takes as its program the reduction of those aspects.

## Expert Systems

In expert systems work the same basic questions arise, that is, for what cases can we expect this system to provide a recommendation and to what extent can we depend on that recommendation? At one level the specification of the population to which an expert system applies is simply a specification of the kinds of cases for which the

---

1. The situation is made more complex by the fact that various outcomes will occur at different points in time. If a child is not placed, one risks the relatively immediate but low probability of death, while if the child is placed the outcome of eventual poor adjustment may be far more likely but much more distant in time. It appears that decision makers in this situation may discount the costs and benefits of future events just as economists discount future costs and benefits.

system provides a recommendation. If the system cannot provide advice on a particular case it should report that fact, that is, it should be honest about the limits of its expertise. As with a human expert, an expert system cannot be expected to have an answer to every possible set of input data, that is, to every possible case. In this sense, the applicability of an expert system is contained in the system and can be made obvious either by examining its programming or by trying it on particular cases.

But the fact that a computer flashes a recommendation on its screen does not guarantee that the case at hand is in fact within the purview of the system, nor does it mean that the recommendation is correct. Many things may affect the applicability and quality of expert system recommendations. As we pursue expert system development, we depend on a small number of experts for our raw data. Questions can be raised about the selection of those experts: Would others consider them "experts?" Are they "representative?" Further, the adequacy of the interviewing has a substantial effect on the quality of the system. In our work interviewing the expert is an intensely interactive affair in which the interviewer is an active participant and shaper. "Interviewer bias" is thus present for good or ill. Finally, there may be problems in the adequacy of our representations of what the experts tell us, culminating in the representation that is the computer program.

Each of these pitfalls has a counterpart in ordinary research. Although I do not want to minimize these problems in expert system development, neither do I want to dwell on them. Instead I want to take up certain other issues that we have encountered which affect the applicability and quality of expert system recommendations.

## Context

Our work has involved the determination of the factors that enter into decisions about child welfare cases and the ways that those factors interact in determining a decision. We have been intrigued by the question of "contextual" factors: those factors that are external to the facts of a particular case. Such factors include organizational and political constraints on decisions, culture, availability of resources (such as particular kinds of treatment programs but also including such things as the worker's time and energy), and caseload factors (the size and composition of the caseload of the worker, office, and agency). We have thought of such factors as sources of "error variance": aspects of the situation that cause variation in decisions from the systematic bases that we are trying to uncover. These elements may also be thought of as affecting the generalizability of the system. A particular system may implicitly assume a certain context and may produce recommendations that conflict with contextual factors in other environments.

Obviously the utilization of research also encounters contextual issues. The most obvious case is when research prescribes an intervention or procedure that is impossible to implement. Less obvious is the situation in which the social circumstances of the case at hand are not the same as those of the research sample and those circumstances have important implications for the outcome of intervention with the case.

The professional culture also affects the utilization of both expert systems and research findings. The possibility of a global shift in views about practice is a major pitfall for both. Our own work has encountered this phenomenon. In the course of our efforts, the State of Illinois has climbed on the "family preservation" bandwagon. A new, large-scale program has been implemented. New services are being made available and workers are being urged to think about cases in a different way. This may cause major shifts in the way a number of decisions are made. We are having to consider the effects of new resources and new ways of thinking in our development of expert systems. The applicability of research findings may be similarly affected by shifts in professional culture.

## Individualization in Expert Systems

The problem of applying aggregate data to individual cases has its counterpart in expert systems. An expert system does not totally individualize a case. It makes a recommendation on the basis of case characteristics that the system elicits from the user. Although our systems deal with several hundred characteristics, there is a limit. Two cases can obviously have the same input data and be different on other characteristics about which the system did not inquire. It is possible that those ignored characteristics will result in the failure of the recommended intervention. In the development of the expert system our experts may have forgotten to tell us about certain infrequently occurring exceptions or may not have known about them. Put in another way, just as in the application of research findings, there may be variability in the outcomes of cases which appear similar to the expert system.

Of course the same thing may happen when you talk to a human consultant. Despite the value placed on "individualization," cases are categorized and the categories do drive intervention decisions. Beyond that, a human consultant may not think to ask an important question or may not know that the question should be asked. But critics of expert systems suggest that the human has at least one advantage over the computer: common sense. In this view, the computer is always subject to gross blunders of the sort that would never be made by a human decision maker. This is because common sense plays such a large role in human decision making in areas such as social welfare. While the computer can be taught some common sense, such a large body of it is relevant that it is impossible to capture all of it in silicon. Blunders by the expert system may be very infrequent but if the system is run on enough cases they will eventually occur.

We have discussed common sense in other papers so I do not want to explore it extensively here. We have suggested that in the end it is an empirical question as to how much common sense is necessary for decisions like those with which we are concerned, and the empirical question is yet to be answered. Nonetheless, these questions about the applicability of the recommendations of a system to a particular case lead us to suggest that the computer system be seen as a consultant providing advice and that as with research results the advice should not be taken uncritically. We insist that the human decision maker retain responsibility for the decision.

## Other Factors Affecting Utilization of Research and Expert Systems Specificity of Prescriptions

Prescriptions vary in their specificity and detail. It is one thing to say that psychotherapy should be used in this case, another to prescribe a particular technique, and quite another to specify exactly what a therapist should say and how he or she should say it in a particular situation. Both expert systems development and research must deal with the problem of determining the prescriptive specificity they wish to achieve.

Our programs have been focused on decisions such as whether to indicate an allegation of abuse and whether to take custody of a child. We have not tried to incorporate advice on the process of actually taking custody of the child. Shortly we will turn to the decision regarding services to be provided to children and their families and there we will need to squarely face the problem of specificity of recommendations.

We are not striving to produce a social work robot, but we do think that we should be as specific as possible in our prescriptions. However, there are undoubtedly limits to how specific we can get in developing social welfare expert systems. One way to think about these limits is in terms of the distinction between knowledge and skill. The performance of most professional activities requires both knowledge and skill. By skill is meant those aspects of performance that are difficult or impossible to capture in verbal description. Knowledge can be taught but skill must be acquired through experience. Knowledge is standardized while skill is spontaneous. Knowledge can be tested while skill must be observed. Skill has elements of "intuition." The successful implementation of recommendations, whether from computers, research, or human consultants, usually requires skill. Skill is also required in the collection of data that the expert system requires, a topic which will be discussed later. It is not yet clear the extent to which expert systems can incorporate skill.

Another issue that arises in determining the level of specificity of prescriptions concerns the amount of information required for various levels of specificity. The recommendation to take custody of a child might be made on the basis of a relatively limited set of data while advice on how to go about taking custody would likely require more information about the family.

### When Do Reasons Matter?

There is a common response by a practitioner to the question of whether a recommendation is appropriate in a particular situation: "it depends." That is, whether the action should be taken depends on other factors that have not been specified. Often "it depends" concerns the reasons for a particular condition, how the condition arose, or the causes of the condition. For example, it may be believed that the way one treats drug addiction depends on the reasons the individual takes drugs.

The question of when reasons matter has plagued practitioners and researchers for a long time. The quest for causes can, of course, lead to infinite regress. We are limited by the state of our knowledge in the extent to which we can pursue this regress and most people would not think it sensible to seek explanations for all interpersonal behavior in the electro-chemical processes of the brain. Short of that, there is much disagreement as to how far to pursue causes.

So far our response to this problem is somewhat tautological: reasons matter when the action to be taken depends on them. However, this response is not totally without meaning. Practitioners often seek a complete diagnostic understanding of a case even when much of that diagnostic formulation has no bearing on decisions about what is to be done. It is clear from our work that extensive exploration of causes is sometimes not necessary for making certain decisions. If a young child has been severely injured by a caretaker, our experts take custody regardless of the family dynamics that led to the injury. If the injury is less severe, the circumstances surrounding the incident are explored. Of course, even in the case of a severe injury where custody is taken, further actions in the case may depend on the reasons for the incident and how it reflects functioning of the family. Hence, we try to keep the various decisions that must be made on a case separate (while recognizing their interactions) and we try to keep straight the specific facts that bear directly on each decision.

So far our systems have very little etiologic knowledge. We are concerned with producing systems that provide recommendations for action. The assumption is that a given set of facts calls for a particular action, hence deep diagnostic understanding is not required. Were we to attempt to develop programs to provide diagnostic formulations we would no doubt have to endow them with understanding of the etiology of human problems.

## Judgments and Data

I want next to take up the question of the kinds of data that are requested of the users of expert system programs. Our programs derive recommendations on the basis of responses to questions they ask. The problem has to do with the level of judgment that the answers require or, alternatively, the level of detail of the questions. For example, do we ask, "Is the client hostile to the worker?" or do we instead ask questions about various indicators of hostility and then let the program determine whether hostility is present?

In our work we have assumed that it is desirable to incorporate inferences into the program. The idea is to open up these inferences to examination and then to standardize them. We hope that the inferences are correct but at least we know how they are being made (that should be evident in the programming of the system). This approach results in our striving for input data that involves as little judgment as possible and thus is fine-grained and detailed.

However, a number of difficulties are encountered in implementing this ideal. A lot of requests for highly detailed specifics may strain the tolerance of the user who might want simply to tell the system that the client is hostile. Beyond that, it is quite difficult to uncover the data that underlie some judgments or a judgment may involve exceedingly complex interactions of data. So far we have dealt with this problem on an ad hoc basis. Where pushing below a judgment appears likely to be fruitful we will do so, while other questions the program asks are left at a relatively abstract level, with the idea that we may come back to them later for further analysis.

In research, similar problems are encountered. Characteristics are measured using indirect indicators and sometimes we even measure "surrogate" variables that we hope are highly correlated with the characteristics we really want. Usually the variables we want are more abstract than the data that we actually gather. Because of the indirectness of the estimation of variable values we must worry about the adequacy of these estimations. Hence we properly obsess about the reliability, validity, and discrimination of measurements.

If our measures pass psychometric evaluation we are then able to go on to look at the central results of our study.

A similar approach might well be taken in expert systems work. The judgments that we ask users to make in responding to the program might be subjected to reliability testing on both a within- and between-judge basis. Such reliability testing is subject to problems similar to those in reliability testing of research instruments, that is, reliability estimates generated in one situation may not apply to others. It is also unclear as to what standards should be adopted for acceptable reliabilities. Since the judgments are being used to determine actions on particular cases, the required reliability should be quite high, just as higher reliability is needed when a psychological test is used for individual diagnosis rather than in research involving a group of cases. Validity determination in judgments required by expert systems may be a more complex matter. In one sense, validity is determined by how the judgment is used by the system and thus has to do with the accuracy of the entire system.

Even with low-level judgments that have high reliability, the data that are provided to an expert system will sometimes be in error. Of course if the user has the facts all wrong there is no way that the system can come up with the right answer. But it is desirable that the system not be too sensitive to small amounts of error (such a system can be said to be "robust" in the face of input error). This can be done by having the system confirm certain key facts or having it require multiple indicators of those facts.

The issue of the character of the data that are input to an expert system again raises the question of the role of skill. As in the implementation of the recommendations (the output) of the system, the quality of the input may be affected by the skill of the user. Skill may enter into the making of judgments that are required in answering the program's questions. At least equally important is the skill involved in gathering the data that the program wants. The process of investigating an allegation of child abuse is a matter of gathering data and then making decisions. Gathering the data takes a lot of skill and it is possible that that is the biggest part of the job. We have not yet attempted to develop programs that will advise on the process of data gathering and as I suggested in the above discussion of skill, there may be substantial limitations to the development of such a program.

### Dynamic Data

The hermeneutic school has tried to impress on us the fact that all observation is interpretative in nature; we dynamically interact with our perceptions in endowing them with meaning. There are no "pristine" facts. While that may be strictly true, as suggested above, some observations are more interpretative than others.

However, we may influence data in another way. Whether or not a child has been abused can be thought of as a fixed fact (although the process of fixing it as a fact is loaded with interpretation) while the "risk" to the child is likely to change. In fact, reducing risk is a major task of the child welfare worker. Hence, as a number of writers have pointed out, the assessment of risk may depend on what can or will be done to affect risk. "Risk" refers to the future, hence, it depends on what will or might happen, including how the worker and the service system respond. Not only are the data dynamic, but we contribute to their changeability. It is not entirely clear how this phenomena should be incorporated into expert systems.

## THE UTILIZATION OF RESEARCH
## IN EXPERT SYSTEMS AND VICE VERSA

I turn now to the utilization of research in the development of expert systems and how work on expert systems can be used in conventional research efforts. Our work in expert systems development has been preeminently qualitative in nature. The data come from intensive interviews with a few expert informants telling us how they make decisions. We have not attempted to systematically study the sources of the knowledge of our experts but it is likely that formal research findings play a relatively small part in that knowledge. The rules the experts give us seem to be based on practice experience (to that extent they are broadly "empirical") and their interpretations of fragments of theory. Law, practices in the agency, and trends in the field of child welfare also play a large role. Of course, formal research findings may well have had at least an indirect impact on all of these sources of knowledge.

Hence, we have not made extensive use of research findings in our work, although we do try to stay abreast of research on risk assessment in child welfare. Some expert system development, in fields in which the science is better developed, is based almost entirely on formally verified empirical findings. In our view, the extent to which decisions in child welfare can be based on existing research findings is limited. Research has uncovered certain factors that are associated with decisions made by workers and with outcomes of cases, but the "R-squares" are not high, that is, there is a lot of unexplained variation in the criteria variables. At times we do ask our experts about factors identified in previous research to make sure that they have considered possibly important aspects, but the research findings are not taken as determinative.

As our work progresses it is possible that we will make more use of existing research findings. In particular, we may use them to help determine "certainty factors." Many expert systems (including those we are building) incorporate the notion that recommendations have varying degrees of certainty attached to them. Certainty enters into the programs in two ways, the certainty of the data provided by the user (the user is asked for the certainty of a response to a question by the program) and the certainty of the conclusions reached by a rule. It is possible that we may utilize research findings to help in setting some of these rule certainties.

Classic research methods will again play a major part when we come to the validation of an expert system. The first step in validation is to determine agreement of the system recommendations with those of a panel of human experts. It would obviously be desirable to go beyond that to study the outcomes of cases in which decisions were based on the system's recommendations. Such a study would, of course, require comparison groups in which other decisions were made. Expert system validation studies of this kind would involve classic large sample designs.

It is hoped that "ordinary" research will benefit from expert systems work as well. Our understanding of the nature of decision making in social welfare should be substantially enhanced by the intensive and detailed examination of decision processes that is the core of expert systems development. Beyond that, the work will uncover many areas needing investigation; in particular, it will uncover critical assumptions and conclusions made by human experts that are not supported by established evidence. Because of the detailed examination involved it should be possible to pose these assumptions and conclusions in crisply verifiable form, thereby facilitating their testing through research.

## *SUMMARY*

Expert systems and research findings as sources of guidance for practice have been compared and a number of considerations that affect utilization of both, sometimes in different ways, have been suggested. Determining whether research findings should be used in a particular case requires consideration of generalizability and the applicability of aggregate findings. The applicability of an expert system to a case depends on whether the case is included in the system's "population" and the degree of individualization of the system. Judgments about applicability may be refined through replication of research and through validation of expert systems.

Other factors affecting utilization of both expert systems and research findings include the specificity of prescriptions, the extent to which cause is explicated or incorporated, and the degree to which judgment is required in determining the "facts" that are used in the decision-making process, whether the decision is aided by research findings or an expert system. Finally, I have suggested ways that expert system development and "ordinary" research might contribute to each other.

## BIBLIOGRAPHY

Dreyfus, Hubert L. and Dreyfus, Stuart E., "From Socrates to Expert Systems: The Limits of Calculative Reasoning," *Technology in Society*, 1984, pp. 217-235.

Dreyfus, Hubert L. and Dreyfus, Stuart E., *Mind over Machine*, New York: Free Press, 1985.

Feissman, James R. and Schultz, Roger D., "Verification and Validation of Expert Systems," *AI Expert*, February, 1988, pp. 26-33.

Johnson, Penny and Stagner, Matthew, "Understanding and Capturing Expertise in Social Work: Developing Expert Systems in Child Welfare," unpublished paper, Chapin Hall Center for Children, Chicago, March 1989.

Marcot, Bruce, "Testing Your Knowledge Base," *AI Expert*, July, 1987, pp. 42-47.

Mullen, Edward J. and Schuerman, John R., "Expert Systems and the Development of Knowledge in Social Welfare," paper presented at the Conference on Empiricism in Clinical Practice, Great Barrington, MA, August 1988.

Schuerman, John R., "Passion, Analysis, and Technology: *The Social Service Review* Lecture," *Social Service Review*, Vol. 61, No. 1, March 1987.

Schuerman, John R., "Expert Consulting Systems in Social Welfare," *Social Work Research and Abstracts*, Vol. 23, No. 3, pp. 14-18, Fall 1987.

Schuerman, John R., Mullen, Edward J., Stagner, Matthew, and Johnson, Penny, "First Generation Systems in Social Welfare," paper presented at the First International Conference on Human Service Information Technology Applications, Birmingham, England, September 1987.

# Evolution and Future Development of Clinical Research Utilization in Agency Settings

Betty J. Blythe

Clinical research is one of several terms which has been employed to denote a number of similar or overlapping concepts. As discussed here, clinical research refers to the process of incorporating research and measurement practices and principles into micro practice by direct service practitioners for the purpose of improving their practice. Further, these applications can occur in any or all phases of direct practice: in assessment, treatment planning, implementation, termination, and follow-up. Because this chapter considers the evolution of clinical research utilization in agencies, however, this definition necessarily shifts a bit as different stages in its evolution are discussed. For instance, the application of single-subject designs by practitioners is a narrower but common conception of clinical research. Empirical clinical practice is another conception of clinical research that typically refers to evaluating one's effectiveness and using practice methods that have empirical support.

This chapter focuses primarily on the past decade and then considers prospects for the future. To put the events of the 1980s into a context, however, activities of the 1970s occasionally will be noted. While the emphasis is on recent events, significant influences on clinical research did occur prior to this time in social work and elsewhere (Tripodi, 1988).

Although the ultimate goal of this clinical research movement is for agency-based social work practitioners to routinely evaluate their practice, to date relatively limited activity in pursuit of this goal has actually occurred in agencies. Most of the support and effort has been put forth by social work academicians. In general, many social work educators were enthusiastic about the idea of integrating research and practice concepts to evaluate social work effectiveness. They responded by writing several papers endorsing the idea and books describing how to apply the single-case methodology. Not all members of the profession were supportive of this movement, however, and a strong debate developed in the literature. Proponents of clinical research also developed curriculum innovations to facilitate the task of teaching clinical research methods. To attempt to institutionalize the ideas, the Council on Social Work Education developed guidelines for graduate education. Methodological changes also occurred over time, although these are less clearly documented. All of these developments are reviewed and analyzed in the following sections. The paper concludes with a discussion of the current situation and suggested directions for the future to enhance the adoption of clinical research methods in agency settings.

## SCHOLARLY WRITING

In the early 1970s, a call for accountability in social work practice provided some of the impetus for our current interest in clinical research (Briar, 1973). At about the same time, an increased application of single-subject designs by researchers investigating the effects of operant behavioral interventions highlighted the availability of the methodology (Agras et al., 1971; Ulman and Krasner, 1965). While behavioral researchers, largely from psychology, psychiatry, and related fields, were applying the single-subject methodology in scientific research, members of the social work professions suggested that the same methodology could be employed by practitioners to evaluate the outcomes of their individual practices (Howe, 1974).

A major response to this call for accountability through the application of single-subject designs was seen in the preparation of several publications. Numerous social work authors have written descriptions explaining the steps to be followed in carrying out single-case evaluations with their clients. Although similar efforts were carried out by psychologists and members of other professions (Barlow, Hayes and Nelson, 1984; Barlow and Hersen, 1984; Kazdin, 1980), much more activity in this regard can be found in social work. An early contribution came from Jayaratne and Levy (1979) who wrote a text aimed primarily at preparing social workers to use single-subject designs in their clinical practice. Several texts followed by other social work educators and researchers (Bloom and Fischer, 1982; Tripodi and Epstein, 1980; Wodarski, 1981).

In addition to these texts, the social work literature also contains considerable debate on the relative merit, appropriateness, and feasibility of empirical clinical practice in general, and of applying single-case methods to monitor client outcomes in particular. From the proponents of empirical clinical practice, several reasons have been given for encouraging and educating social workers to apply single-case methodology in their work with clients. The two more general arguments are that the methodology allows them to determine their effectiveness with individual clients or client units, and to design and validate new, effective social work methods by repeatedly testing specific interventions with similar clients (Blythe and Briar, 1985). Several other, more specific reasons also have been suggested. Levy (1983), among others, argues that the methodology is helpful in requiring that workers clearly specify their interventions and in providing continuous feedback on client progress toward goal attainment. Taken together, these two sets of information allow practitioners to more quickly and easily revise their treatment plans, when necessary. Levy further asserts that the continuous feedback to clients may serve as an intervention itself, insofar as it encourages them to continue their work or to work harder. Nelson (1988) observes that the process of applying single-case designs to a particular case has several indirect benefits. The worker needs to think about goals and select interventions more systematically and carefully than often is the case. In addition, the client problem is understood in great detail, as the worker attempts to clearly define it so that it can be measured. Finally, this continued monitoring of the client problem may help the worker and/or client to uncover patterns that help to explain fluctuations in the problem. It should be noted that, for the most part, these suggested benefits may seem to be sound, but have not been empirically tested. Ivanoff and her colleagues have summarized the position of those favoring empirical clinical practice as follows:

(They) believe ethical, effective, and ultimately efficient service can be provided only through applying empirically derived interventions, systematically collecting data, and specifying goals, objectives, and intervention methods. The information gained through this process enables practitioners to build a sound body of practice knowledge. (Ivanoff, Blythe, and Briar, 1987, p. 293)

Meanwhile, the case against empirical clinical practice is based on several arguments. Heineman-Peiper (1985), among others, suggests that single-case research design is not appropriate for clinical practice. Others raise concerns about relying on quantitative research, arguing that qualitative methods can be just as informative, if not more so (Ruckdeschel and Farris, 1981). Davis (1985) suggests that the empirical clinical practice movement reflects the "male voice" and is another example of the suppression of the "female voice" in social work. In her view, qualitative research reflects this female voice and is more congruent with social work practice. Others such as Thomas (1978) and Kagle (1982) contend that applying single-subject designs in practice will yield a distorted view of practice and may even compromise service itself. To summarize:

opponents of empirical-practice models cite philosophical incongruities between evaluation and clinical work, criticize the logical empiricist model of science as an appropriate model in social work research, and express concerns about sacrificing methodological rigor and services. (Ivanoff, Blythe, and Briar, 1987, p. 293)

### Current Situation

The production of texts on single-subject design seems to be slowing down. There may be a trend toward research texts that take a broader, or at least different, view of clinical research (see for example, Blythe and Tripodi, in press; Hudson and Nurius, in press). It is hoped that these new offerings will not simply summarize or repeat the work of the past, but will advance our thinking with regard to the needs of practitioners who are attempting to apply clinical research methods in practice.

The debate about empirical clinical practice seems to be slowing. One review suggests that the debaters have tended to adopt extreme positions, which primarily serves to intensify the debate (Ivanoff, Blythe, and Briar, 1987). Unfortunately, it appears that there has been little resolution of differences. Since most of the debate was carried out by educators, it is likely that these differences influence efforts to prepare practitioners to conduct clinical research.

## CHANGES IN CURRICULUM

Another related set of activities observed in social work, and also aimed at encouraging the application of clinical research methods by practitioners, was carried out in schools of social work. Here, several schools developed curriculum innovations to prepare social workers to use the methodology. The intent of most of these curricula was that the trained workers, sometimes referred to as clinician scientists, practitioner-scientists, practitioner-researchers, or personal scientists, would routinely evaluate their practices, (Blythe, 1988; Briar, 1980; Conte and Levy, 1980; Grinnell, 1985). Several of these educational programs are described in a monograph by Weinbach and Rubin (1980), one of the products of the Project on Research Utilization in Social Work Education conducted by the Council on Social Work Education in the late 1970s.

Downs and Robertson (1983) outlined, in general terms, the four possible approaches to teaching students to use research methods in practice. These are (1) pair the required courses in research methods and practice; (2) offer research and practice courses separately, but emphasize empirically based practice (presumably in both sequences); (3) teach research courses tied to a specific practice focus; and (4) teach a special course on the "clinician-researcher" model. Similar to the first approach, the University of Washington School of Social Work has offered what may be the most comprehensive and longest running program attempting to prepare students to evaluate their practice (Gottlieb and Richey, 1980; Levy, 1987). Here, students in the master's program enroll in combined methods and research courses for the second and third quarters of their first year.

The two courses attempt to integrate single-subject research methods into the practice content. In addition, these two courses are tied to specific field practicum sites that provide opportunities for students to carry out single-case evaluations in their practice.

During the later 1970s and into this decade, much of the activity around teaching clinical research methods involved experimental programs such as the University of Washington's. In addition, several attempts were made to evaluate the effectiveness of these curriculum innovations. Some studies examined the curriculum innovations in terms of their effects on attitudes or beliefs, yet the question of central importance seems to relate to their effect on behavior (Richey, Berlin, and Jaffee, 1979; Siegel, 1985). In other words, do workers trained in these integrated research and practice courses evaluate their practice? While the results are somewhat mixed, the general consensus of the research is that these courses have a short-term effect. Whether this effect is maintained over time apparently relates, in part, to the amount of support for clinical research in the worker's agency environment (Blythe, 1984; Richey, Blythe, and Berlin, 1987; Simons, 1987).

### Current Situation

Since the effect of changes in curriculum are virtually impossible to separate from the effect of changes in educational policies, the current situation with regard to curriculum issues will be discussed after the following section.

## CHANGES IN EDUCATIONAL POLICIES

Another educational development related to clinical research occurred in the first part of the last decade, the adoption of a new set of Guidelines for Graduate Schools of Social Work Curriculum by the Council on Social Work Education. In the area if research preparation, these guidelines stipulated that "the professional foundation content in research should thus provide skills that will take students beyond the role of consumers of research and prepare them systematically to evaluate their own practice and contribute to the generation of knowledge for practice" (Council on Social Work

Education, 1982). Subsequent debate questioning the feasibility of the second goal embedded in those guidelines, the generation of knowledge for practice, resulted in its being omitted in 1986 (Commission on Accreditation, 1987).

The actual impact of this move by the Council remains largely unknown. Given the disagreement within the profession regarding the relative merits and appropriateness of evaluating practice with quantitative methods, some unevenness in operationalizing the guidelines is to be expected (Smith, DeWeaver, and Kilpatrick, 1986). Moreover, some schools are just now completing their first reviews under these guidelines. Nonetheless, a recent study sheds some light on how well those guidelines are accepted by graduate schools of social work (Fraser, Lewis, and Norman, 1989). Data were collected from all 90 graduate schools accredited in 1987. With regard to the Council on Social Work Education requirement that students be prepared to evaluate their own practice, a little over 80% of the respondents agreed with this requirement "quite a lot" or "completely." The new guidelines have, in some way and in varying degrees, changed social work education at the master's level, with 61.5% of the respondents indicating that curriculum revisions were made in response to the guidelines. Unfortunately, the preliminary report of this study does not clearly define the nature of these revisions, nor does it adequately specify how the guidelines are being implemented by schools. Thus, some deans or research sequence chairs (the respondents in this study) may personally agree with the guidelines, yet their personal beliefs may have had only a limited effect on the curriculum.

### Current Situation

Although the guidelines should have "institutionalized" the testing of practice evaluation methods into social work curricula, a more pessimistic possibility is that the guidelines simply led some schools to relegate the content to already crowded, required research courses. While the above-cited data do not appear to directly address this question, Fraser and his colleagues do note that only a little over one-third (or 35) of the schools have practice faculty involved in planning or delivering some of the research content. Does this mean that nearly two-thirds of the schools have left the task of teaching students to evaluate practice to research instructors who *may* know little about practice and often have more interest in and greater knowledge of more traditional approaches to research and evaluation? Moreover, it is more difficult although not impossible, to teach students to integrate research methods into practice in research courses which typically spend less time dealing with practice issues and more time on research principles and methods.

In general, one hears less about schools mounting new, innovative methods of preparing students to conduct clinical research. In fact, some schools have abandoned their experimental efforts to combine classes on research and practice (sometimes in combination with the field), usually because it is difficult to staff the courses. There simply are not enough instructors who are qualified to teach both research and practice in an integrated fashion to meet the demand. Or, in other cases, faculty and/or administration find it too confining to tie up so many faculty work load credits in just one area of the curriculum.

Finally, there is some anecdotal evidence to suggest that faculty at many schools still do not share a common understanding of the intent of these guidelines. For instance, discussions among faculty preparing for reaccreditation by the Council on Social Work Education often conclude that since practice classes teach empirically based and theoretically based methods, the above-mentioned guidelines are met. Yet this in no way means that their graduates are prepared "systematically to evaluate their own practice." In part, this lack of clarity can be traced to the unfinished debate over the merits and appropriateness of preparing practitioners to carry out clinical research.

## *CHANGES IN THE METHODOLOGY*

Interestingly, it seems that as they tried to prepare students to use single-subject design methods, particularly in classes requiring that students actually evaluate one or more of their clients, educators realized that some of the earlier "requirements" of the methodology had to be modified for clinical practice. In retrospect this is not surprising, given that our initial teaching and writing about single-subject methods was primarily based on the experiences of behavioral researchers applying the methodology in situations allowing more control over both the manipulation of the independent variable and the collection of data related to the dependent variable. Since we had not fully pilot tested the methods we were teaching our students, several mistakes were made. Some of these have been identified, some may still be continued in some classrooms.

An early example of one of these errors relates to the discussion of design. Because we were basing our teaching and writing on the experiences of experimental researchers, we tended to emphasize more rigorous designs allowing greater control over threats to internal validity. As our students described their frustrating experiences or even their surprise that we would make certain suggestions, we educators came to realize that designs such as the withdrawal design rarely fit clinical practice. If a client has found some relief, presumably due to a worker's intervention, the client and often the worker are hesitant to intentionally withdraw the intervention to see if the problem returns and can once again be controlled by reintroducing the intervention. Moreover, many interventions cannot be withdrawn. Thus, over time, we tempered our remarks regarding the application of more rigorous designs and began to promote the basic AB design as the design of choice. Nonetheless, we undoubtedly lost some earlier "converts" who found our suggestions to be out of touch with practice. For programs in which the methodological concepts were only discussed theoretically (perhaps by instructors who had not tried to use the methodology themselves), and students were not required to apply the concepts in their field work, it is likely that some "misguided" guidelines were allowed to perpetuate.

Another problem experienced by individuals attempting to teach and apply the methodology in social work practice relates to the issue of measurement. Essentially, practitioners find it difficult to assess known measures that are easy to use in a clinical setting and sensitive enough to discern modest improvements or deterioration with regard to treatment goals. In fact, there are some data to suggest that this is a major stumbling block encountered by workers attempting to evaluate their practice (Blythe, 1984; Richey, Blythe, and Berlin, 1987). Similar to the problem in the area of designs, practitioners have received some mixed messages about the necessity of having rigorous measures. Teachers and methodologists have advocated for direct measures with high reliability and validity that are sensitive to the client problem. Often standardized paper-and-pencil measures have established reliability and validity, but may not be closely enough related to the treatment goals to detect client change. Behavioral measures may be more direct, but reliability may be difficult to establish. And, behavioral measures usually are not helpful when goals relate to client feelings or cognitions. Meanwhile, other social work goals only require a dichotomous measure, such as a goal "to enroll a child in YMCA swimming classes" or "to place a client in a nursing home" (Blythe and Tripodi, in press). Our teaching and writing on evaluating practice typically overlooks such goals, possibly leading practitioners to conclude that these goals are less important indicators of success or outcome, an incorrect conclusion in the opinion of this author.

### Current Situation

These are only a few examples of the methodological concerns that have been uncovered. While some of these "realizations" and improvements that occurred as single-subject methods were being taught did find their way into the literature, many more did not. Many innovations have been developed to facilitate the use of the methodology by students and practitioners, but these innovations rarely are disseminated through conventional means such as professional journals (Blythe et al., 1985). For example, instructors have developed guidelines for dealing with concerns that clients are "fudging" data and for making data recording procedures unobtrusive. These innovations were developed in response to difficulties workers and students faced as they attempted to implement the methodology. While most practitioners would likely find this information helpful, it rarely is disseminated to a large audience in the profession.

More importantly, much work remains in this area. To some extent, educators and authors probably are continuing to overlook application problems posed by the existing methodology and to promote some procedures that do not fit with most agency practice. These errors can be perpetuated because so much of the activity has been conducted in the laboratory-like conditions of the classroom rather than in actual agency conditions.

## *ACTIVITIES IN AGENCIES*

As noted earlier, the bulk of the profession's efforts to advance clinical research activity has occurred in educational settings. A few researchers have set up interesting, laboratory-like experiments in agencies, but these rarely last beyond the involvement of the researcher (Dolan and Vourlekis, 1983; Mutschler, 1984).

Nonetheless, there have been some notable efforts initiated by agency staff to systematically conduct some type of clinical research. Boysville provides a prime example of this in its management information system known as BOMIS (Grasso, Epstein, and Tripodi, 1988). Among other things, this system routinely collects client demographics, family assessments, staff ratings of client behavior, intervention information, and client change information to evaluate their structural family treatment intervention. Follow-up data are collected up to 18 months following termination. Information gathered by the system is "fed back" to treatment staff and supervisors for their use. In addition to meeting some information needs of line staff and managers, BOMIS also yields data for ongoing research on practice within the agency.

Another example is the Sage Hill Camp Behavior Rating System which is used at the Sage Hill Camp in Vermont and (in a modified version) at Childhaven in Seattle, Washington. This system monitors, on a daily basis, children's moods and interpersonal relations with peer and staff (Durkin, 1988). The system was developed because traditional clinical records, which were problem-oriented, were found not to be helpful clinical tools. Moreover, the rating system was developed expressly for these populations, so that it is more likely to fit the needs of staff. In addition to clinical applications, the data resulting from the system can be aggregated to serve managerial and program evaluation needs.

### Current Situation

Some notable and significant examples of clinical research, especially that which is institutionalized within agencies, can be found. Overall, the incidence of individual practitioners evaluating their practice is a spotty occurrence. There seems to be some increased interest on the part of agencies, at the level of both clinical and administrative staff, to develop methods of evaluating their work. This interest appears to be independent of the urging and exhortation from the literature, or our educational efforts.

## FUTURE DIRECTIONS TO ADVANCE
## AND PROMOTE CLINICAL RESEARCH

While considerable activity has occurred in the area of promoting clinical research in agencies, more work remains. This section considers future endeavors that might encourage the wider application of clinical research methods in agency settings. Suggestions are made for scholarly writing, graduate education, computer technology, agency activities, and methodological development.

### Scholarly Writing

Much more of the professional literature needs to reflect and document the experiences of agencies and agency-based practitioners who are conducting clinical research. Despite an acknowledged need, the profession has not developed a newsletter or other easily accessed publication outlet that would allow practitioners to readily share the results of their clinical research efforts. It also would be helpful to hear about the experiences of both individual practitioners and agencies with regard to the types of clinical research activities they are engaging in, the perceived benefits of such activities, the stumbling blocks, and any supports that enable them to conduct clinical research.

Other writing needs to move beyond simply describing how practitioners can go about carrying out single-case evaluations and reflect a broader orientation to clinical research. Moreover, these "new" descriptions of clinical research should emphasize the research and measurement tools that are most useful in agency work, as indicated by the experiences of those actually applying the methods in agencies or field placement settings. The experiences of practitioners and teachers of clinical research with regard to techniques and aids for dealing with potential implementation problems also need to be published. The literature contains some examples of information systems and ways in which computers can support clinical research efforts, yet there probably is more activity in the field. Perhaps a special issue of a journal could be devoted to reporting agency examples of these applications. Finally, case studies and guidelines for using clinical research data in case decision-making and in analyzing treatment failures would be helpful contributions to the literature.

### Agency Activities

In general, I believe that much more of our efforts and activities should be focused here. There is some difficulty with this suggestion insofar as the group of people most concerned about clinical research come from academia, yet the intended target is agency practitioners. With some notable exceptions, it has been difficult for academicians to become involved in agency practice to the extent that they can influence research operations beyond the stage of a demonstration project. One area in which academics can participate is in conducting research on clinical research activity in agencies. For example, agencies which are already involved in considerable clinical research activity could be used to examine some of the hypotheses about the ways in which clinical research potentially improves practice.

More of the leadership in this area may have to come from agencies. To the extent that there actually is an increased interest among agency staff in evaluating their work, the activity level will increase. It would be desirable if agencies with more experience, such as Boysville, could provide consultation to other agencies. A conference for those agencies involved in clinical research and those interested in developing a clinical research agenda would be one avenue for encouraging some cross-agency exchange of information.

## Education

Despite having an ultimate goal of preparing practitioners to routinely evaluate their individual practice in agency settings, educators have rarely focused their efforts on the agency and, in particular, on agency administrators. The importance of educating administrators about the arguments in support of clinical research as well as the administrative and agency benefits of such research have been explicated (Briar and Blythe, 1985). Yet, educational efforts to promote clinical research have not taken into account the fact that administrative support of practitioners' research efforts is important, if not crucial. In short, the logic and approach has been somewhat simplistic and narrowly focused. Crudely stated, social work practice will benefit from the routine application of clinical research tools (whatever they might be). Therefore, we should teach social work students how to use these tools and expect that they will do so upon graduation, thereby revolutionizing the profession. In fact, we have overlooked a crucial ingredient — the involvement of administrators from both academia and practice. Administrative students need to be informed that this technology exists, how it potentially affects direct practice, and how the results of clinical research efforts can be used to inform agency planning and evaluation efforts (Briar and Blythe, 1985).

Since computerized information systems seem to be a logical outcome of more elaborate clinical research activity in agencies, educational efforts should focus on both direct practice and administrative involvement with such systems. Direct practice students need to be aware of some of the computer applications and information system components that could assist them in their daily work. Such knowledge would help them influence agency decisions as computer systems are being developed and expanded. Administrative students also need to be exposed to content explaining how information systems can and should be sensitive to treatment issues and practice decisions. Moreover, administrative students need to realize the pitfalls in using information systems to evaluate staff performance. For example, Boysville's system is generally well-received by staff, yet staff are somewhat reluctant to have their efforts evaluated by the measurement tools providing data to the system

(Grasso, Epstein, and Tripodi, 1988). When such systems actually are used to evaluate staff performance and this evaluation has a somewhat punitive connotation, staff typically begin to provide less reliable information to the system.

Ideally, educators will emphasize clinical research tools and methods that are directly applicable to agency practice. Clinical research should encompass, but go beyond, single-case evaluation methods. To the extent possible, this content should be taught in practice courses or from the perspective of applying them in direct practice, to enhance practice.

### Computer Technology

Since so much of the activity in this area has involved development of technology to meet the individual needs of a specific agency or to address a particular application, we do not have a general sense of our knowledge level, the areas of strength, and the gaps. An overall review and evaluation of the developments in this area would be helpful. There likely are more ways in which clinical research activities could be supported and enhanced by computer technology, but it would seem useful to avoid haphazard development and "reinventing the wheel" many times over in several agencies by systematically evaluating the available knowledge and technology in some way.

### Methodology

Methodologists could assist these efforts by specifying some of the areas and ways in which practitioners can depart from standard prescriptions for using research tools and yet not overly compromise the research aspect of their efforts. As one example of such a contribution, Hayes discusses conditions under which multiple-baseline studies can occur using clients seen at different points in time (Hayes, 1981).

While it often has been suggest that qualitative research methods are well suited to clinical practice, there are few specific descriptions of how that might occur. Again, methodological work explicating the possible applications of qualitative methods in direct social work practice in agencies would further our efforts here.

Methodologists also could develop additional tools to assist administrators in using the results of clinical research efforts to inform planning and program evaluation efforts. While the suggestions for aggregating single-case data with meta-analysis strategies are helpful, more work remains in this area (Gingerich, 1984). Guidelines for interfacing clinical research data with program evaluation activities and case examples would be informative (Jayaratne, Tripodi, and Talsma, 1988).

## CONCLUSION

Clearly, those of us who envision agencies routinely using clinical research data for decision-making at all levels will have to exercise patience for some time to come. We should not grow overly frustrated with the pace of development and abandon our efforts. As stated repeatedly here, it is critical that we redirect our efforts toward agencies. Everything that is proposed and taught with regard to clinical research should be examined in light of its applicability for agency-based practitioners. Exemplary agency experiences with clinical research also should be studied carefully to identify lessons for other agencies. Thus, if we always keep in mind the intended uses of these clinical research methods and, whenever possible, pilot test these methods in agency settings, we are more likely to develop and support methods that can be applied in practice.

## REFERENCES

Agras, W. S., Leitenberg, H., Barlow, D. H., Curtis, N. A., Edwards, J. A. & Wright, D. E. (1971). Relaxation in systematic desensitization. *Archives of General Psychiatry, 25*, 511-514.

Barlow, D. H., Hayes, S.C., & Nelson, R. O. (1984). *The scientist practitioner: Research and accountability in clinical and educational settings*. New York: Pergamon Press.

Barlow, D. H., & Hersen, M. (1984). *Single-case experimental designs: Strategies for studying behavior change* (2nd ed.). New York: Pergamon Press.

Bloom, M., & Fischer, J. (1982). *Evaluating practice: Guidelines for the accountable professional*. Englewood Cliffs, NJ: Prentice-Hall.

Blythe, B. J. (1984, November). An examination of practice evaluation activities among social workers. Paper presented at the 18th Annual Convention for the Advancement of Behavioral Therapy, Philadelphia, November 1984.

Blythe, B. J. (1988). Applying practice research methods in intensive family preservation services. In J. K. Whittaker, J. Kinney, E. M. Tracy, & C. Booth (Eds.), *Improving practice technology with high risk families: Lessons from the "Homebuilders" Social Work Education Project* (pp. 147-163). Seattle, WA: University of Washington Center for Social Welfare Research.

Blythe, B. J., Ivanoff, A. M., Jayaratne, S., & Richey, C. A. (1985, March). Teaching social work students to evaluate their practice. Paper presented at the Annual Program Meeting of the Council on Social Work Education, Detroit, MI.

Blythe, B. J., & Briar, S. (1985). Developing empirically based models of practice. *Social Work, 30,* 483-488.

Blythe, B. J., & Tripodi, T. (in press). *Measurement in direct social work practice: Guidelines for practitioners.* Newbury Park, CA: Sage.

Briar, S. (1973). Effective social work intervention in direct practice: Implications for education. In *Facing the Challenge* (pp. 17-30). New York: Council on Social Work Education.

Briar, S. (1980). Toward the integration of practice and research. In D. Fanshel (Ed.), *Future of social work research.* Washington, DC: National Association of Social Workers.

Briar, S., & Blythe, B. J. (1985). Agency support for evaluating outcomes of social work services. *Administration in Social Work, 9*(2), 25-36.

Commission on Accreditation. (1987). *Handbook of accreditation standards and procedures* (rev. ed.). New York: Council on Social Work Education.

Conte, J. R., & Levy, R. L. (1980). Problems and issues in implementing the clinical-research model of practice in educational and clinical settings. *Journal of Education for Social Work, 16*(3), 60-66.

Council on Social Work Education. (1982). Curriculum policy statement for the master's and baccalaureate degree programs in social work education. *Social Work Education Reporter, 30,* 5-12.

Davis, L. V. (1985). Female and male voices in social work. *Social Work, 30,* 106-113.

Dolan, M. M., & Vourlekis, B. S. (1983). A field project: Single-subject design in a public social service agency. *Journal of Social Service Research, 6*(3/4), 29-43.

Downs, W. R., & Robertson, J. F. (1983). Preserving the social work perspective in the research sequence: State of the art and program models for the 1980s. *Journal of Education for Social Work, 19*(1), 87-95.

Durkin, R. (1988). The Sage Hill Behavior Rating System: Some of its clinical, administrative, and research uses. *Journal of Child Care,* Spring Special Issue, 19-29.

Fraser, M. W., Lewis, R. E., & Norman, J. L. (1989, March). Research education in M.S.W. Programs: Four competing perspectives. Paper presented at the Annual Program Meeting of the Council on Social Work Education.

Gingerich, W. J. (1984). Meta-analysis of applied time-series data. *Journal of Applied Behavioral Science, 20,* 71-79.

Gottlieb, N., & Richey, C. (1980). Education of human services practitioners for clinical evaluation. In R. W. Weinbach, & A. Rubin (Eds.), *Teaching social work research: Alternative programs and strategies* (pp. 3-12). New York: Council on Social Work Education.

Grasso, A. J., Epstein, I., & Tripodi, T. (1988). Agency-based research utilization in a residential child care setting. *Administration in Social Work, 12*, 61-80.

Grinnell, Jr., R. M. (1985). Becoming a practitioner/researcher. In R. M. Grinnell, Jr. (Ed.), *Social work research and evaluation* (2nd ed.), (pp. 1-15). Itasca, IL: F. E. Peacock

Hayes, S. C. (1981). Single-case experimental design and empirical clinical practice. *Journal of Consulting and Clinical Psychology, 49*, 193-211.

Heineman-Peiper, M. (1985). The future of social work research. *Social Work Research & Abstracts, 21*(4), 3-11.

Howe, M. W. (1974). Casework self-evaluation: A single-subject approach. *Social Service Review, 48*, 1-23.

Hudson, W. W., & Nurius, P. S. (in press). *Computer-based practice: Theory, methods and software*. Belmont, CA: Wadsworth.

Ivanoff, A., Blythe, B. J. & Briar, S. (1987). The empirical clinical practice debate. *Social Casework, 68*, 290-298.

Jayaratne, S., & Levy, R. L. (1979). *Empirical Clinical Practice*. New York: Columbia University Press.

Jayaratne, S., Tripodi, T., & Talsma, E. (1988). Methodological observations on applied behavioral science. *Journal of Applied Behavioral Science, 24*, 119-128.

Kagle, J. D. (1982). Using single-subject measures in practice decisions: Systematic documentation or distortion? *Arete*, 1-9.

Kazdin, A. E. (1980). *Research design in clinical psychology*. New York: Harper & Row.

Levy, R. L. (1983). Overview of single-case experiments. In A. Rosenblatt & D. Waldfogel (Eds.), *Handbook of clinical social work* (pp. 583-602). San Francisco: Jossey-Bass.

Levy, R. L. (1987). Single subject research designs. In *Encyclopedia of Social Work* (18th ed.). Silver Spring, MD: National Association of Social Workers.

Mutschler, E. (1984). Evaluating practice: A study of research utilization by practitioners. *Social Work, 29*, 332-337.

Nelson, J. C. (1988). Single-subject research. In R. M. Grinnell, Jr. (Ed.), *Social work research and evaluation* (3rd ed.) (pp. 362-399). Itasca, IL: F. E. Peacock.

Richey, C. A., Berlin, S. B., & Jaffee, B. (1979). The integrated educational unit: A three-year evaluation of an approach to combining methods, research, and field instruction. Paper presented at the Annual Program Meeting of the Council on Social Work Education, Boston, March 1979.

Richey, C. A., Blythe, B. J. & Berlin, S. B. (1987). Do social workers evaluate their practice? *Social Work Research & Abstracts, 23*(2), 14-20.

Ruckdeschel, R. A., & Farris, B. E. (1981). Assessing practice: A critical look at the single-case design. *Social Casework, 62*, 413-1419.

Siegel, D. H. (1985). Effective teaching of empirically based practice. *Social Work Research & Abstracts, 21*(1), 40-48.

Simons, R. L. (1987). The impact of training for empirically based practice. *Journal of Social Work Education, 23*, 24-30.

Smith, M. L., DeWeaver, K. L., & Kilpatrick, A. C. (1986). Research curricula and accreditation: The challenge for leadership. *Journal of Social Work Education, 22*(2), 61-70.

Thomas, E. J. (1978). Research and service in single-case experimentation: Conflicts and choices. *Social Work Research & Abstracts, 14*, 20-31.

Tripodi, T. (1988, October). A typology of research knowledge for relating research to social work practice. Paper presented at the 90th anniversary of the Columbia University School of Social Work.

Tripodi, T., & Epstein, I. (1980). *Research techniques for clinical social workers*. New York: Columbia University Press.

Ulman, L. P., & Krasner, L. (Eds.) (1965). *Case studies in behavior modification*. New York: Holt, Rinehart, and Winston.

Weinbach, R. W., & Rubin, A. (1980). *Teaching social work research: Alternative programs and strategies*. New York: Council on Social Work Education.

Wodarski, J. S. (1981). *The role of research in clinical practice: A practical approach for the human services*. Baltimore: University Park Press.

# Strategies for the Analysis of Databases in Social Service Systems

David Fanshel
Paul A. Marsters
Stephen J. Finch
John F. Grundy

## *INTRODUCTION*

The social services are now on the verge of an important development in service delivery made possible by the new information technology epitomized by the development of management information systems. We can anticipate the phenomenon of data routinely gathered in the course of service operations, routinely organized into aggregated tables for various service entities, and probed by analysts using advanced statistical techniques to extract the intelligence required for sound management of the programs. The new thrust will have important implications for monitoring the adequacy of service provision by public and voluntary agencies and will provide an underpinning of information about service operations heretofore denied policy makers and funding sources. It is difficult to exaggerate the importance of this development.

The focus of this chapter is stimulated by an awareness that a major problem has stood in the way of adequate exploitation of the information technology. The resistance of social workers to the burden of the ever-increasing demands upon them for documentation is obvious to all. Many current examples of management information systems suffer from a profound case of the "database syndrome" (Fanshel, Finch, and Grundy, 1987). An administrator of a social

---

The research reported here was funded by a grant from the William T. Grant Foundation and the Robert Sterling Clark Foundation.

service organization collects data using a large staff of data collectors, data entry personnel, and computer programmers. This center regards the data as "information," and because we are in the "information age," no further justification or work is required. The database gets larger and larger as more and more staff members are required to fill out ever more forms, with no one analyzing or interpreting the forms already collected. No effort is made to perform a statistical analysis to extract operationally meaningful measures of system performance.

For the purpose of illustrating a general approach to dealing with social service data, we have chosen to focus on the burgeoning area of child welfare prevention services. This is an important feature of permanency planning brought into being by Congressional enactment under the Adoption Assistance and Child Welfare Act of 1980 (Public Law 96-272).

Jones (1985, p. 37) has commented on a major shortcoming of all the preventive service studies she reviewed:

> They fail to report the characteristics of all the clients served, the services provided, or differential outcomes by either client characteristics or service patterns. Consequently no assessment can be made of differential patterns of success within a program, and no progress is made in trying to ascertain the important indicators of risk or the important components of the intervention.

It is well known that many poor families living in distressed areas of cities are beset with a plethora of personal and social problems. It all can be dealt with by social agencies. Ripple and Alexander (1956) use the phrase "problems at issue" to distinguish between those problems the client and the social worker agree represent phenomena that are to be the object of joint effort to change, and those difficulties that might represent sources of stress or dysfunction for the family although not targeted as something to be worked on. The latter might represent areas being dealt with through informal sources available to the family, e.g., the main provider's unemployment, or problems not readily changed such as crowded housing. In examining the experience of agencies, it becomes important to take into account the fact that each client family can bring its own mix of problems that are targeted for service.

## THE LOWER EAST SIDE FAMILY UNION INFORMATION FORM

This chapter focuses on analysis of data reporting the outcome of service encounters involving 160 client families known to the Lower East Side Family Union (LESFU). These cases were those initiated at LESFU between April 15, 1982 and March 15, 1983. This agency is a social service organization serving the Lower East Side area of Manhattan and has as its purpose the provision of preventive services to families whose children are at risk of placement in foster care. The program, founded in 1974, has received national recognition for its innovative approach to problems of the urban poor and has been described by Weissman (1978) and Beck (1979). Its catchment area is characterized by extreme poverty. It includes the famous Bowery section, "Alphabet City" (in recent years a notorious center for the wholesale drug trade), Chinatown, and the original Jewish settlement areas of Hester Street and Orchard Street. The range of problems faced by the clientele is far wider than those usually encountered by family service agencies.

The agency has as part of its professional practice a view that service work with its clients progresses sequentially through seven stages. This sequence is the "LESFU Model":

1. Intake (Pre-work Agreement): The LESFU worker and the client mutually come to an understanding of the problems the family faces. As many as three interviews with the client may be needed before an understanding of the client's problems is obtained.
2. Work Agreement: Both client and worker agree on the specification of the problems that they will work on together. The "work agreement" is a clear statement of the focus of the working agenda.
3. Goal Statement: This is a joint statement with the client of "expectations" about how or how much the problem can be resolved. The principle is that the client is entitled to know

what the chances are of achieving the case goals, e.g., obtaining public housing in the face of long waiting lists.

4. Convening: Since LESFU "high risk" clients have more than one problem, there are often a number of service providers involved with the family. "Convening" is a meeting or other means of gathering together the client and client's providers to begin the process of coordinating services to the client.

5. Contract: Through the process of convening, the client, LESFU, and other providers should come to agreement about what each party will do to strengthen the family. Contracts are written statements by which these parties formally agree to their roles and responsibilities.

6. Monitoring: In monitoring, LESFU continually reviews the extent to which LESFU, the client, and providers are living up to the terms of the contract and whether circumstances have changed so that the service contract should be changed.

7. Follow-Up/Termination: Since contracts are only established for high risk clients, monitoring each case against its contract may not be possible. However, LESFU associates are responsible for "following-up" with the client and/or provider to insure that the correct services are made available and that additional problems have not arisen for the family. For "high risk" cases, termination could occur if the client's problems have been resolved or are under control, or for other reasons (e.g., joint LESFU/client decision that LESFU was not assisting the client).

We are able to examine data describing service operations because LESFU had in place a computerized management information system (the LESFU MIS) that collected information about the kinds of problems a client brought to the agency, and provided for indication as to whether reported problems are resolved or not. Figure 1 is a one-page form that the worker[1] for a case fills out once a month for each family in the worker's caseload. After a case was opened and the first MIS form had been filled out, the worker categorized each of the client's problems for which help had been sought into a set of numeric codes. The major problem areas are listed in Table 1 and reflect the spectrum of problems that a family might face. Each of these areas was elaborated into a more specific group of problems. Here we report only at the overall problem area level.

We sought to make use of the fact that there was continuous reporting on cases on a monthly basis over the life of each case, thus making possible the creation of a time-series data file. We were particularly interested in the social worker's identification of the problems being worked on with each client family and which of these had been resolved in the past month. Given the mix of problems brought by the families in many of the cases, we sought to determine which kinds of problems ever got solved.

Every month, the worker reported whether the problems previously reported for the client were still open or had been resolved, and which problems were being actively worked on that month. Newly emerging problems could be identified on any reporting occasion. On each MIS form, a problem was described as "open" (meaning that the worker had identified it as an area requiring service and put this problem on the agenda of the case) or "resolved" (meaning that the problem had been successfully dealt with to the extent possible within the constraints of LESFU's mission). The concept must be seen in relative terms. The definition of "resolved" may vary from worker to worker or from problem type to problem type.[2]

Each submission of the form listed a reported time spent working on the case during the month covered by the report and a listing of the problem codes reported as actively worked on. These reports were consolidated for each case to generate a record that contained the total amount of time spent, the number of months in which a problem was worked on, and the problems that were reported. Each month, the worker was asked to record the stage of the model reflecting the status of work on the case.

## ISSUE OF BIAS IN REPORTING ABOUT CASES

Before discussing findings we must mention that we recognize that all of the data we have been discussing has come from a single source: the social work associate filling out a monthly report for the LESFU MIS for each case on her or his caseload. The degree of error stemming from the bias of the observer is a source of legitimate concern. We have analyzed this matter using two debriefing

FIGURE 1. Monthly Case Summary Form Filled Out by Social Work Associates

## CASE SUMMARY

MONTH:

WORKER

CLIENT:

OPENED: ___ / ___ / ___    CLOSED: ___ / ___ / ___

**TYPE**

___ HIGH RISK    ___ NON-HIGH RISK    ___ LIMITED SERVICE    ___ UNCLASSIFIED

**STATUS**

___ PRE-WORK AGREEMENT    ___ WORK AGREEMENT    ___ GOALS    ___ CONVENE

___ CONTRACT    ___ MONITOR    ___ FOLLOW-UP

**NUMBER OF ACTIONS TAKEN THIS MONTH:** _____

**TIME SPENT ON CASE:** _____ HOURS    _____ MINUTES

**PROBLEM AND ISSUE CODING**

STATUS: ID = IDENT.    O = OPEN    R = RESOLVED

CHANGE: + = IMPROVE    0 = SAME    − = WORSE

ASTERISK (•): CHECK (✓) COLUMN IF ADDRESSED DURING THIS MONTH.

| | PROB. CODE | STATUS | CHANGE | (•) | | PROB. CODE | STATUS | CHANGE | (•) | | PROB. CODE | STATUS | CHANGE | (•) | | PROB. CODE | STATUS | CHANGE | (•) |
|---|---|---|---|---|---|---|---|---|---|---|---|---|---|---|---|---|---|---|---|
| 1 | | | | | 5 | | | | | 9 | | | | | 13 | | | | |
| 2 | | | | | 6 | | | | | 10 | | | | | 14 | | | | |
| 3 | | | | | 7 | | | | | 11 | | | | | 15 | | | | |
| 4 | | | | | 8 | | | | | 12 | | | | | 16 | | | | |

| ISSUES | STATUS | CHANGE (*) | PROBLEM AREAS AFFECTED | | | | | |
|---|---|---|---|---|---|---|---|---|
| | | | 1 | 2 | 3 | 4 | 5 | 6 |
| PROVIDER NOT AVAILABLE | | | | | | | | |
| PAYMENT ELIGIBILITY | | | | | | | | |
| LANGUAGE | | | | | | | | |
| TRANSPORTATION | | | | | | | | |
| CHILD CARE | | | | | | | | |
| RECOGNIZING PROBLEMS | | | | | | | | |

| ISSUES | STATUS | CHANGE (*) | PROBLEM AREAS AFFECTED | | | | | |
|---|---|---|---|---|---|---|---|---|
| | | | 1 | 2 | 3 | 4 | 5 | 6 |
| TAKING ACTION | | | | | | | | |
| NEGOTIATING WITH PROVIDERS | | | | | | | | |
| KEEPING APPOINTMENTS | | | | | | | | |
| FOLLOWING SERVICE PLAN | | | | | | | | |
| OTHER: | | | | | | | | |
| OTHER: | | | | | | | | |

STATUS (A-E):
A = INITIAL APPOINTMENT SET
B = ASSESSMENT FOR SERVICES
C = ACCEPTED FOR SERVICES
D = SERVICE ON-GOING
E = SERVICE TERMINATED

ISSUES (0-6):
0 = SERVICE UNAVAILABLE
1 = REFUSES TO SERVE CLIENT
2 = NOT PROVIDING SERVICES
3 = POOR QUALITY SERVICES
4 = RESISTS CONTRACT
5 = RESISTS MONITORING
6 = OTHER

PROVIDER CODING

| No. | PROVIDERS | STATUS | ISSUES | PROBLEM AREAS AFFECTED | | | | | |
|---|---|---|---|---|---|---|---|---|---|
| | | | | 1 | 2 | 3 | 4 | 5 | 6 |
| 1 | | | | | | | | | |
| 2 | | | | | | | | | |
| 3 | | | | | | | | | |
| 4 | | | | | | | | | |
| 5 | | | | | | | | | |
| 6 | | | | | | | | | |

LESFU-2

TABLE 1. LESFU Management Information System—Major Groups of Problem Codes

```
0:  Family Relations, Adult
1:  Social Relations, Adult
2:  Income and Employment, Adult
3:  Housing and Environment, Family
4:  Health, Adult
5:  Family Relations, Child
6:  Social Relations, Child
7:  Educational and Vocational Training, Child
8:  Life Skills, Child
9:  Health, Child
```

interviews with the social work associates and in-person research interviews with the clients. We are now preparing a manuscript for publication on this aspect of our study. At this time we can report that we are encouraged by the degree of agreement we find between the clients and their social workers on important characteristics of the client's experience with LESFU.

Among the areas in which significant agreement has been established are the following: (1) Specification of child behavior problems as an important agenda item for service, and reports about changes that have taken place in the child since case opening. (2) Depiction of the father's involvement or lack of involvement in the family's current living situation. (3 Identification of housing problems as occupying the attention of client and worker with associated case actions. (4) The nature of contacts between worker and client and the breadth of problems dealt with. (5) Extent of the mother's motivation to seek changes in the family's situation. (6) The evidence of improvement in the adjustment of family members. (7) Concern about the financial problems facing the family. (8) The extent of attention given to family relationship problems.

## BASIC SUMMARY STATISTICS

The median length of time for case activity was 11 months. The median number of problems reported for the cases was eight a minimum of two and a maximum of 24. The median number of problems reported resolved in these cases was two, the maximum number was 13, and overall 33% were reported resolved. Of the 160 cases, 77% had at least one problem reported resolved.

In Table 2, we present the prevalence rate[3] and the rate of reported resolution[4] for each of the ten problem groupings. Between two-thirds and three-quarters of the 160 cases had problems in adult family relations, adult income and employment, family housing and environment, and child educational and vocational training. The least frequently occurring problem groups were the adult social relations group and the child life skills group.

The highest percentage of problems reported resolved were in the adult income and employment group, with a percentage of 57%. Helping to restore families to public assistance eligibility status after abrupt termination of income maintenance payments was a major activity of the LESFU staff. Child educational and vocational training problems were resolved at a rate of 49%, and adult family relations problems were resolved at a rate of 41%. Adult social relations problems were the least likely to be resolved, with a per-

TABLE 2. Prevalence of Problems and Rate of Reported Resolution by Problem Grouping

| | Problem Group | Prevalence Rate (number)[a] | Reported Resolution Rate [b] |
|---|---|---|---|
| 2 | Adult Income and Employment | 74.3%(119) | 56.7% |
| 0 | Adult Family Relations | 73.7 (118) | 40.8 |
| 3 | Family Housing and Environment | 68.7 (110) | 36.6 |
| 7 | Child Educational and Vocational Training | 68.7 (110) | 49.2 |
| 9 | Child Health | 56.2 (90) | 36.1 |
| 4 | Adult Health | 53.7 (86) | 36.1 |
| 6 | Child Social Relations | 36.8 (59) | 36.1 |
| 5 | Child Family Relations | 36.2 (58) | 32.0 |
| 1 | Adult Social Relations | 31.2 (50) | 25.0 |
| 8 | Child Life Skills | 16.8 (27) | 30.3 |

Notes: a. The prevalence rate of a problem group is the percentage of the 160 cases that had at least one problem in the group.

b. The resolution rate of a problem group is the percentage of all of the problems in that group reported in the MIS reported resolved at the end of the case.

centage resolution rate of 25%. Other problems were reported resolved at a rate of about 33%.

## One Measure of Reported Case Success:
## Reported Resolution Ratio

We created a summary measure for each case called the reported
resolution ratio using the problems present in a case and the calculation of the problem-specific rates of reported resolution for all cases
in the study. This is the ratio of the number of problems reported
resolved at the end of a case to the number of problems expected to
be reported resolved based on the problem-specific rates observed.
It is an example of an indirectly standardized ratio (Fleiss, 1981,
pp. 240-247), called the reported resolution ratio.[5] Its average value
is roughly 1. Values greater than 1 indicate that more problems
were resolved than expected given the problems present in the case;
values less than 1 indicate that fewer problems were resolved than
expected. The value of this measure is that it incorporates information about the relative difficulty of resolving the problems presented
in a case because it includes the expected number of problems reported resolved based on the outcomes for all cases in the study
where the problem was identified as present.

For example, consider a case that has four problems reported:
002 (conflicts between adult family members), 205 (adult public
assistance problems), 704 (child not enrolled in school), and 910
(child's other health problem). Since the reported resolution rate for
problem 002 was 30% on the average for each individual case, we
expect 0.30 of a problem reported resolved from each case that has
a problem 002. Similarly we expect 0.64 of a problem reported
resolved from each case that has problem 205 because the rate of
reported resolution for this problem was 64%. Finally, we expect
0.61 of a problem reported resolved from each case that has problem 704 and 0.41 of a problem reported resolved from each case
that has problem 910. For the example case, then, we would expect
1.96 problems reported resolved (1.96 = .30 + .64 + .61 + .41).
Thus, if the example case had three problems reported resolved,
then the reported resolution ratio would be 3/1.96 = 1.53, indicat-

ing that this case had more success than would be expected based on the history of reported problem resolution in the LESFU MIS.

As must be true mathematically, the mean reported resolution ratio was close to 1 (i.e., 0.96) for 160 cases. The standard deviation was 0.78, the upper quartile point was 1.63, and the lower quartile point was 0.23.

There is modest evidence in support of the hypothesis that a case that progressed further in the sequence of stages in the LESFU model had more problems reported resolved then expected ($p < .05$). The number of problems reported resolved was less than expected for cases that remained within the first two stages of the LESFU model. The number reported resolved was somewhat more than the number expected for cases that advanced to the goals stage or beyond.

## *Summary Statistics on Worker and Team Effects*

Our first analysis to determine whether there was a worker effect was a one-way analysis of variance using as the dependent variable the indirectly standardized reported resolution ratio and as the independent variables the worker responsible for a case. The worker variables explained 31% of the variability of the indirectly standardized reported resolution ratio ($p < .001$). The worker effects ranged from a highest value of 0.88 to a lowest value of $-.96$. Thus, the worker with the highest average indirectly standardized reported resolution ratio resolved almost twice as many problems as would be expected based on the problem mix in that worker's caseload and the reports of resolution throughout the agency. The worker with the lowest average indirectly standardized reported ratio reported no resolutions of problems among the cases assigned.

These results strongly suggest the hypothesis that the individual workers vary in effectiveness. The reason might be that some workers are genuinely more effective than others or more ready to report a problem as resolved, or it might be that some workers have caseloads that are less easy to guide to resolution and hence have systematically lower average indirectly standardized reported resolution ratios. There was a relatively large turnover of staff during the study period, and this phenomenon might well affect these esti-mates.

Each client is assigned to one of four teams of workers located at different sites, and these teams are identified on the MIS. There were no overall differences among the teams significant at the 5% level. In addition, there were no differences significant at the 1% level of significance for any rate of reported resolution among any problem type compared.

### Summary Statistics for Time Analysis

The total time reported in the records analyzed was 11,000 hours (1,571 seven-hour worker days). The times reported for each case were summed to give the total time reported spent on a case. The average time reported spent on a case over the total period it was active was 68.75 hours (requiring 9.8 worker days). The standard deviation of the time reported spent on a case was 47.32 hours (6.8 worker days).

We used multiple regression to identify those problem areas that consumed a large amount of the organization's time reported spent. The unit of analysis was the case, and the dependent variable was the total estimated time ($T$) reported spent on a case as before. The independent variables were the counts of the number of times each problem area was worked on for each case (represented by $N_{ij}$ for the $i$th client, where $i$ was between 1 and 160, and $j$th problem area, where $j$ was between 1 and 10). The regression model used was

$$E(T_i) = u_0 + u_1 {}^* N_{i1} + u_2 {}^* N_{i2} + \ldots + u_{10} {}^* N_{i10} \qquad (1)$$

The coefficient $u_j$ is the unit coefficient that estimates the average amount of time spent on problem area $j$ each time that a worker reported working on that problem area. When these coefficients are multiplied by the number of periods the $i$th problem area was ac-tive, the model estimates the total amount of time reported spent on each problem area.

The model fit the data relatively well. When the coefficients were estimated by Ordinary Least Squares (OLS) regression the model reduced the standard deviation of the estimated time spent on a case to 31 hours from the original standard deviation of 47 hours. That is, the multiple correlation coefficient was 0.59.

We also ran the model with the intercept term set to 0 to determine roughly the degree of sensitivity of the results to reasonable changes in the specification of the model. For these data, the results using the model with the intercept term not set to 0 seem slightly more reasonable. The model with the intercept term set to 0 had slightly less explanatory power and had a standard error of estimate equal to 32, an increase of only 3% over the results of the model with the intercept. Residual plots indicated no obvious model inadequacies for either model.

Table 3 presents the estimated amount of time spent on each major problem area using the two models. It is an example of the type of report that could be routinely produced from this database each month. It provides management with a reasonable accounting of the expenditure of staff time to the major problem groupings. A similar table could be produced for each staff member.

Based on the value of the intercept, we estimated that a total of 2,400 hours of the 11,000 total staff hours went to general case activity not related to a specific problem (15 hours per case). We could speculate that time spent with the client not related to the specific problems being worked on might include orientation of the client to the agency, filling out forms, and discussion designed to

TABLE 3. Estimated Hours Spent by Problem Group

| Problem Group | Estimated Hours (intercept in model) | Estimated Hours (no intercept) |
|---|---|---|
| Child Educational and Vocational Training | 1685 | 1904 |
| Adult Income and Employment | 1443 | 1917 |
| Adult Family Relations | 1321 | 1527 |
| Child Health | 1254 | 1396 |
| Adult Health | 957 | 957 |
| Family Housing and Environment | 707 | 1084 |
| Child Social Relations | 627 | 643 |
| Child Family Relations | 333 | 561 |
| Adult Social Relations | 226 | 296 |
| Child Life Skills | 26 | 71 |

put the client at ease and to determine what was happening in the client's life.

Four problem areas consumed the greatest fraction of time as estimated by the model. The two largest areas were child educational and vocational training and adult income and employment. The staff spent slightly less time on adult family relations and child health problems. The areas of child life skills, adult social relations, child family relations, and child social relations received relatively less attention.

## Comparison of Time Allocated to Problem and Rate of Reported Resolution

How much time is spent per problem resolved based on the reports filed in the MIS database? We calculated the average amount of time estimated per problem resolved as a measure of average staff time "cost" associated with the resolution of the problem area. Table 4 presents the number of problems reported resolved in each problem group and the ratio of the hours estimated spent on a problem area to the number of resolutions reported. The time esti-

TABLE 4. Estimated Hours Spent Per Problem Reported Resolved by Problem Group

| Problem Group | Estimated Hours Per Problem Resolved (intercept in model) | | Estimated Hours Per Problem Resolved (no intercept) |
|---|---|---|---|
| Child Educational and Vocational Training | 98 | 17.2 | 19.4 |
| Adult Income and Employment | 114 | 12.7 | 16.8 |
| Adult Family Relations | 85 | 15.5 | 18.0 |
| Child Health | 22 | 57.0 | 63.5 |
| Adult Health | 51 | 18.8 | 18.8 |
| Family Housing and Environment | 63 | 11.2 | 17.2 |
| Child Social Relations | 35 | 17.9 | 18.4 |
| Child Family Relations | 25 | 13.3 | 22.4 |
| Adult Social Relations | 15 | 15.1 | 19.7 |
| Child Life Skills | 11 | 6.5 | 2.4 |

mated spent per problem reported resolved is around 17 hours for each of the problem groups using the results of the model with an intercept term (19 hours per problem reported resolved using the model without an intercept term).

Three aspects of this table struck our attention. The estimated time per problem reported resolved was very high for child health problems — roughly 60 hours per problem reported resolved for both models used. The estimated time per problem resolved was about two hours less than average for adult income and employment problems and family housing and environment problems.

These calculations suggest that the staff has a rather sensitive eye to the bottom line issues of productivity and control their investment of time that they invest in areas where they can accomplish some definable objective. They appear willing to expend considerable effort in child-health related problems with relatively small prospects for resolution. Of course, we cannot tell from this data whether their efforts were defensible, but given the sensibility of the statistics elsewhere we have to presume that the efforts were appropriate responses. The relatively lower values for adult income and employment problems and family housing and environment problems may reflect an efficiency developed from long practice and the reduced internal effort required from the staff because other governmental agencies have to perform tasks to resolve these problems.

## Association of Time Reported Spent and Increased Success

We used multiple regression to explain the reported resolution of problems as a function of the time investment in a case, the expected time invested based on the problems reported present and the normative data available for the agency, and the degree to which they match. More specifically, if a worker invests more time in a case than would be expected to be invested, is there an association with greater success as measured by the number of problems reported resolved at the end of the case?

Since there was potential to have correlations artificially induced by the use of rates (Neyman, 1952), we used the number of problems reported resolved at the end of a case as the dependent variable in regression analysis with the number of problems expected to be resolved as an independent variable. The unit of analysis was the case. The dependent variable was the logarithm (base e) of 1 plus the number of problems reported resolved. The choice of the logarithm was made because the techniques of exploratory data analysis as described in Tukey (1977) indicated that the logarithm of the number of problems reported resolved was the appropriate variable to use. We added 1 to the number of problems reported resolved to avoid the possibility of taking a logarithm of a zero count or generating a prediction of a negative number of problems resolved.

The most important independent variable was the logarithm (base e) of the number of problems expected to be reported resolved based on the rates of reported resolution as defined above.

Our next set of variables was additional general structural factors. They were the logarithm (base e) of 1 plus the number of actions reported in the case, the logarithm (base e) of the sum of the time spent on the case, the logarithm of the sum of the number of problems reported to exist over the case's history, the logarithm of the number of months the case had time reported spent on it or actions taken on it, the logarithm of the time expected to be reported, and the logarithm of the ratio of the sum of the time reported spent on a case to the time expected to be spent on the case. We also used variables that indicated whether a case reached a specified stage of the LESFU model or higher.

The time expected to be spent on a case is the amount of time that we would predict to reported spent on this case using the problems present in each case, the number of months each problem was reported, and the regression coefficients from the model. That is, let $ET_j$ represent the time expected to be reported spent on the $j$th case and let $N1_j, N2_j, \ldots, N10_j$ be the number of times the $i$th problem ($i = 1, \ldots, 10$) was worked on in the $j$th case.

$$ET_j = cb_1{}^*N1_j + cb_2{}^*N2_j + \ldots + cb_{10}{}^*N10_j,$$

where $cb_1, cb_2, \ldots, cb_{10}$ are the calculated regression coefficients.

Our next set of variables indicated which worker was responsible for the case. That is, we ask the question whether there are workers whose cases have significantly greater numbers of problems reported resolved, controlling for other important variables.

Formally, this regression analysis used the following model:

$$E[\ln(NR_j+1)] = b_1^* + \ln(ER_j) + b_2^*\ln(A_{j+1}) + b_3^*\ln(T_j)$$
$$+ b_4^*\ln(N_j) + b_5^*\ln(M_j) + b_6^*\ln(ET_j)$$
$$+ b_7^*\ln(T_j/ET_j)$$
$$+ c_1^*I(\text{stage 1 or higher})$$
$$+ c_2^*I(\text{stage 2 or higher})$$
$$+ c_3^*I(\text{stage 3 or higher})$$
$$+ \ldots + c_7^*I(\text{stage 7 or higher})$$
$$+ d_1^*I(\text{first worker on case was worker 1})$$
$$+ d_2^*I(\text{first worker on case was worker 2})$$
$$+ \ldots + d_{19}^*I(\text{first worker on case was worker 19}),$$

where $NR_j$ represents the number of problems reported resolved on the $j$th case, $ER_j$ the number of problems expected to be resolved on the $j$th case, $A_j$ the number of actions reported taken in the $j$th case, $T_j$ the sum of the time reported spent on the $j$th case, $N_j$ the number of problems reported for the $j$th case, $M_j$ the number of months that the case was reported to be active, $ET_j$ the expected time predicted for the $j$th case, and ln the natural logarithm (logarithm to the base e). The variable $I$ (stage 1 or higher) is a variable with the value 1 if a case reached stage 1 of the LESFU model or a higher stage and the value 0 otherwise. Similar definitions hold for the other indicator variables used.

The fitted equation for $\ln(NR_{j+1})$ was:

$$0.70^*\ln(ER_j) + 0.89^*\ln(I(\text{level 3 or higher} + 1))$$

(se = 0.08)     (se = .14)
(t = 8.0)       (t = 6.4)

$$- 1.08^*I(\text{worker A})$$

(se = .26)
(t = -4.1)

$$- 0.76^*I(\text{worker B})$$

(se = .21)
(t = -3.5)

$$- 1.59*I(\text{worker C})$$
$$(se = .58)$$
$$(t = -2.7)$$

$$- 0.43*I(\text{worker D})$$
$$(se = .17)$$
$$(t = -2.4)$$

$$+ 0.22*\ln(T_j/ET_j)$$
$$(se = .09)$$
$$(t = 2.4)$$

The mean squared error for this model was .33, corresponding to a percentage of variance explained equal to 43%.

## CONCLUSIONS

Our first concern was documenting whether or not this organization complied with its mandate. Examination of Table 2 shows that the agency's caseload did in fact have problems that might well lead to the placement of a child in foster care. Further, the rates of reported resolution measured the effectiveness of the organization with regard to problem resolution. The time estimates in Table 3 provide an important characterization of which problem areas receive the attention of the staff, and the time per reported resolution in Table 4 are estimates of the cost in professional staff time for reported resolution of a problem for each problem area. The descriptive picture that has emerged from these analyses offers objective and replicable details of the inner workings of this agency.

Given the service mission of the agency which requires it to help prevent the disruption of families, the revelation that much agency effort is being expended in work on child education, adult income and employment, and adult family relations supports the view that mission objectives to deal preventively with problems likely to lead to placement are being followed.

One of our principal concerns was to determine whether there are aspects to the LESFU approach to work with its clientele that were associated with greater success in a case. After the obvious, the next most significant association was that those cases that had progressed to stage 3 or higher of the LESFU model again had a greater number of problems reported resolved. This finding confirms the simple analysis of variance findings reported earlier.

Do some workers have different patterns of success in cases? There were significant worker effects with four workers associated with lesser numbers of problems resolved than the comparison worker (the comparison worker was the one with the greatest number of cases).

Was the investment of additional time in a case associated with a greater degree of reported problem resolution in a case? Once the worker effects had been included, the logarithm of the indirectly standardized time ratio was a significant variable. The association was positive, indicating that those cases receiving greater amounts of time than that projected had greater numbers of problems reported resolved. The value of the coefficient was 0.22, indicating that an increase in the time reported spent on a case equal to 10% of the time expected to be spent on the case was associated with a 2.2% increase in the number of problems reported resolved.

## DISCUSSION

The practice example we have examined here involves use of a relatively simple form filled out by a social work associate every month on each case for which service is being rendered. If an agency such as LESFU has a staff of 20 workers, each of whom is carrying an average of 15 cases, we would have about 300 forms submitted per month. If a case remains open on average six months, we would have an accumulation of 3,600 forms over a year's time. Without analysis, this volume of paper flow, even in an agency of modest size, would swamp the agency without any yield of useful findings.

Analysis of routinely gathered data such as the LESFU MIS can serve as an administrative tool identifying features of strong performance in problem resolution as well as less effective ones. Routinely collected data from such a system are observational data rather than data from a randomized experiment, and the interpretation of the results must always duly consider the principle that these findings are associations and not necessarily causations. For example, we have used variables specifying the individual worker responsible for a case. We are aware that many readers might infer that a worker with a low coefficient was not as successful as other workers. While such an inference may be valid, we have no guarantees that the workers have comparable caseloads, and so we must be appropriately cautious in our interpretation of these results.

Such caution should not extend to ignoring the findings. Our method of analysis did control for the number of problems expected to be reported resolved, and so there is at least a first order correction for differences in the difficulty of the caseloads of the various workers compared. An appropriate response would be to examine the work of individuals identified to determine whether a worker had unusually effective techniques and practices. An individual worker who is unusually successful in achieving agency goals can be identified and modes of work related to such outcomes can be used as prototypes in creating training programs. On the other hand, staff who achieve less adequate outcomes can be identified for training and other forms of supportive help to overcome deficits in performance.

Such analysis may also provide useful information about caseload assignments. Workers assigned very difficult cases where more time investments can result in higher success rates might be assigned smaller caseloads. It is also possible to compare preventive service agencies with respect to inherent difficulties of caseloads and to have the support required from funding sources adjusted to meet the realities of variation in clientele served.

The reader might wonder about the practical use of this effort to develop a higher degree of exactness in the understanding of the time distribution expended by social work associates in meeting the needs of families at high risk, such as those served by the Lower East Side Family Union. There are three major contributions to be made by improving the quality of the estimates of time involved in such service operations. First, the internal administration of service organizations can be strengthened by enabling managers to better understand the nature of the time invested in cases. There is no area of social service administration that poses greater difficulty for boards of directors and administrative staff than the need to establish caseload sizes that can be considered appropriate for the service mission and the tasks at hand. Staff time is perhaps the most important ingredient among agency resources and understanding how it is spent can lead to more rational establishment of work norms. Time estimates must be made repeatedly since the nature of clientele coming to the agency is likely to shift over time, reflecting a dynamic social environment. Accounting for worker efforts on an ongoing basis by estimating service time demands can make possible a more rational organization of work.

A second contribution of this effort is in the area of public monitoring of social programs that receive federal and state funding. In New York State, there are about 100 social agencies like the Lower East Side Family Union that receive support for their activities from funds made available as a result of the New York State Child Welfare Reform Act of 1979. Between 1980 and 1989, preventive child welfare services expenditures by the state rose from $9.3 million to $70.5 million. Such services have a mission to help vulnerable families support their children at home and spare them placement in the foster care system. How does the state monitoring agency, the New York State Department of Social Services, and its counterpart, the New York City Human Resources Administration, account for how these funds are being used? How can the experiences of many agencies be understood in an integrated manner? How can service providers be compared with respect to the kinds of cases, they are carrying, the investments made in cases and the results of their service efforts? Time allocation according to defined problem categories can provide data that permit comparison among providers as well as trend data for the entire package of preventive services brought into being by the enabling legislation.

A third contribution is the development of management assistance tools for the individual professional for the handling of individual cases. The focus of management information systems and reports has virtually always been the production of tools to evaluate staff performance and give guidance on fundamental executive responsibilities. Although these functions are vitally important, the management information system and its developers have a responsibility to provide tools to help those who deliver the services in their day to day work. The reports discussed here can be used by the individual worker in planning personal time to be distributed among cases. The worker can be provided with a prediction of the amount of time that should be budgeted for a case. The utility of this for planning workload and case handling over the short range is clear. Further, the worker can compare the investment made on a case to date with an expected investment based on the rest of the agency's experience. Such a comparison can have many rewards. The worker can keep time investments in line with the parameters established by all of the workers in the agency or understand why this is not possible in the individual case. Such information can also assist agency administration in determining how many new cases to assign to individual staff each month, depending on the ongoing time commitments shown for a given caseload.

## NOTES

1. Service in this agency is rendered by social work associates drawn from the neighborhood and trained on the job. Educational backgrounds vary for those serving in this position and can include individuals with less than a college degree. The team leader is usually a person with a graduate social work degree.

2. It is recognized that conditions faced by clients can be such that "problem resolution" would not be feasible. The MIS form allows for the worker to show categories in which change may have taken place (improve/same/worse) even if the problems are not resolved. This aspect of case information is the subject of a doctoral dissertation at Columbia University undertaken by Amelia Chu.

3. The prevalence rate of a class of problems is the percentage of the 160 cases with at least one problem reported from the class.

4. The rate of reported resolution of a class of problems is the percentage of problems that were reported resolved at the end of the case.

5. The definition of the number of problems expected to be resolved in the $j$th case (called $NE_j$) is

$$
\begin{aligned}
NE_j = \; & R_1 * I(\text{case } j \text{ has problem 1}) \\
& + R_2 * I(\text{case } j \text{ has problem 2}) \\
& + \ldots \\
& + R_{10} * I(\text{case } j \text{ has problem 10}),
\end{aligned}
$$

where $R_1, \ldots, R_{10}$ are the problem-specific rates of reported resolution and where $I$ (case $j$ has problem $k$) is a variable that has the value 1 if problem $k$ were reported for case $j$ and has the value 0 if problem $k$ is not reported for case $j$.

## REFERENCES

Beck, B. M. *The Lower East Side Family Union: A social invention*. New York: Foundation for Child Development, 1979.

Fanshel, D., Finch, S. J., & Grundy J. F. *Collection of data relating to adoption and foster care*. Washington, DC: Administration for Children, Youth and Families, U.S. Department of Health and Human Services, 1987.

Fleiss, J. L. *Statistical methods for rates and proportions*, 2nd ed. New York: John Wiley and Sons, 1981.

Jones, M. A. *A second chance for families: Five years later*. New York Child Welfare League of America, 1985.

Neyman, J. *Lectures and conferences on mathematical statistics and probability*, 2nd ed. Washington, DC: Graduate School, U.S. Department of Agriculture, 1952.

Ripple, L., & Alexander, E. Motivation, capacity and opportunity as related to the use of casework service: Nature of the client's problem. *Social Service Review*, 1956, 30, 38-54.

Tukey, J. W. *Exploratory data analysis*. Reading, MA: Addison Wesley, 1977.

Weissman, H. H. *Integrating services for troubled families: Dilemmas of program design and implementation*. San Francisco: Jossey-Bass, 1978.

# Computers in Agency Settings

Elizabeth Mutschler

## *INTRODUCTION*

Much has been written about the transformation of the United States and other technologically advanced nations from industrial societies to information societies. In an industrial society a majority of the work force is employed in manufacturing occupations, and the key element is energy. An information society is a nation in which a majority of the labor force is composed of information workers and in which information is the most important element (Bell, 1973; Mariem, 1984). One indication of the rapid speed of the information revolution is the number of computers in use. Starting in the 1950s, according to Rogers (1986), the number of computers in the U.S. went from 600 in 1956, to 30,000 in 1966, 400,000 in 1976, and over 8 million in 1986. It is expected that in the early 1990s, 50% of American households will have a home computer (Rogers, 1986).

Human service agencies are participating in this transition to an information society and are affected by the use of information technology in dramatic and substantive ways. During the 1960s and 1970s computer applications in human services have been limited mostly to fiscal and administrative functions, e.g., budget control, client billing, staff scheduling, or planning and monitoring the use of resources (Hedlund, Vieweg, and Dorg, 1985). Increasingly, however, information technology is also used in clinical practice, such as providing information for quicker and more effective intake and referral services, client-based information systems, programs supporting client assessment, treatment planning, monitoring and evaluation, or expert and consultation systems able to generate recommendations for human service decision makers (Gingerich, 1990a; Finn, 1988; Mutschler, 1987).

As human service agencies are expanding their use of computers, one important area of research is how information technology innovations are adopted and implemented; a subsequent research issue relates to the impact of information technology on human services. Adoption and implementation of information technology can be described using the theoretical framework of diffusion of innovations. Information technology and its potential for data processing and decision support are the innovations; human service providers, both individual professionals and organizations, are the users of the new tools. The technology and the users are inextricably intertwined and are likely to influence each other in the diffusion process.

This chapter addresses issues related to the implementation of information technology in human services. It briefly describes the evolution of computer applications in human service agencies, presents a model of diffusion theory to address current issues about adoption and implementation, and suggests further research regarding the effects of information technology on human services. Data from a 1987 survey of human service professionals regarding the utility of computer technology in their own practice will illustrate some of the issues addressed here.

## COMPUTER APPLICATIONS
## IN HUMAN SERVICE AGENCIES

Computer applications can be described by the objects they process (see Figure 1). Blum (1984) suggests three types of objects: (1) Data are uninterpreted items (collections of facts) given to the user. Examples are lists of client names, addresses, or services provided. (2) Information is a collection of data (or information) elements that contain meaning. The data are usually stored in a permanent database. Examples are selected reports about client or service characteristics, information about community resources available to clients, or computer-generated scores of assessment instruments. (3) Knowledge is the formulation of the relationships, rules, or practice experience by which information is formed from data. An expert or consultation system, for example, can generate informa-

FIGURE 1. Information Technology Innovations in Human Service Agencies

| Type of Innovation | 1950's | 1960's | 1970's | 1980's | 1990's |
|---|---|---|---|---|---|
| Data Applications | Agenda Setting | Matching | Redefin- ing | Clarifying | Routinizing |
| Information Applications | - | Agenda Setting | Matching | Redefin- ing | Clarifying |
| Knowledge Applications | - | - | Agenda Setting | Matching | Redefin- ing |

tion or recommendations for decision makers by combining the professional's input of client data with a predefined knowledge base and a rule base (Blum, 1984).

## Data and Information Applications

The listing of unsorted facts (data) typically represents the raw material for more complex information applications. We will describe four examples of information applications that have been developed and are currently being used by human service agencies.

*Management Information Systems.* This management tool systematically collects data through input documents, accumulates these data in organized data files, and processes and summarizes various aspects of the database in on-line or special reports. An MIS usually focuses on administrative tasks such as accounting and fiscal management, inventory, personnel matters, and generating external and internal reports. Recent emphasis has been placed on the development and use of integrated client and fiscal information systems that can serve such multiple functions as accounting, billing, client-tracking, planning, and evaluating client services (Grasso and Epstein, 1989; Newkham, 1986; Fanshel and Finch, 1985). Easy-to-use software for integrated database management has become available with the advent of smaller, less expensive, but more powerful interactive computers. So called "general application packages" permit noncomputer specialists (with relatively small amounts of training) to create and use sophisticated computerized databases (Hedlund, Vieweg, and Dong, 1985).

*Computerized Client Assessment and Monitoring.* Among the earliest computer applications in clinical practice was direct client interviewing (Greist and Klein, 1980). Research in many different settings, covering varied client problems, has clearly shown that computer interviews are reliable, accurate, and highly acceptable to most clients (Slack and VanCura, 1978). Early concerns about the presumed impersonal nature of computer interviews have been refuted by the findings that most clients find the interviewing process enjoyable and the interview content relevant to their problems. In fact, several studies have suggested that as the subject becomes more sensitive, such as counseling for alcohol and drug problems or sexual dysfunctions, respondents appreciate the computer interview even more (Greist and Klein, 1980; Erdman et al., 1981). Studies have found that 85% or more of psychiatric in-patients can be interviewed at the time of admission (Erdman et al., 1981). Hudson (1988) developed a computerized package of client assessment and monitoring instruments which is successfully used by human service agencies. The computerized instruments, which include monitoring of self-esteem, marital satisfaction, and parental attitudes, can be graphed and a printout of past and current client functioning can be obtained by the client and the social worker at the end of each session.

Figley (1985) reviewed the uses of computers in family therapy. The computer graphs and compares, for example, how different family members perceive closeness or distance among themselves. The computer's capability in handling complex data sets allows the graphic assessment of family interactions at the beginning, during, and at the end of treatment, thus contributing to assessment, treatment planning, and monitoring in family therapy.

So far, computer programs have typically been used to create computerized versions of already available interview schedules and instruments. However, the challenge is to develop new assessment tools that are designed to take advantage of the computer's special strengths. Johnson (1979) and his colleagues developed the Psychological Systems Questionnaire, a personality inventory, and similar work is underway by Greist et al. (1987) to develop a computerized version of the DSM III. Both instruments are designed specifically for interactive administration, computer scoring, and interpretation. Questions are presented according to a logical interrogatory branching sequence as opposed to a fixed linear sequence of questions. Through the use of this flexible system design, a large pool of items is reduced and individualized to allow a comprehensive, detailed and efficient assessment of each person who is tested.

*Computer-Based Client Education.* In a recent review, Gambrill and Butterfield (1988) pointed out how computer-based client education offers the advantages of cost-effectiveness, accessibility, added coverage to compensate for the shortage of counselors, and a way to provide information to clients in an anonymous format on topics that potentially are embarrassing. Examples include health awareness games in the waiting area of a medical clinic that serves a low-income, culturally diverse neighborhood (Hakanson, Ellis, and Raines, 1983). Other education programs provide information to clients about entitlements for which they are qualified, give female teenagers information about birth control, and help the elderly find available housing (LaMendola, 1985). An interactive computerized program about lithium, its potential side effects, and its interaction with other medications is being made available to patients in treatment for depression or related mental health problems (Jefferson, Greist, and Marcetick, 1979). More recent programs, particularly those that use videodisk technology, have the ability to branch and adapt according to the viewer's response (Denton, 1988). These interactive programs have great potential for letting the clients decide which aspects of the program best fit their own needs.

*Computer Applications Serving the Disabled.* A rapidly expanding area are computer innovations for disabled clients. Information technology can bridge gaps in two major ways: The first (and of most interest in this context, since it is an information application) enables the individual to gain access to different types of information which would not otherwise be accessible, e.g., "reading" a book for those who cannot see. The second enables the individual to control a mechanical device which substitutes a physical function, such as steering a wheelchair (Hales, 1987; Hawkridge, Vincent, and Hales, 1985). Reports of information applications range from a language program combined with video tapes for learning-impaired children (Kreis, 1979), to improving the written expression of learning-disabled students through specifically designed word processing programs (Kerchner and Kistinger, 1984), to a computer that can produce a braille version of a text that is entered by a typist with no knowledge of braille (Gill, 1982).

### Knowledge Applications

Knowledge applications are different from information applications. The latter retrieve, organize, and process information but they cannot go beyond the data stored in the database. Knowledge applications apply and evaluate data against a knowledge base and a set of rules in order to tell more; they can generate new conclusions. One example of a knowledge application is an expert or consultation system. Expert systems have evolved from a field of study called "artificial intelligence," which is concerned with giving computing systems the capabilities normally associated with human intelligence such as reasoning, learning, and self-improvement (Schoech et al., 1985). In general, expert systems consist of three parts: (1) an inference mechanism, (2) a knowledge base associated with decision rules, and (3) a set of facts. The inference mechanism applies rules to facts and thereby generates new facts and recommendations. This first component of the expert system assumes that complex decision tasks can be broken down into concrete decisions that can be represented in the form of if-then rules. The inference mechanism has control functions that determine under what conditions which rules should be applied to which facts; it also provides the "interface" with the user, that is, it asks questions of the user and reports conclusions.

A major part of developing an expert system consists of working with experts and professionals in specific knowledge areas to uncover the rules underlying their decisions (Schuerman, 1987). The rules in a decision support system thus embody specific knowledge of a particular domain. They typically indicate how strongly a given inference can be drawn when specific observations are made. An example of a rule from an experimental consulting system for child placement is:

IF: placement is needed, and
    relatives are available to care for the child, and     Premise
    relatives are willing,
THEN: PLACE THE CHILD WITH RELATIVES     Conclusion

(Schuerman, 1987)

The premise is the conditional portion of the rule and is formed by the conjunction of a set of conditions, all of which must be true for the rule to hold. When the premises of a rule are true, there is reason to believe that its conclusion is true.

As described by Schuerman (1987), the third component of an expert system refers to the facts of a specific situation; in clinical practice it is usually a particular client case. Some expert systems have the capability to deal with uncertainty by attaching probability values or uncertainty factors to facts and rules. For example, if it is almost certain that relatives are willing and able to care for the child, the probability would be .95; if it is questionable, the probability might be .60. The inference mechanism combines the certainty values of all facts and rules to determine the certainty (or probability) of the conclusion or recommendation generated by the system.

To summarize, an expert system consists of a knowledge base associated with decision rules, and an inference mechanism that is triggered by the practitioner's input of specific facts about clients and/or their problem situations. As more experimental expert systems are developed (Schoech et al., 1985; Gingerich, 1990b), their potential as well as their limitations need to be examined in practice settings.

The described development in information and knowledge applications is at once exciting and complex, challenging and diverse. Some of the emerging issues as well as potential future research directions in the application of information technology and its effects on human services will be addressed in the next section. The framework for discussion will be the diffusion of innovations model, developed by Rogers (1986).

## ADOPTION AND IMPLEMENTATION OF INFORMATION TECHNOLOGY IN HUMAN SERVICES

### Diffusion of Innovations Model

Everett M. Rogers has done extensive work studying the diffusion of innovations in contexts ranging from the introduction of boiling water in a Peruvian town to examining the effects of information technology in Silicon Valley (Rogers, 1962, 1986). Rogers' diffusion of innovations model, adapted for human service organizations by Larsen (1987) will be summarized briefly and will serve as framework for our subsequent discussion (see Figure 1).

Rogers defines diffusion as the process by which an innovation is communicated through certain channels over time among the members of a social system. The characteristics of an innovation (e.g., relative advantage, compatibility, work complexity), as perceived by the members of a social system, determine its rate of adoption. The diffusion process consists of a sequence of five stages, two of the stages occurring before and three stages after the decision to adopt the innovation.

*Agenda Setting.* This includes general organizational problems which may create a perceived need for an innovation. Most human service agencies are aware of computers and their potential. Their questions at this stage include: What tasks should the computer perform? How do we introduce the technology into the organization? What computers fit our needs? In many human service organizations we can also observe the reverse: They are beginning with a solution (the computer technology) but are not sure of the problem (Larsen, 1987).

*Matching.* At this stage the problem is matched with the proposed technological solution. This is a kind of assessment in which the human service organization decides which tasks could be done more efficiently and/or more effectively with the help of information technology. At this point a decision is made whether to adopt, perhaps on a trial basis, or to reject the new technology.

*Redefining/Restructuring.* The application of the information technology often differs from the users' plan before adoption. The initially designed information system must be adjusted to fit the organization. In addition, the structure of the human service organization may need to be changed. A new administrative group having responsibility for the computer system may be created, or the information technology may affect the power structure of the entire organization, such as when the new system creates access to information for different people of the agency staff.

*Clarification.* As more and more staff members begin to use the computer technology, the capabilities of the system become apparent throughout the organization. As this stage unfolds, more stable arrangements may be determined for the computer's use and applications. This is essentially the process of embedding the innovation into the organization.

*Routinizing.* The last stage in the implementation process is routinization. At this stage the computer has been incorporated into the regular activities of the organization, and no longer is considered to be an "innovation." The information system becomes part of the organization's established operating tools and procedures.

These stages do not always occur in neatly arranged sequences, nor is one stage completely finished before the next begins. Yet some element of each usually occurs during the implementation process (Larsen, 1987; Rogers, 1986).

## EMERGING ISSUES IN THE DIFFUSION PROCESS

As described earlier, we are currently observing a rapidly growing and potentially far-reaching process of computer applications in human service agencies. Computer use is moving from fiscal and administrative applications to a wide range of applications in treatment planning, patient education, and consultation or expert systems. In our discussion we are particularly interested in how practitioners in human service organizations perceive the accelerating implementation of information technology and how its use affects human service organizations and practice. In 1987 we did a survey of 60 experienced human service professionals who attended continuing education workshops on a variety of topics. The professionals were asked to complete a questionnaire about their agency's and their own use of computers, and their views about computer applications. While it is not a random sample, the respondents represent a fairly typical group of social service practitioners working in small, medium, to large human service agencies, serving urban and rural client populations (see Mutschler and Hoefer, 1990, for a more detailed description of the study).

## Matching Task Structure and Information Technology

During the initiation of the diffusion process, represented by agenda-setting and matching, the perceived needs for computer technology are defined and plans for implementation are developed. One question at this stage is which type of tasks are best served by the new technology. We asked the practitioners in our survey to indicate for which tasks their agencies and they personally used computers.

The results in Table 1 confirm earlier findings that in both administrative and clinical areas structured tasks are more likely to be computerized than unstructured tasks (Mutschler, 1987; Schoech et al., 1985). The agencies used the computer for accounting (76%), generating reports (72%), and recording client data (46%), as compared to much less structured tasks like treatment planning (9%), and clinical decision making (7%). A similar pattern was true for practitioners' own use of computers, except on a more restricted level. Practitioners' computer use at work was highest for word processing (16%), report generation and recording data (both 9%), clinical decision making (4%), and treatment planning (2%). Similar patterns of administrative and increasing clinical computer applications on an agency basis were found in recent surveys of computer use in private, nonprofit agencies (Finn, 1988), and in agencies serving as MSW training sites (Nurius, Hooyman, and Nicoll, 1988).

Relating these results to our earlier discussion of information versus knowledge applications, we find that at present information applications match a much larger number of tasks in human service agencies than knowledge applications. Studies concerned with the development of expert or consultation systems suggest that in human services decisions are often based on experience, intuitive judgments, and attitudes. As yet, we know too little about practi-

TABLE 1. Computer Applications by Human Service Agencies and by Professionals (n = 54)

| Applications | Computer Use | | | |
|---|---|---|---|---|
| | My Agency | | Myself (at work) | |
| | n | % | n | % |
| 1. Accounting | 41 | 76 | 2 | 4 |
| 2. Statistics/Reports | 39 | 72 | 5 | 9 |
| 3. Word Processing | 38 | 70 | 9 | 16 |
| 4. Management Information | 26 | 49 | 2 | 4 |
| 5. Recording Client Data | 25 | 46 | 5 | 9 |
| 6. Payroll | 23 | 43 | 1 | 2 |
| 7. Graphs/Charts | 19 | 36 | 2 | 4 |
| 8. Communications | 19 | 35 | 0 | 0 |
| 9. Quality Assurance | 14 | 26 | 1 | 2 |
| 10. Client Intake | 12 | 22 | 1 | 2 |
| 11. Education/Instruction | 11 | 20 | 2 | 4 |
| 12. Outcome Monitoring | 10 | 19 | 1 | 2 |
| 13. Literature Search | 8 | 15 | 0 | 0 |
| 14. Treatment Planning | 5 | 9 | 1 | 2 |
| 15. Clinical Decision-Making | 4 | 7 | 2 | 4 |
| 16. Interviewing Clients | 3 | 6 | 2 | 4 |

tioners' decision making, the underlying rules, and the knowledge base practitioners use (Schuerman, 1987; Schoech et al., 1985).

Regarding the match between tasks and information technology, Christensen (1986) suggests that researchers and practitioners need to ask a number of critical questions, including: Should an intake interview be transferred from an intake worker to a computerized assessment interview administered by a data entry clerk? Should social workers agree to use an expert system when they do not understand or know about the underlying rules, or if they believe the resulting recommendations are inappropriate for a particular client? Should clients be asked for their informed consents prior to their records being entered into the agency's information system, which can be accessed by a number of agencies via remote terminals? For which tasks are expert or consultation systems appropriate, and for which tasks should they not be used?

## Assistance for Users in the Redefining and Implementation Stages

Once the decision is made to adopt the new technology, it often is difficult to have it accepted and used in an organization. This is true even when the innovation has apparent advantages (Larsen, 1987). Many human service organizations have gone through the frustrations of failed or only partly implemented computer systems (Mutschler and Cnaan, 1985; Greist and Klein, 1980). It is often asserted that computer systems are more likely to be accepted if they are responsive to the needs of practitioners, and if users are well trained in the application of information technology (Hedlund, Vieweg, and Dong, 1985; Schoech et al., 1985).

We asked respondents in the survey about their training for using computer hardware or software. As Table 2 indicates, 44% of the respondents had no training at all, 32% had received training at college or a university, 19% through in-service training, 3% through computer stores, and 25% from a variety of sources. There was a significant relationship between training and computer use. Of those who had some training, 79% used personal computers at work. Of those without training, only 30% used personal computers (chi square $= 13.09, p < 001$).

When we asked respondents about their views on several issues related to computer use, an interesting finding emerged. As Table 3 shows, we found rather negative attitudes toward computer use. The majority of the respondents believe that the negative aspects of computers outweigh the positives. Only 12% think the computer can help with paperwork, and 9% think that it can aid in their work with clients. It is remarkable that concerns about the confidentiality of client data, which are frequently cited in the literature (Geiss and

TABLE 2. Training of Human Service Professionals Using Computers or Computer Software ( n = 60)

| Questions | n | Percent* |
|---|---|---|
| 1. Never have taken a course. | 26 | 44 |
| 2. Course on computing at college or university. | 19 | 32 |
| 3. Computing store course. | 2 | 3 |
| 4. In-service training on use of computers. | 11 | 19 |
| 5. Other | 15 | 25 |

\* Since some professionals participated in more than one type of training the total is greater than 100%.

Viswanathan, 1986; Erdman et al., 1981) were not evident in this survey. The participants' rather negative view may be based on current or past experience where they had to bear the heaviest burden in generating the input for new information systems but only rarely reaped significant benefits from large information systems (Mutschler and Hasenfeld, 1986).

The most surprising result, however, was that despite the relative negative attitudes toward computers, these attitudes did not seem to affect who uses computers. When we compared users and nonusers for each of the four items in Table 3, there were no statistically significant differences in the attitudes between those who are computer users and those who are not. It seems then that practitioners' attitudes toward computer technology alone do not determine the actual use of the technology. The findings of this study suggest that the amount of training, closely followed by easy access to a computer (Mutschler and Hoefer, 1990), are the most important factors related to computer use. Grasso, Epstein and Tripodi (1988) report

TABLE 3. Computers in Human Services: Views of Professionals (n = 60)

| Questions | Strongly Disagree/ Disagree | | Not Sure | | Strongly Agree/ Agree | |
|---|---|---|---|---|---|---|
| | n | % | n | % | n | % |
| 1. Computers can help me with "paperwork" (e.g., statistics, reports). | 42 | 72 | 9 | 16 | 7 | 12 |
| 2. The negative effects of computers and their potential costs are greater than their contribution to my work. | 8 | 14 | 16 | 30 | 31 | 56 |
| 3. Computers can improve my work with clients. | 33 | 58 | 19 | 33 | 5 | 9 |
| 4. The use of computers in human service agencies will breach confidentiality of client information | 51 | 97 | 2 | 3 | 0 | 0 |

similar findings regarding the effect of users' attitudes. Studying the utilization of a computerized information and program evaluation system in a residential child care agency, Grasso et al. found that users' attitudes explained only 3.5% of the utilization variance. The most powerful predictor (explaining 27.7% of the variance) was the users' perception of facilitators, such as timeliness of information, comprehensibility, and usefulness of reports. While administrators may not have much direct influence on workers' attitudes, they can provide training and make hardware and software available to users. Similarly, the importance of on-the-job training has been emphasized by recent findings. When Grasso et al. (1988) compared in-service training with computer training received outside the agency, they found that agency-based on-the-job training was significantly more effective.

Finally, human service practitioners also have to be aware that the implementation of information technology is an incremental process. Users frequently learn about the potential of a computerized system after some initial experience (Keen, 1988). The database, system design, and software, therefore, have to be flexible enough to be responsive to the skills and evolving needs of the users and the organization.

## *Implementation Effects on Users, Organizations, and Practice*

We asked respondents in our survey about general computer use on an agency level and whether or not they themselves used computers. Ninety-one percent of the agencies are currently using a computer. On an individual level, 65% of the respondents use a computer, while 35% do not use a computer at all (Mutschler and Hoefer, 1990). These findings indicate that, compared to surveys only a few years ago (Hedlund, Vieweg, and Dong, 1985; Schoech, 1982) where most of the applications were in the fiscal and administrative areas, we now have a much broader use of computers, including clinical applications (Mutschler and Hoefer, 1990; Finn, 1988; Nurius, Hooyman, and Nicoll, 1988). We can conclude from this survey, as well as from the literature review earlier in this chapter, that many information applications have reached the clarifying stage in the diffusion process, or have already become part of the routine procedures of a human service organization.

So far, few studies have addressed the significant and potentially far-reaching implications for human service organizations and practice. Larsen (1985), for example, describes three parallel effects or trends, all resulting from the implementation of computers. The first trend is substitution. The pattern of investing in information technology is similar to that previously observed in manufacturing, where there was an attempt to substitute capital in the form of technology for increasingly costly labor (Tornatzky and Fleisher 1990).

Some human service settings may plan to use computers to perform tasks now done by clerical aides. Greist and his colleagues (1980) also addressed fears of human service practitioners that some of their tasks might be done by computers. The degree to which this substitution is cost efficient, or what long-range effects it might have, needs to be explored.

The second trend is expansion of capacity, particularly that related to communications and information storage and retrieval. Human service users may realize the opportunities computers provide for extending activities, processing information, providing novel services through patient education, or to disabled patients, and through increasing awareness of programs and computer skills. Such information applications, as described earlier, are available at constantly decreasing costs if human service professionals know how to apply them to their day-to-day tasks.

The third trend is the movement toward end-user computing. This means that computers, and especially microcomputers, are no longer the property of computer professionals, but are found in the hands of those who actually perform the work of the organization. Data entry, report generation, and accessing information for decision making, for example, are increasingly performed by professionals interacting with their terminals rather than by remote clerks. Of specific interest is whether and in what areas end-user computing can improve the efficiency and/or effectiveness of human services.

The extent to which these trends are occurring and their potential effects on human services are only beginning to be studied. One of the few human service agencies that uses an integrated computerized information system on all levels of the organization and has begun to study its effects is Boysville of Michigan, a family treatment and residential child care setting for children and adolescents. Practitioners have been trained to use a computerized family assessment tool to document and monitor family functioning in relation to a number of outcome measures (Grasso and Epstein, 1989).

The authors note that in human service agencies the most commonly used clinical measures involve number counts of staff activity (e.g., client contacts, services provided, etc.) and client outputs (e.g., cases closed, type of program completion, satisfaction with service, etc.). The agency conducted a study examining the effects of regularly obtaining such quantified client information from all practitioners. The authors warn that quantitative measures of effectiveness and efficiency can result in a number of unintended goal distortions (Grasso and Epstein, 1987). In an earlier study, Conrad (1983) has shown, for example, that the assessment system applied in a New York foster care agency encourages foster care workers to put more emphasis on accomplishing a certain number of parental visits or placing the child in an adoptive home by the required date, rather than on the way these goals are accomplished. Grasso and Epstein (1988) cautioned in their report that the introduction of an effects management system alone places pressure on staff to conceal their practice problems or to hide their professional doubts. But for social workers to learn and to encourage professional growth, they must be free to doubt. The authors conclude that even the most sophisticated information system and computer technology will fail to produce beneficial effects without concurrent commitment of management to improve staff skill in integrating the information system into their daily tasks (Grasso & Epstein, 1987, p. 100).

Related questions need to be raised about the emerging potential of knowledge applications. For example, what is the role of expert or consultation systems? Will professionals be free to disagree with the rules selected for a specific knowledge domain? Under what conditions (if at all) can an expert system be used to perform tasks in human services (Gingerich, 1990b), or if a consultation system gives inappropriate or incorrect advice, who is legally responsible? (Schuerman, 1987).

## CONCLUSION

So far, human service agencies have implemented information technology mainly to realize gains in efficiency, using the computer's inexhaustible capacity for rapid, accurate, and consistent data processing and retrieval. As human services move into the information age we can expect greater emphasis on asking how information technology can contribute to making human services more effective. As a consequence we need to explore how information technology may alter those processes rather than simply supporting existing decision-making processes, since the creative use of computer support is hypothesized to improve existing service patterns. However, as has been shown here, we cannot assume that more information automatically improves the service effectiveness. Without specific training in how to use data, and how to creatively develop and implement decision support models which explicitly incorporate data, decision makers may frequently reject computer support innovations. Finally, we need a better understanding of the computer technology's intended and unintended effects on human services so that we can expand our knowledge about technology dissemination, and can facilitate the adoption and implementation of innovations.

# REFERENCES

Bell, D. (1973). *The Coming of Post-Industrial Society: A Venture in Social Forecasting*. New York: Basic Books.

Blum, B. I. (1984). "Why AI." In G. S. Cohen (Ed.) *Proceedings: The Eight Annual Symposium on Computer Applications in Medical Care*. Washington, DC: Institute of Electrical and Electronics Engineers, 3-9.

Christensen, K. E. (1986). "Ethics of Information Technology." In G. R. Geiss & N. Viswanathan (Eds.) *The Human Edge*. New York: The Free Press, 72-91.

Conrad, K. (1983). "Promoting Quality of Care: The Role of the Compliance Director," *Child Welfare*, Nov.-Dec., 639-649.

Denton, L. (1988). "Mental Health Field Begins to Interact with New Technology," APA Monitor, *19*(2), 20-21.

Erdman, H. P., et al. (1981). "The Computer Psychiatrist: How Far Have We Come? Where Are We Heading? How Far Dare We Go?" *Behavior Research Methods and Instrumentation*, *13*, 383-398.

Fanshel, D., & Finch, S. J. (1985). "Computerized Information Systems and the Quest for Permanency for Children in Foster Care: Observations from the New York Experience." In M. J. Cox & R. D. Cox (Eds.) *Foster Care: Current Issues, Policies, and Practices*. Norwood, NJ: Ablex Publishing, 73-112.

Figley, C. R. (Ed.) (1985). *Computers and Family Therapy*. New York: The Haworth Press.

Finn, J. (1988). "Microcomputers in Private, Nonprofit Agencies: A Survey of Trends and Training Requirements," *Social Work Research and Abstracts*, *24*(1), 10-14.

Gambrill, E., & Butterfield, W. (1988). "Computers as Practice and Research Tools," *Social Work Research and Abstracts*, *24*(1), 4-6.

Geiss, G. R., & Viswanathan, N. (1986). *The Human Edge: Information Technology and Helping People.* New York: The Haworth Press, Inc.

Gill, J. M. (1982). "Microcomputer Aids for the Blind," *Computer Education,* *42*, 21.

Gingerich, W. J. (1990a). "Developing Expert Systems." *Computers in Human Services,* *6*(4), 251-263.

Gingerich, W. J. (1990b). "Expert Systems and their Potential Uses in Social Work." *Families in Society,* *71*(4), 220-228.

Grasso, A. J., & Epstein, I. (1989). "Integrating Management Information, Program Evaluation, and Practice Decision Making: The Boysville Experience." *Computers in Social Work,* 4, 85-94.

Grasso, A. J., & Epstein, I. (1987). "Management by Measurement: Organizational Dilemmas and Opportunities," *Administration in Social Work,* *11*(3/4). 89-100.

Grasso, A. J., Epstein, I. & Tripodi, T. (1988). "Agency-Based Research Utilization in a Residential Child Care Setting." *Administration in Social Work,* *12*, 61-80.

Greist, J. H., & Klein, M. H. (1980). "Computer Programs for Patients, Clinicians, and Researchers in Psychiatry." In J. B. Sidowski, J. H. Johnson, & T. A. Williams (Eds.), *Technology in Mental Health Care Delivery Systems.* Norwood, NJ: Ablex Publishing Co, 165-166.

Greist, J. H., Klein, M. H., Erdman, H. P., & Bires, J. K. (1987). "Comparisons of Computers — and Interviewer — Administered Versions of the Diagnostic Interview Schedule." *Hospital and Community Psychiatry*, 38, 1304-1311.

Hakanson, N., Ellis, L. B. M., & Raines, J. R. (1983). "The Computer Health Education Projects: The First Four Years," *Health Education,* *14*(6), 54-57.

Hales, G.W. (1987). "The Disabled." In F. Blackler & D. Osborne (Eds.) *Information Technology and People.* London: British Psychological Society, 149-166.

Hawkridge, D. G., Vincent, T., & Hales, G. W. (1985). *New Information Technology in the Education of Disabled Children and Adults.* Beckenham, England: Croom Helm.

Hedlund, J. L., Vieweg, B. V., & Dong, W. C. (1985). "Mental Health Computing in the 1980s: General Information Systems and Clinical Documentation." *Computers in Human Services,* *1*(1), 3-33.

Hudson, W. W. (1988). "Computer-Based Clinical Practice: Present Status and Future Possibilities." Paper presented at Conference on "Empiricism in Clinical Practice: Present and Future," Great Barrington, Massachusetts.

Jefferson, J. W., Greist, J. H., & Marcetick, J. R. (1979). "The Lithium Information Center." In T. Cooper et al. (Eds.), *Lithium: Controversies and Unresolved Issues.* Amsterdam: Excerpta Medica, 958-963.

Johnson, J. H. (1979). "Technology." In T. A. Williams & J. H. Johnson (Eds.) *Mental Health in the 21st Century.* Lexington, MA: D. C. Heath.

Keen, P. G. W. (1988). "Decision Support Systems: A Research Perspective."

In G. Fick & R. H. Sprague (Eds.) *Decision Support Systems: Issues and Challenges.* New York: Pergamon Press, 24-37.

Kerchner, L. B., & Kistinger, B. (1984). "Language Processing/Word Processing: Written Expression, Computers and Learning Disabled Students," *Language Learning Quarterly, 7,* 329-335.

Kreis, M. (1979). "Project Video Language: A Successful Experiment," *American Annals of the Deaf, 124,* 542-548.

LaMendola, W. (1985). "Introducing Computers into the Mainstream of the Human Services," *Computer Use in Social Services Network, 5,* 6.

Larsen, J. (1987). "Implementing Computers in Mental Health Settings." In J. H. Greist, J. A. Carrol, H. P. Erdman, M. H. Klein, & C. Wurster (Eds.) *Research in Mental Health Computer Applications: Directions for the Future.* Rockville, MD: National Institute of Mental Health, 110-122.

Mariem, M. (1984). "Some Questions for the Information Society," *Information Society, 3,* 181-187.

Mutschler, E. (1987). "Computer Applications." In *Encyclopedia of Social Work* (18th ed.). New York: National Association of Social Workers, 316-326.

Mutschler, E. & Cnaan, R. (1985). "Success and Failure of Computerized Information Systems: Two Case Studies in Human Service Agencies," *Administration in Social Work, 9*(1), 67-79.

Mutschler, E., & Hasenfeld, Y. (1986). "Integrated Information Systems for Social Work Practice," *Social Work, 31*(5), 345-349.

Mutschler, E., & Hoefer R. (1990). "Factors Affecting the Use of Computer Technology in Human Service Organizations," *Administration in Social Work,* in press.

Newkham, J. (1986). "Information Technology Applied to Facilitating Practice." In G. R. Geiss & N. Viswanathan (Eds.) *The Human Edge.* New York: The Free Press, 168-182.

Nurius, P., Hooyman, N., & Nicoll, A. E. (1988). "The Changing Face of Computer Utilization in Social Work Settings," *Journal of Social Work Education, 2,* 186-197.

Rogers, E. M. (1986). *Communication Technology.* New York: The Free Press.

Rogers, E. M. (1962). *Diffusion of Innovation.* New York: The Free Press.

Schoech, D. J., Jennings, H., Schkade, L. L., & Hooper-Russell, C. (1985). "Expert Systems: Artificial Intelligence for Professional Decisions," *Computers in Human Services, 1*(1), 81-115.

Schoech, D. J. (1982). *Computer Use in Human Services: A Guide to Information Management.* New York: Human Sciences Press.

Schuerman, J. R. (1987). "Expert Consulting Systems in Social Welfare." *Social Work Research and Abstracts, 23*(3), 14-18.

Slack, W. V., & VanCura, L. J. (1978). "Patient Reaction to Computer Based Medical Interviewing," *Computers and Biomedical Research, 1,* 527-531.

Tornatzky, L. G., & Fleisher, M. (1990). *The Process of Technological Innovation.* Lexington: Lexington Books.

# Development of an Empirically Based Practice Framework for Facilitating Family Involvement in Services to People with Developmental Disabilities

Melvyn C. Raider
David P. Moxley

This chapter describes an agency-based research project designed to determine the variables associated with the multiple dimensions of family involvement within an agency serving people with developmental disabilities. The project evolved out of the concerns of the agency's utilization review committee, comprising representatives of several disciplines of line staff and middle-level supervisors. The intended outcome of the project was to provide empirical information with which the delivery of services could be enhanced.

The utilization review committee of the agency was struggling with the issue of family involvement within its residential service delivery system. Although the agency served people who have been removed from their natural homes, center staff felt it was critical that family members maintain contact with their disabled relatives. Family members were encouraged to participate in many ways, including becoming involved in service planning, visiting the client in his/her home, and being involved with the client in community activities.

Subsequently, the administration of the agency became concerned that they did not really understand the extent to which family members were involved with their disabled relatives. The administration did not understand why some family members were involved and frequently participated with their relatives while others did not sustain contact. In addition, the administration did not understand

*345*

the barriers to family involvement. Without such information the administration was not comfortable in developing a broader base policy on the involvement and participation of family members. Consequently, the agency staff members did not have a clear programmatic direction for promoting family involvement.

The utilization review committee, with the support of administration, embarked upon a collaborative research project with Wayne State University Developmental Disabilities Institute and the Wayne State University School of Social Work. The faculty members from these units of the university saw the project as an opportunity to develop an applied research program in the area of consumer participation in human service delivery and recognized that the project held promise for involving social work graduate students in agency based-research practice.

Consistent with the author's commitment to service delivery-focused, agency-based research, line staff were extensively involved in every step of both the qualitative and quantitative phases of the study. The service delivery-focused approach to program evaluation and agency-based research is a process of collecting agency data and using it to answer research and/or evaluation questions of interest to workers and administrators. It is intended that by conducting such research the agency can improve the quality of services it provides (Raider, 1987).

The service delivery-focused approach involves a number of major steps, the three most pertinent of which describe the process used to conduct this research project. These are: (1) identification of the primary user, (2) establishing a research team and procedures, and (3) achieving consensus on research design.

## IDENTIFICATION OF THE PRIMARY USER

In the service-delivery approach to evaluation and/or research, the direct service worker is viewed as the primary user of research results. In addition, the primary purpose of the evaluation or research is to facilitate quality service provision. The impetus for initiating this research originated with staff and middle management, who are on the utilization review committee. This is rather unique in as much as the focus for initiating evaluation or research traditionally has been with top management. The authors welcomed the initiative of the utilization review committee and viewed it as a step forward in operationalizing the service-delivery approach to research and evaluation. Although the impetus for the research project originated with the utilization review committee, top management quickly came to support the initiative.

## ESTABLISHING THE EVALUATION TEAM AND PROCEDURES

The second step in implementing the service-delivery approach involves establishing a team to plan and coordinate all the activities necessary to implement the research or evaluation project. This team is usually quite active during the early stages of research, although, once the research project is substantially underway the team's work diminishes. For this project the utilization review committee served as both the research team and a focus group to help determine the research methodology. The team helped gain support and arranged logistics of meetings with each interdisciplinary case management group in the agency and arranged for a meeting of all the agency's staff. In regular periodic meetings the team planned for resources needed to carry out the project and specified logistics. A critical task for the research team was specifying detailed procedures to protect the rights of respondents. Respondents were to be assured that if they chose not to participate it would in no way affect services provided to them or the disabled relative. Confidentiality was guaranteed since participants' comments and/or responses would not be identified for agency staff. Further, participants would have the right to cease participation at any point in the process.

## ACHIEVING CONSENSUS ON EVALUATION FOCUS

In order to carry out this step of the service-delivery focused approach to research and evaluation, it is necessary to establish a process to enable both workers and administrators to agree on evaluation focus issues such as the research questions to be asked, the ways in which data will be collected to answer these questions, and how these questions may be operationalized so as to be measured.

The utilization review team served as a focus group for the purpose of conceptualizing research questions. The authors met with all individual interdisciplinary teams to gain their input and contributions. An open-ended, heuristic approach was taken throughout this process by constantly modifying research questions and the research methodology based on feedback from the various agency groups. Throughout this process the authors acted as "lynchpins" between the utilization review committee and the interdisciplinary teams.

## THE LITERATURE

The literature on family involvement in services provided to people with developmental disabilities is very limited. Much of the available literature does not view family members as active participants. When families are discussed it is typically in terms of parents, siblings, or others being a source of problems for the professionals who have the charge of working with the identified client.

The importance of involving families in services to people with developmental disabilities has been acknowledge for many years. As long ago as 1968, Congress incorporated parent involvement into the Handicapped Children's Education Program. Public Law 94-142 (Turnbull, 1983) has encouraged family involvement by specifying the role of family members in formulating, planning, and evaluating services to students with handicapping disabilities (Weintraub et al., 1976).

The rationale for involving family members is well known in the field of developmental disabilities. Shearer and Shearer (1977) identified reasons for promoting the involvement of family members. First, family members are consumers of services and so they should have input into which and how services are provided. Second, family members can advocate for the program and promote community support for its continuation and development. Third, family members can identify relevant service goals and objectives for the disabled person. Last, involvement of family members in programs can result in higher functional achievement by the person with developmental disabilities.

The nature of family involvement is often defined and prescribed by human service agencies and professionals rather than by family members themselves. Paradoxically, family members have not participated actively in specifying the nature of family involvement, nor have their needs been considered in prescribing appropriate forms of involvement with their family members who are developmentally disabled.

## *PROJECT GOALS*

The research project was guided by seven project objectives that cut across the domains of research, education, dissemination, and utilization. The objectives were to:

- develop a conceptual and operational definition of family involvement utilizing qualitative and quantitative measures that may be useful to the assessment of involvement within agency settings,
- identify and operationalize independent variable measures that may influence family involvement,
- assemble a database of information on involvement by families with a developmentally disabled relative,
- develop programmatic and administrative practice guidelines leading to the improvement of family involvement within an agency setting, and
- develop the skills and capacities of graduate social work students conducting the agency-based research.

## *THE RESEARCH SETTING*

At the time the research project was carried out, this nonprofit agency had a total budget of approximately 7 million dollars. The agency was working with over 100 community or specialized residential alternatives, serving about 734 clients who represented all severity levels of developmental disability. The agency served these individuals through the development, maintenance, and monitoring of foster care, group home, independent living, and nursing home residences. The majority of residents, however, resided within foster homes of from one to two clients.

As a means of assuring appropriate delivery of quality habilitative and residential care, the agency offers an extensive training program for its residential providers. In addition, the agency coordinates licensing and financial reimbursement of providers. The system makes use of an interdisciplinary team model. Teams of professionals composed of nursing, social work, psychology, clerical assistance, and administrative personnel deliver clinical services and provide case management to all clients. Approximately 80% of the agency's funding comes from the county mental health authority, with the balance being generated from contracts with the Michigan Department of Social Services.

## THE QUALITATIVE STUDY

### Defining Involvement and Development of the Questionnaire

Our research began with a pilot study, the purpose of which was to define family involvement in a manner which was as sensitive as possible to an array of potential involvement activities. A review of the literature enabled us to identify a conceptual framework guiding our definition of involvement which we used to develop a structured interview schedule. Stringent protections were built into the research protocol to assure clients of confidentiality and guarantee that nonparticipation would in no way jeopardize their receiving services. We then proceeded to conduct 40 in-depth interviews of family members who were randomly selected from the rosters of the agency.

From these qualitative interviews we identified a number of potential involvement activities that were both formal and informal in nature. Formal activities required the involvement of family members in administrative or programmatic activities like participating in quarterly team meetings. Informal activities included such things as gift giving, telephone contacts, and outings. These finding enabled us to empirically define family involvement as follows:

The participation of family members as active agents in promoting the well-being of a person with developmental disabilities and/or the well-being of developmentally disabled people as a group within our communities. Family members can collaborate effectively with professionals in all phases of service provision to affect beneficial outcomes for persons with developmental disabilities.

This conceptualization incorporates the idea of multiple levels of involvement within the service system and different roles that can be assumed by family members.

## *Levels of Family Involvement*

Family involvement can occur at multiple levels in the system, starting with the individual who is disabled, and extending to the general society or even to policy levels. The first level of involvement is person-focused. Here, family members seek to directly enrich people with developmental disabilities. The family can be involved in assisting its disabled member in learning new skills and capacities, working collaboratively with professionals in developing a realistic habilitation plan, advocating for the specific interests of the disabled member, evaluating the care provided to the person, and educating providers about the person's needs. An interview we conducted with an adult sibling of a person with a severe disability illustrates involvement at this level:

> It's important for me to keep up with how my brother's care is going. For me, involvement means keeping track of this plan. Whether it is really being done by professionals is important. More important is whether he is actually learning things. I keep a notebook of my observations and I record his progress in learning how to dress, use the transportation system, and whether he seems to be happy. I review these observations with professionals, especially the case manager.

The second level of involvement is program-focused, and seeks to enhance the design and delivery of services to persons with developmental disabilities. Usually this form of involvement takes place within an agency or within a service system. Family members can work with staff to assess the needs of developmentally disabled persons served by the program. They can also advocate for the program and evaluate its impact on the well-being of individuals with developmental disabilities. At this level forms of involvement are diverse. They include participation in advisory activities, agency governance (e.g., serving on the board of directors), and development of the agency's service delivery program. According to one family member:

> My personal definition of involvement is being active within my son's agency. I serve on an advisory committee that is looking at the needs of all clients within the program. We're trying to make some recommendations about using more community resources in the services the agency offers.

Community-focused involvement is a third level at which family members' participation can be identified. It enhances the responsiveness of agencies which provide generic services and stimulates them to provide additional services and benefits for developmentally disabled persons as a means of promoting their social integration (Heal, Haney, and Amado, 1988). Family members undertaking involvement at this level may work to promote community understanding of developmental disabilities, to encourage generic community agencies to make their services accessible to developmentally disabled persons, and to monitor and evaluate the accessibility and appropriateness of generic services.

One family member shared with us her efforts to make her church accessible to people with developmental disabilities:

> It wasn't that my church was against people with disabilities. They just don't understand them. I decided that my brother and the people he lived with should have a chance to worship at my church if they wanted to. I talked this over with my pastor and he helped me to get the congregation to make some changes. We had to make the church easy to get into with a wheelchair. So we did this and we had people with disabilities coming over to the church for services.

Finally, family involvement can focus on society's treatment of people with developmental disabilities. Family members have long made contributions to the field through involvement with voluntary associations (Dybwad, 1982). Family members pioneered the availability of many services that were later incorporated into government programs (Dybwad, 1982). At this fourth level of involvement, family members seek to influence social policy in the field of developmental disabilities. Testimony before governmental bodies, service on commissions or task forces, and participation on citizen committees can all be means by which family members protect and promote the interests of people with developmental disabilities. Involvement of family members is crucial at this level. Legislators and other government officials may give more legitimacy to family members' identification of the needs of persons with developmental disabilities than they do to professionals, who may be seen as promoting their own interests rather than those of disabled people.

Comprehensive family involvement, therefore, addresses the many levels at which involvement can take place as part of the greater effort of serving people with developmental disabilities. Professionals and agencies serving people with developmental disabilities can plan to incorporate family members at one or all levels of involvement.

The qualitative study also enabled us to develop a closed-ended instrument that could be used to quantitatively measure family involvement. The first section included a set of questions regarding the relationship of the informant to the disabled member as well as background questions regarding the person's disability. The second section involved questions about the circumstances that led up to the person's placement out of the natural home. A third section introduced questions pertaining to the accessibility of involvement activities to the informant and covered such issues as transportation, available time, motivation, and availability of professionals and providers to interact with the family member. Covered by the fourth section were questions about specific involvement activities and questions pertaining to the informant's knowledge of the person's disability and his or her habilitative program. A final section obtained demographic data. All questions were closed-ended and designed in a Likert format. Possible response categories ranged from strongly agree to strongly disagree.

## THE QUANTITATIVE STUDY

### Selection of Respondents and the Resulting Sample

Potential respondents were identified through the automated record system of the agency based on the criteria that their disabled member was an adult (defined as 18 years of age or older), the informant was related to the disabled family member, and the disabled person was residing within a community residential alternative, either a group home, foster home, or independent living situation. A large number of disconnected telephone numbers prevented a more systematic process of sampling. A total of 86 interviews were conducted with family members who could be contacted by telephone and who gave consent to participate in the study.

Of the 86 informants the majority were parents (74.4%), with the balance consisting of siblings (9.3%), grandparents (1.2%), and other kin (15.1%). Most respondents were Caucasian (67.4%), while the balance were Black (26.7%), Hispanic (3.5%), or other (2.3%). The majority of respondents were employed full-time (41.9%) or retired (27.9%), while 6.9% worked part time and 23.3% were unemployed. The mean age of respondents was approximately 56, and the mean years of education was 11.85.

The average time that the disabled member lived with natural family members was 11.85 years (S.D. = 10.14). Most of the developmentally disabled relatives of the informants were considered to have a disability which placed them in the moderate to severe range of functioning.

### Data Collection and Analysis Procedures

Interviews were conducted during the winter of 1987. To preserve confidentiality, the interviews were conducted by an employee of the agency who was trained by the researchers in the appropriate interview protocol. The interviewer contacted the informants by telephone, explained the nature of the study, and completed an informed consent procedure with the family member.

After consent was given the interviewer read each question and solicited the informant's rating. Each interview required approximately 45 minutes to complete.

Completed questionnaires were coded and read by an optical scan procedure into MIDAS, a statistical package developed and maintained by the University of Michigan. For the purpose of this study simple frequencies were generated for key questions. To test the statistical significance of each question for which frequencies were reported, the Kolmogorov-Smirnov Test was used. Correlational analysis was also undertaken.

## OVERVIEW OF RESULTS

### Description of Involvement Activities

Family members were most likely to agree with those items dealing with informal involvement activities rather than more formal involvement activities; informants were more likely to agree with activities such as sending gifts to the disabled family member, visiting with the disabled member in the home of the family member, and being very involved in making purchases. All of these activities achieved statistical significance using the Kolmogorov-Smirnov Test. According to this statistical test, family members were more likely to respond to these items in the direction of agreement.

It is important to identify those items that did not achieve statistical significance. For the most part, these items reflect formal involvement activities that professionals may indicate as being of some importance (Fullan, 1982). These activities involve: (1) making telephone contact with program staff, (2) participation in individual staffings, (3) visiting the disabled member in his or her residential placement, and (4) arranging recreational or leisure activities for the disabled member.

### Perceived Accessibility of Involvement

Accessibility in this context means the extent to which family members have time to be involved and whether it is easy to contact the disabled member or the residential providers, case managers, and administrators working with the disabled family members.

Informants tended to agree with the statements that they had time to be involved with their disabled family members, it was easy to contact the disabled family member, and it was easy to contact the member's residential provider and case manager. In addition, informants tended to disagree with the two statements about being able to discuss the disabled member's situation with the interdisciplinary team and with the agency supervisor. It is important to also note that most informants felt they were obligated to be involved with their disabled member.

Only one item did not attain statistical significance: the question asking whether it was easy for them to attend the agency meetings regarding the family member. However, according to open-ended comments of a number of family members ($N = 30$), staffings, clinical meetings, and planning sessions were not held at convenient times so that family members could attend. Overall, formal family involvement activities were seen as accessible to our informants. In only one instance — that is formal agency meetings — did qualitative findings reveal barriers to family involvement.

What activities did our informants tend to identify as important? To answer this question we asked our informants to provide an overall rating of involvement and we then correlated this rating with discrete involvement activities. The correlations with the highest magnitude were obtained for formal involvement activities. The informants who rated themselves as involved also said they were involved in staffings ($r = .4357$), support groups ($r = .5450$), and formal educational activities ($r = .5329$). Of lesser importance were more informal activities like telephone contact ($r = .3443$), sending gifts ($r = .2050$), visiting in the disabled person's home ($r = .3792$), participation in counseling ($r = .3041$), and providing financial support ($r = .2751$).

The results of the quantitative study, in combination with insights from the professional literature, enabled us to develop an administrative policy and practice model for facilitating family involvement. The model may be viewed as having two broad components: overcoming barriers to family involvement and interventions to promote family involvement.

## OVERCOMING BARRIERS TO FAMILY INVOLVEMENT

We identified three broad categories of barriers: (1) resource barriers involving the need for time, opportunity, and supports to make it possible for family members to participate; (2) training and skill barriers involving concrete knowledge and skills family members require to successfully carry out involvement roles; and (3) communication barriers relating to the knowledge and understanding families and professionals have of each other's subjective experience that can result in divergent views and expectations of involvement (Fullan, 1982).

In overcoming resource barriers professionals working with low-income persons must consider the extent to which family involvement can be sustained by people who have limited resources. Such an analysis is necessarily pragmatic and takes into consideration whether family members have time to become involved, whether family members will be "docked" for time taken away from work (if they are hourly wage earners), whether they have transportation, and whether the family can make arrangement for adequate child care to have the freedom to become involved with the developmentally disabled person. Providing convenient times, making child care arrangements, and coordinating transportation are just some of the supports the agency should consider when planning a program of family involvement (Reimenschneider, 1980).

In overcoming training and skill barriers it is especially important to equip family members with the skills to execute involvement roles successfully. For instance, becoming an advocate for a developmentally disabled family member requires not only detailed knowledge of individual planning, agency systems, and community political structure, but also the ability of family members to relate to professionals in different ways. Family members may need to learn to asset themselves and to deal with professionals in conflictual situations. By assessing what parents want from training, providing comprehensive training opportunities which address the diverse involvement roles family members can assume, and providing a flexible schedule of training, professionals can assist family members in building requisite skills for involvement.

Family members learn to be effective in influencing decisions and improving services if a training program assists them in developing the skills of gathering information, mastering techniques for intervening when necessary, and developing skills in providing support to one another (Moore et al., 1981).

Professionals can also benefit from a training and educational program aimed at the development of skills and capacities that are relevant to working with families (Fullan, 1982). A program of this sort should include content in areas such as listening actively, assessing family needs, negotiating expectations regarding involvement, and reaching out to families who are experiencing resource difficulties. Remeinschneider (1980) demonstrated that it is possible to equip professionals with the skills and capacities to understand the individualized needs of low-income and minority families and to design an effective program of family involvement where their resource needs are met.

Family members and professionals must reconcile their often divergent assumptions, views, and expectations of involvement to overcome communication barriers. It is critical to reach such reconciliation before attempting to recruit family members into a family involvement program. First, professionals and families can come together and define their different assumptions, views, and expectations. Second, family members and professionals can actively negotiate with each other to attain a joint understanding of how they can be involved and what activities each will undertake. Finally, professionals should not adhere firmly to "ritualistic" forms of involvement. There are many levels of involvement and many roles that family members can assume. Professionals should be concerned especially with reaching a "shared definition" of involvement and establishing mutual expectations based on this shared definition. This is especially important when families do not have abundant resources to support their involvement.

## INTERVENTIONS TO PROMOTE
## FAMILY INVOLVEMENT

Our approach to the promotion of family involvement considers the perspective of family members themselves and not merely the need for their involvement in formal administrative activities. There are three components of our proposed process: (1) contracting for family involvement; (2) developing a support system for involvement; and (3) monitoring and evaluating involvement.

### Contracting

The promotion of involvement begins with the professional and the family members joining to identify the preferences of family members. During this initial period, the professional must work with family members to understand the family's structure, needs, and resources. Professional-family collaboration is crucial in this phase because professionals and family members must come to a joint decision about an individualized definition of involvement and the possibilities for involvement available to family members. These options are:

1. *Treatment Agent.* Family members can be involved in the direct provision of habilitative services to people with developmental disabilities. Family members can offer skill-building opportunities in the home setting, work within classrooms, and implement key aspects of the person's habilitation plan.

2. *Planner.* Family members can serve a distinctive role in helping to identify and define appropriate goals and in selecting appropriate strategies for attaining these goals. They can be actively involved in collecting and imparting relevant information. Planning at the "person-focused" level of involvement may involve the family member working with the interdisciplinary team to identify habilitative needs and goals. Family members may have vital information about the person with developmental disabilities that professionals do not possess. This information may include historical, longitudinal, and naturalistic knowledge of the person's development and functioning. The involvement of family members as planners becomes especially crucial if an ecologically valid habilitation plan is to result. Family members can assist agency staff to plan services and to work with community agencies to plan and design generic service delivery.

3. *Advocate.* Family members can promote the interests and needs of the developmentally disabled person as if these interests are their own. This can take place at an individual level by promot-

ing the interests and needs of the specific family member, at the agency or program level by promoting the interests of the family as a group, at the community level by promoting within local government the interests of developmentally disabled people in general, and at a societal level by advocating social policies.

4. *Evaluator.* Family members can also assume the role of evaluator or monitor. Three basic evaluation questions are: Do people with developmental disabilities have adequate supports to help them develop? Do people with developmental disabilities benefit from the services or supports they receive? Are services provided in a manner that results in community integration of the person? At an individual level, family members can evaluate the effectiveness of individualized plans of services, while within the agency, family members can critically assess whether programs of service are actually making a difference in the lives of the clients served by the agency.

The evaluator role is also relevant at the community and societal levels. For instance, the family member-evaluator can help to define whether services and supports provided by generic agencies are appropriate and accessible to people with developmental disabilities. The family member also can advise on whether benefit programs are having a positive impact on people with developmental disabilities.

5. *Consultant/Educator.* This role takes advantage of the special knowledge that family members may have concerning the developmentally disabled person in the family. Family members' experiential knowledge can be incorporated into the education of professionals about the needs of a client. Such knowledge can also assist the education of staff about the perspectives, concerns, and ideas of family members, in providing consultation to generic providers, and in the education of state and national leaders about the needs of persons with developmental disabilities.

Once involvement roles have been agreed on, the involvement contract may be formalized. An involvement contract should be based on family preferences and desires concerning time commitments and on the types of roles and activities the family wishes to undertake. Professionals are likely to increase the probability that family members will follow through with such a plan and realize success if they collaborate with the family as early as possible in efforts to define involvement.

It must be recognized by professionals during the contracting phase that forms of involvement will vary among and between families. For example, one family may decide to be active in the process of individualized habilitation planning. Another family may become involved at home in teaching daily living skills. And another family may become involved in contracting agency professionals by telephone on a monthly basis to discuss the developmentally disabled person's progress and needs.

The process of contracting for family involvement must consider the possible barriers to involvement and the resources discussed earlier. Professionals must, therefore, conduct their needs assessment with family members to review and identify resource concerns. Linking an assessment of the needs of an individual family to a periodic needs assessment of all families participating in the agency provides a data base which can be useful in planning an agency-wide family involvement program.

## *Developing a Support System*

The development of a support system for family involvement is a second crucial aspect of our process. Support system development follows an ecological approach to family involvement and includes: (1) making the agency accessible; (2) recognizing the role of informal support; and (3) making normalized support services available to families. Gearing an agency to family involvement requires the organization to review its hours of operation, its proximity to transportation, and the attitudes of staff toward families. Steps that an agency can undertake include: (1) developing a broad agency policy on involvement, (2) building staff awareness of the importance of family involvement through in-service education, and (3) bringing families and staff together for joint educational and socialization opportunities.

Many families are embedded within extended families and/or have friendship networks that can support them in their involvement. These natural support systems can be adjuncts to family members' involvement through which they can obtain resources such as transportation and child care. These informal social support resources also can buffer the stress experienced by families of developmentally disabled persons by providing emotional support, information about how to cope, and crisis intervention for family members.

General support services may need to be provided to families to assist them in coping with problems not directly related to developmental disabilities, but which left unresolved may disrupt the involvement of family members (Slater and Wikler, 1986). Linking families to social, income maintenance, health, or mental health services may be a means of lowering their stress levels so they can invest energy in involvement activities. Employing these normalized resources within a comprehensive program of family involvement can be an important part of the strategy used to enhance the coping capacities of the families serviced by an agency.

## Monitoring and Evaluation

The process of promoting family involvement must also incorporate regular opportunities for professionals and family members to review and discuss family involvement activities. The needs and capacities of families will change over time. At certain periods families may be actively involved, while at other times, because of other life demands, their involvement may taper off. Monitoring this "ebb and flow" of involvement will allow professionals and families to renegotiate and modify involvement expectations. Such monitoring may also reduce the "role strain" families can experience by having to balance other life demands with the needs of the family member who has a developmental disability. The monitoring process, therefore, should be sensitive to how the needs and preferences of families change over time.

Evaluation of involvement takes place on a periodic basis. As emphasized by Shearer and Shearer (1977), a rationale for involvement is that it can increase the functioning of the developmentally disabled person. This is the major evaluative question professionals and family members should ask when reviewing the effectiveness of an involvement program: vis, has it made an impact on the life of the developmentally disabled person? An evaluation conducted with this as the paramount question keeps the developmentally disabled person at the center of all involvement activities.

This chapter has illustrated an approach which used research to provide a framework with which a model for practice was developed. Contributing to the success of the project was the collaboration of an agency committed to systematic planned change with a university. The agency benefited by obtaining empirical data to facilitate development of new policies and procedures to enhance involvement and participation of family members. The university benefited by having the opportunity to involve social work graduate students in "hands-on," agency-based research practice. Finally, consumers of service benefitted by having a direct impact on the policies and procedures which affect their lives and the lives of their developmentally disabled family members.

## REFERENCES

Dybwad, G. (1982). The Achievements of Parent Organization. In J. A. Mulick, and S. M. Pueschel (Eds.). *Parent-Professional Partnerships in Developmental Disability Services*. Cambridge, MA: Academic Guild Publishers.

Fullan, M. (1982). *The Meaning of Educational Change*. New York: Teachers College Press.

Heal, L. W., Haney, J. I., and Amado, A. R. (1988). *Integration of Developmentally Disabled Individuals into the Community*. Baltimore: Paul H. Brookes.

Moore, D., Weitzman, S., Steinberg, L., and Manar, U. (1981). *Child Advocacy and the Schools*. Chicago: Designs for Change.

Raider, M. (1987). "A Service Delivery-Focused Approach to Evaluation of Group Work Intervention in Residential Agencies." *Residential Treatment for Children and Youth*, 4 (4).

Reimenschneider, A. (1980). Parent-Professional Interaction: Key to Parental Involvement. Unpublished Project Report. Columbus, Ohio: Ohio State University School of Social Work.

Shearer, M. S., and Shearer, D. (1977). Parent Involvement. In J. B. Jordan, A. H. Hayden, M. B. Kaines, and M. M. Woods (Eds.). *Early Childhood Education for Exceptional Children*. Reston, VA: Council on Exceptional Children.

Slater, M., and Wikler, L. (1986). "'Normalized' Family Resources for Families With a Developmentally Disabled Child." *Social Work 31*(5), pp. 385-390.

Turnbull, A. (1983). Parental Participation in the IEP Process. In J. A. Mulick, and S. M. Pueschel (1983). *Parent-Professional Partnerships in Developmental Disability Services*. Cambridge, MA: Academic Guild Publishers.

Weintraub, F. J., Abeson, A., Ballard, J., and LaVor, M. (1976). *Public Policy and the Education of Exceptional Children*. Reston, VA: Council for Exceptional Children.

# INTRODUCTION TO SECTION V

# Educating for Research Utilization

Leon W. Chestang

Social work education finds itself peculiarly challenged in the matter of research utilization. On the one hand, our position in the academy encourages faculty to engage in research and scholarship. Moreover, accreditation standards related to research teaching combine with tenure requirements to push faculty members to place a high priority on research. At the same time, the pull of student interest and the demands of other areas of curriculum present countervailing forces to the motivation generated by these standards and requirements. This results, for some faculty members, in the single-minded pursuit of tenure and, for others, in rationalization of their failure to devote time to the integration of research in their teaching.

Neither of the above strategies contributes to the development of teaching approaches that foster research utilization. This is because faculty research dedicated to winning tenure often does not address the needs and interests of agencies and practitioners working in the field or because of their own interests and orientation, some faculty members fail to model for students their own convictions about the relevance of research to practice issues and problems.

For their part, social agencies and practitioners focused on dealing with the day-to-day problems of clients frequently fail to see the relevance of research to the tasks before them. It is important to note, however, that requirements for accountability by federal funding agencies and private foundations have resulted in significant changes in the expectations of both agencies and schools of social work. The expectation of collaboration between agencies and schools as a prerequisite for grant applications has the potential for increasing the partnership between agencies and schools of social work. Although much remains to be done, we are already seeing improvements in these relationships.

This development is important, because, as Jenkins observes in this volume, the probability of utilization of research finds is increased when the work is undertaken jointly by agencies and educators. Joint research activity also has the potential for addressing the problem of the frequently observed disjuncture between university-generated research and research generated by agencies.

In spite of the above issues, higher education for the social work profession is uniquely positioned to advance the utilization of research in our field. Certain obvious steps are implied by our role in the academy. We can, of course, teach about research and the use of findings in the field. What we have not done with sufficient emphasis is to call attention to the impact of research findings on practice. Such emphasis is particularly important today when public social services are wanting for trained professionals and when the commitment of so many students is to the private practice of their profession.

Although the findings of social work research do not offer a panacea for the pressing problems facing society, the do, in many instances, point the way to useful strategies for dealing with some of these problems. The field of child welfare is a case in point. The current emphasis on permanency planning as an alternative to foster care is, in large measure, a direct result of research in the field of child welfare.

Other issues cry out for new, innovative, databased approaches, including teenage parenting, alcohol and drug abuse, and school dropouts. Higher education in social work can lead the way in reaching out to agencies to develop research proposals addressing problems such as these.

While the opportunity and the potential for meaningful collaboration between schools of social work and agencies are present, this will not occur without their mutual commitment to the research enterprise. Funding agencies have provided the impetus by requiring joint activity. It is left to the partnership to approach each other and to begin the challenging work of designing practice-relevant studies from which educators, practitioners and the profession can benefit.

The following chapters raise many of the critical issues of which educators must be aware as they pursue this challenge. Rubin raises an important question as to whether our expectations of social work students, particularly those at the BSW level, are realistic. Jenkins stresses the importance of shared responsibility and participation in research if findings are to be used by practitioners. Kirk and Penka alert us that even with the new emphasis on research in the last decade, we can hardly be confident that graduates of MSW programs are reading more research articles or using their research skills, once they complete their education. And Rosenblatt cautions against the loss of creativity to which we can fall prey in the over-zealous commitment to research.

Each of these social work educators has provided a thoughtful analysis of a key issue facing professional education as we move toward the 21st century. The progress of our profession, the careers of our students, and the lives of the public whom we serve will be affected by the quality of the response we make to these and related challenges before us.

# Education for Research Utilization in BSW Programs

## Allen Rubin

A decade ago the social work profession was showing signs of an increased commitment to resolving long-standing problems in its production and utilization of research. It was not the first time such signs had emerged (Zimbalist, 1977; Kirk, 1979), but several developments — including increased public demands for accountability and related worries about job declassification, the growth of doctoral level social work education, the emergence of two new social work research journals, and the recognition of the applicability of single-subject designs to the evaluation of social work practice — fostered the optimistic view that this time significant progress in strengthening the profession's empirical knowledge base and its integration with professional practice might really ensue (Briar, Weissman, and Rubin, 1981).

Also fostering optimism was the convening by our professional organizations of national and regional conferences to address problems in the production and utilization of research. The proceedings of those conferences showed that despite the growing optimism, there was much indeed about which to be concerned. Studies were showing that social workers by and large rarely consulted research studies to guide their practice. They attached little value to research and seemed to lack the level of understanding of research methods needed to utilize research appropriately. Social work agencies were virtually devoid of support systems fostering research utilization. Moreover, social work practitioners holding negative attitudes about research could point correctly at the scarcity in our professional journals of research studies with implications that they were likely to find useful in guiding their practice (Fanshel, 1980; Briar, Weissman, and Rubin, 1981; Dea, 1981).

At the same time, low priority was being assigned to research in the education of social work practitioners. The 1969 Curriculum Policy Statement of the Council on Social Work Education (CSWE) downgraded research from a method to a content area (Meyer, 1986) and lacked specificity concerning research content in graduate programs. No curriculum policy statement existed at that time for undergraduate programs. Earlier accreditation standards regarding the research curriculum in graduate programs had been relaxed in the paradoxical belief that deleting research requirements would spur curriculum experimentation and innovation in research, which in turn would result in a stronger research curriculum that would be better integrated with practice and more relevant to students. But instead of promoting practice-research integration, this relaxation merely resulted in the widespread diminution of research requirements without any accompanying systematic infusion of research content into other parts of the curriculum (Rubin and Zimbalist, 1981).

What progress have we made during the past decade toward resolving these problems? What more needs to be done? My assignment is to address these questions in connection to education for research utilization at the undergraduate level.

## SIGNS OF PROGRESS

It is evident that *some* progress has been made in recent years regarding the role of research in social work education. Perhaps the most significant sign of progress is the increased emphasis on research and its integration with practice in the CSWE accreditation standards and Curriculum Policy Statement that took effect in 1983. The changes adopted in 1983 acknowledge the responsibility of graduate and undergraduate educational programs to prepare students to evaluate their own practice systematically, to show how content on research relates to the knowledge and skills that are included in the practice curriculum, and to impart an "understanding and appreciation of the necessity of a scientific, analytic approach to knowledge building and practice" in every part of the professional foundation curriculum (Meyer, 1986). These changes led Smith, DeWeaver, and Kilpatrick (1986) to remark:

Nowhere have more significant changes been made than in the philosophy and expectations governing the role of research in the social work curriculum. Research—perhaps the most troubled and troubling sequence in a social work curriculum—is now expected to assume much greater prominence within the curriculum and more adequate integration with other curricular areas. These changes both reflect and direct a new conceptualization of the professional social worker as one who incorporates more of the scientific method in practicing the art and science of social work. (pp. 61-62)

Other signs of progress can be found in the literature on social work education. Many more articles on research and its integration with practice have been appearing in the *Journal of Social Work Education* (formerly called the *Journal of Education for Social Work*) during the past ten years than had been appearing earlier. Also, more research methodology textbooks authored by social workers and filled with social work practice applications have recently appeared.

But these signs of progress do not mean that social work education is anywhere near an adequate resolution of its long-standing problems in preparing students to produce or utilize research. It is nice that more articles on research and its integration with practice are appearing in the social work education literature, but this trend may not represent what is happening in the mainstream of social work education. Although these articles have been identifying a variety of innovative ways to integrate practice and research (Kraybill, Iacono-Harris, and Basom, 1982; Barth, 1984; Rabin, 1985), and some of these integrative approaches seem to be having a somewhat positive impact on students (Reinherz, Regan, and Anastas, 1983; Dean and Reinherz, 1986), their appearance does not imply that these innovations are being adopted by others and/or that we are moving in general toward a widespread incorporation of research into practice courses or practice into research courses by instructors and programs that previously showed little interest in such integration.

## PROBLEMS

Moreover, the results of attempts to integrate research and practice have not been uniformly positive. Fortune (1982), for example, evaluated a research course that attempted to integrate research and practice and concluded that her negative findings suggested that a single course is not enough, "especially when other courses may not value a scientific approach" (p. 11). Some raise questions about the feasibility of more comprehensive approaches to integrating research and practice. Siegel (1983) evaluated a comprehensive strategy in one MSW program and found that students' attitudes about research worsened after the integrative experience. Siegel concluded that one plausible explanation for this deterioration can be found in the "limitations of the idea of empirically based practice" (p. 12). Among the problems she cited were difficulties in locating research studies whose findings could be used to inform practice, time and cost constraints involved in evaluating one's own practice effectiveness, and lack of support by agency administrators. Students' experiences in attempting to implement empirically based practice may have made them more aware of these problems and therefore made them more skeptical about the feasibility of empirically based practice. Similar problems have been identified in studies that have found that most of those MSW students who have been trained in empirically based practice do not actually conduct practice evaluation after graduation (Robinson, Bronson, and Blythe, 1988; Poulin, 1987; Simons, 1987; Siegel, 1983).

As for new accreditation policies, we all like to see our favored policies adopted, but our understanding of social policy analysis also tells us that adopting a policy is no guarantee that it will be interpreted properly or implemented appropriately. Many social work educators are not interested in research (Faver et al., 1986) and value it less than other curriculum areas (Griffin and Eure, 1985). Those educators who lack a research orientation or who doubt the wisdom of the new policy's aims regarding integrating what they teach with research may seek ways to resist complying with the policy. A recent content analysis by LeCroy and Goodwin (1988) of the course syllabi of practice courses in MSW programs suggested that only a small proportion of these courses appear to be in compliance with the 1983 CSWE curriculum policy stipulation that recent research be taught in practice courses. Thus, we might wonder whether the new policy will matter very much if the educators expected to implement it lack enthusiasm about research and about the policy. With these issues in mind, let us now look more closely at progress and problems in the research curriculum of undergraduate social work programs.

## THREE BSW PROGRAM SURVEYS

Three national surveys of the research curriculum in undergraduate social work programs were conducted during the past decade. A comparison of their results provides some clues about the progress that has been made during the decade, the impact of the new curriculum policy statement, and problems that remain unresolved.

The major finding of the first survey (Bogal and Singer, 1981) was that 43% of undergraduate research courses were being taught by a non-social work faculty member. This study also found that when social work faculty teach the research course a much stronger emphasis is placed on the relationship between research content and social work issues and practice principles. Its authors concluded that the findings illustrated the need for undergraduate research courses to be taught by social work faculty, arguing that: "Research taught as a separate discipline — often by non-social work faculty — cannot help but be seen as an 'extra' rather than an integral part of undergraduate social work education" (p. 49).

The second survey (Lawson and Berleman, 1982), conducted in 1980, also had troubling findings. Whereas the Bogal and Singer survey found that 43% of research courses were being taught by a non-social work faculty member, the Lawson and Berleman survey found that in a majority (53%) of undergraduate programs the research requirement was taught by non-social work faculty members, usually sociologists. More than two-thirds (69%) of the instructors teaching the research requirement reported that the social work students in their course were mixed with "students majoring in other disciplines, primarily sociology and psychology" (p. 90), and only a handful of the instructors teaching these mixed-major classes held separate expectations for the social work majors. Respondents attempted to justify this situation on grounds of a shortage of social work faculty (many programs had five or fewer faculty members) and the greater competence in research of other departments.

Lawson and Berleman also found in the course outlines submitted by the surveyed instructors that the required textbooks in the large majority of courses were interdisciplinary in nature. Two-thirds of the instructors reported the perception that good materials which integrated social work practice and research were unavailable. Lawson and Berleman also observed great variation in course objectives, ranging from the ability to read articles in journals to completion of a research project and multivariate data analysis. In addition, they found that 52% of undergraduate programs required only one research course and that in most of these programs this course did not cover statistics. Most of the remaining programs required two research courses, including one on research methods and one on statistics.

Thus, the above two surveys showed that as of 1980 there were serious problems in the undergraduate research curriculum. The situation they found was, in some respects, similar to that of MSW programs, particularly in terms of the number of research courses required, confusion regarding appropriate objectives for those courses, and inadequate integration of practice and research (Rubin and Zimbalist, 1981). But the latter problem, inadequate practice-research integration, seemed even more troublesome in undergraduate programs. Not only were instructors commonly removed from the practice curriculum, but about one-half of them were outside the field of social work altogether and affiliated with another department. Moreover, the social work students often were mixed with other majors in research courses that had no distinct social work expectations.

The third national survey of the undergraduate research curriculum was conducted by Poulin in 1987, four years after the first curriculum policy statement applicable to undergraduate programs was adopted—a curriculum policy statement that attaches great importance to the undergraduate research curriculum, emphasizes practice-research integration, and calls on BSW programs to go beyond the role of preparing consumers of research and to prepare entry level practitioners who are capable of evaluating their own practice, knowledgeable about program evaluation, and able to contribute to the generation of knowledge for practice (Poulin, 1987).

A comparison of Poulin's findings with those of Lawson and Berleman must take into account the differences in response rates to the mailed questionnaires that the two surveys experienced. Lawson and Berleman achieved a response rate above 50%, and the attributes of their respondent programs were consistent with national data on program attributes reported by CSWE. Poulin, however, obtained a response rate of 39.8% of BSW program directors (which perhaps has something to do with complaints from deans and directors about the increasing number of surveys they are being asked to participate in these days. I had thought about surveying BSW program directors to obtain additional and updated data for this report, but decided not to after reading Poulin's paper). More important than Poulin's smaller response rate was the fact that his respondents, in comparison with the CSWE data, underrepresented smaller BSW programs, which are most likely to feel that they lack the resources needed to implement a research curriculum consistent with the aims of the 1983 Curriculum Policy Statement.

Nonetheless, Poulin's findings suggest that undergraduate social work programs have a long way to go if they are to meet the ambitious aims of the 1983 statement. For one thing, there does not appear to have been any increase in the extent of the required research curriculum, which in Poulin's 1987 data accounted for a smaller percentage of course credits than in the 1980 data of Lawson and Berleman. For another, Poulin found that 42% of the responding programs have their research course taught by non-social work faculty. This is hardly any improvement over the 43% and 53% figures found in the earlier two surveys, particularly in light of the underrepresentation of smaller programs in Poulin's survey. Indeed, even if Poulin's figures are representative, one could argue that having 42% of the research courses taught by non-social work faculty four years after adopting the expanded objectives of the 1983 policy statement is less defensible than the 53% figure in the context of no curriculum policy statement. (Although these percentages may be unacceptably high, we should bear in mind that the percentage of BSW students who enroll in research courses taught by non-social work faculty is probably lower than these percentages, since the BSW programs with non-social work faculty teaching research tend to be the smaller ones with lower enrollments.)

The argument that the new curriculum policy statement makes farming out required research courses to other departments *less* defensible does not imply that this phenomenon was ever okay in the first place. Even without the expanded research aims of the new policy, we can decry farming out the required research courses simply on grounds that this is no way to help students see the utility of research to social work. That is, even if one rejects the aim of preparing undergraduate students to evaluate their practice or to produce research, one might insist on having research taught by social work faculty simply in order to more adequately prepare students to understand research, appreciate its value, and consume it. As noted above, the widespread farming out of required undergraduate research courses was observed and decried by Bogal and Singer (1981) and by Lawson and Berleman (1982) before the new curriculum policy statement was developed.

Returning now to the 1987 survey, Poulin also asked his respondents to rate the extent to which their students graduated with a mastery of each of eight research curricular goals derived from the 1983 Curriculum Policy Statement. Most respondents felt that their programs were at least moderately successful in preparing students to evaluate their practice effectiveness, but they ranked their success on this goal lower than most of the other eight research goals. Factors that were associated with perceived success on the practice evaluation goal were: (1) whether non-social work faculty members teach research; (2) whether practice evaluation content is covered in the research courses; and (3) whether practice evaluation content is included in the field work sequence. Poulin noted that the second of the above three factors did not hold up in a multivariate analysis since practice evaluation content is almost always covered in research courses taught by social work faculty.

Interestingly, almost 90% of Poulin's respondents indicated coverage of practice evaluation content in the practice sequence. This is in stark contrast to the LeCroy and Goodwin (1988) finding cited earlier that only a small percentage of MSW practice course syllabi mention content on research and practice evaluation. In considering this discrepancy we must remember that Poulin's data were on BSW program directors' perceptions only. Those perceptions might not accurately reflect what is actually being covered. It is not entirely inconceivable that many directors who reported adequate coverage of practice evaluation content were being influenced in their responses by a social desirability bias and may privately believe that the practice evaluation objectives of the Curriculum Policy Statement are not feasible at the BSW level.

Of course, the LeCroy and Goodwin data from course syllabi may not precisely reflect actual coverage either. All we can say at this point is that either the MSW course syllabi are grossly understating the extent to which MSW practice instructors are actually covering this content, BSW program directors are grossly exaggerating the extent to which their practice instructors are covering it, or BSW practice instructors are covering it much more than are MSW practice instructors. If we take the data reported by BSW program directors seriously, then their perceived success in preparing BSWs to evaluate their practice would seem to be maximized by the strategy of covering practice evaluation in practice courses, having social work faculty teach required research courses, and incorporating practice evaluation content in the field work sequence.

Yet Poulin also found that program directors perceived that three of the four most problematic obstacles to preparing students to evaluate their practice are related to field work. (Lack of student interest was the fourth.) These included the lack of field instructor expertise and interest in practice evaluation and the lack of opportunity in field placements for students to do practice evaluation. If we doubt the validity of the BSW program directors' self-reports as to the extent of practice evaluation content in the practice sequence, and believe that the LeCroy and Goodwin content analysis of practice course syllabi in MSW programs may more accurately reflect what practice instructors are really doing in BSW programs, then we might be skeptical of integrative strategies, such as the one suggested by Lukton (1988) that recommends deleting separate research courses and relying primarily on practice instructors to incorporate relevant research content into the practice sequence.

## ISSUES IN THE RESEARCH CURRICULUM

### Compliance with Curriculum Policy

Poulin's findings suggest that there may be some gaps between how the research curriculum is being operationalized in many BSW programs, particularly the smaller ones, and the expanded aims of the current CSWE curriculum policy governing the research curriculum in those programs. (The LeCroy and Goodwin findings suggest similar gaps concerning MSW practice courses.) That these gaps were observed four years after that policy took effect raises questions about how that policy is viewed by those educators who are expected to comply with it or who are expected to monitor such compliance. When those who are assigned the role of ensuring that organizational policies are implemented do not understand or do not like the policies they are expected to implement or enforce, they often interpret those policies in ways that fit their own needs or predilections and find ways to resist complying fully with the policies (Tropman and Dluhy, 1976). How have CSWE accreditation site visitors and commissioners, for example, reacted in accreditation reviews of those BSW programs that have non-social work faculty teaching the required research course or that lack practice evaluation content in the research, practice, or field work sequence?

I posed this question to Nancy Randolph, CSWE's staff director of accreditation. She responded that the commissioners view it as a problem when non-social work faculty teach the required research course, but not one that automatically means that a program is not in compliance with accreditation policy. In order to be approved for accreditation, programs with this arrangement would have to show that they have an adequate relationship with the external discipline, one that ensures that the research content will be related sufficiently to social work practice concerns. Randolph claimed that programs that cannot demonstrate such a relationship, or that lack practice evaluation content, are either being denied accreditation or are instructed to make needed improvements and report back within a year in order to obtain approval. Still, we might wonder how many schools that *appear* to have adequate relationships with an external discipline teaching the required social work research courses really are ensuring sufficient integration in the teaching of those courses. How many of them are just giving lip service to such relationships in order to get around a policy that they find undesirable or infeasible? Should we really accept these relationships as a substitute for having the research courses taught by social work faculty?

According to Randolph, programs having problematic attributes in their research curricula may have less to do with CSWE's enforcement of its policies governing research than with the fact that many faculty members pay no attention to those policies until their program's reaccreditation review is imminent. Furthermore, even then they may not fully understand what the policy means. Since programs come up for accreditation every seven years, it is conceivable that many of the ones with the problematic research arrangements are simply those that had been accredited just before the new curriculum policy took effect and therefore had not yet gotten around to paying attention to it.

## Is the Curriculum Policy Realistic?

Some, however, have questioned whether the aims of the current curriculum policy governing research are unrealistic. Smith, De-Weaver, and Kilpatrick (1986), for example, have noted that the new policy has raised anxiety among undergraduate faculty members who see it as requiring more than small programs can accomplish. The mean number of full-time social work faculty members in undergraduate programs is five (Rubin, 1986). Many programs have only one or two. And these faculty members may not be adequately prepared to teach research. According to Randolph, the CSWE commissioners take this into account when reviewing small programs for accreditation.

Meyer (1986) has reported a varied faculty response to the curriculum policy statement on the question of whether students at both the undergraduate and graduate levels should be expected to learn more than to be consumers of research. Some, such as Smith et al. (1986), have questioned whether the new policy requires more of undergraduate students than they are able to achieve. Perhaps many BSW program directors, who are in a special position to influence the implementation of the policy, feel the same way.

One director of a small undergraduate program confided that her chief criterion in hiring part-time instructors to teach the required research course was whether the instructor would nurture students, grade easily, and keep the course content and expectations at a very low level so as to avoid arousing anxiety and discontent among students in the program, whom the director portrayed as terrified of research and statistics. Moreover, the director questioned the wisdom of teaching research methods to undergraduate students, believing that simply assigning review articles that identified what interventions received some empirical support, such as the one by Reid and Hanrahan (1982) or by Rubin (1985), was adequate research preparation for undergraduate students ridden with math anxiety.

This conversation, combined with the LeCroy and Goodwin (1988) findings, made me wonder what would happen if we adopted at the BSW level the strategy proposed by Lukton (1988) for the MSW level that we delete research courses and rely primarily on practice instructors to cover practice-relevant research content. How many BSW program directors and non-research faculty members would operationalize this strategy in a manner that would fall far short of preparing students with the knowledge and skills needed to evaluate critically the designs and methodologies of research studies? How many would imply that all students have to do is read the conclusions of those studies?

Although the above comments came from just one director and were not part of any survey, we know that BSW program directors tend to value research less than other curriculum areas (Griffin and Eure, 1985). How many other BSW program directors share her views about students, hiring research instructors, and curriculum policy? We will probably never know, since most directors are not likely to be as candid as she was. Too bad; the answer would help illuminate whether the current curriculum policy is realistic.

### Will BSWs Evaluate Their Practice in Agencies?

An issue bearing on how realistic the curriculum policy is pertains to obstacles to BSW students conducting research, including evaluating their own practice, in social work agencies, and how those obstacles bear on what can be done in field work as well as in practice after graduation. The data available on what happens to BSWs after graduation are limited. The little data we do have are based mainly on responses to mailed surveys and contain potentially serious biases associated with nonresponse. It seems reasonable to suppose that BSW graduates who are not social work-employed and who have the weakest identification with the profession are greatly underrepresented in the data. Of the BSW graduates who did respond, almost 30% did not obtain social work employment and about one-fifth did not seek such employment, and these numbers seem to be increasing (Hardcastle, 1987; Attinson and Glassberg, 1983). One survey found that only 18% of them belonged to any social work professional association, as compared to over two-thirds of recent MSW graduates (Attinson and Glassberg, 1983).

We do not know how many graduates of BSW programs with the strongest curricula on practice evaluation are actually evaluating their social work practice after graduation. But studies of the same question among graduates of MSW programs with such curricula have had mixed results (Gingerich, 1977, 1984; Richey, Blythe, and Berlin, 1987; Welch, 1983; Simons, 1987; Robinson, Bronson and Blythe, 1988). Some of the findings have been encouraging, although our encouragement ought to be diluted by the likelihood that the real amount of practice evaluation may be exaggerated due to obvious response rate and social desirability biases. Most of the findings have been disappointing.

Even when BSWs succeed in attaining social work employment they conceivably may be less likely than MSWs to have roles that are conducive to employing practice evaluation technology. Their work with clients might be less likely to involve clinical objectives that can be plotted longitudinally or therapeutic interventions of sufficient duration for conducting single-case experiments. They may be more commonly expected to provide crisis intervention and case management services focusing on linkage and referral functions and resource provision objectives—services and objectives that do not fit easily with establishing baselines and monitoring variation over time in client behaviors or cognitions.

In light of the proportion of BSW graduates who do not even obtain social work employment, the lack of demand for research tasks in the role expectations of those who do obtain social work employment (Nelson, 1983), and the assumption that, by and large, BSWs seem to have less professional autonomy and identification with the profession than MSWs and are less likely to have opportunities to do practice evaluation, it seems reasonable to suppose that the proportion of BSW graduates utilizing research procedures to evaluate their practice is, at best, miniscule. (This reasoning, of course, does not pertain to those BSW graduates who go on to earn their MSWs. I should also point out that I am not disparaging undergraduate social work education here. It is easy to find serious problems at *every* level of our educational continuum. I am focusing on problems in research-practice integration at the BSW level simply because that is my assignment.)

Numerous obstacles to conducting practice evaluation in clinical practice in agency settings have been identified. Commonly mentioned are: the lack of organizational supports; disinterest in practice evaluation (and even hostility to it) among agency staff and field instructors; difficulties in applying scientifically valid methods with some case situations; difficulties in obtaining careful, unbiased, and nonreactive measurements, particularly in connection to the many repeated measures required in valid single-case designs; practitioner inexperience and uncertainty in using practice evaluation technology; and heavy time demands placed on practitioners (Robinson, Bronson, and Blythe, 1988; Poulin, 1987; Simons, 1987; Siegel, 1983). These obstacles are usually mentioned in the context of discussions about why so few MSW practitioners evaluate their practice. We can assume that such feasibility problems are even greater for BSW level practitioners.

## Ambiguity in Distinguishing Purposes
## of MSW and BSW Research Curricula

In light of the foregoing problems, it is understandable that some social work educators deem the curriculum policy governing research in undergraduate programs to be unrealistic. What is more, the policy is vague as to how to distinguish the different purposes of the research curriculum at the BSW and MSW levels. The same expectations—that students will be prepared to evaluate their own practice, use program evaluation, and contribute to the generation of knowledge for practice—are stipulated for both levels. Smith, DeWeaver, and Kilpatrick (1986) criticize this ambiguity, noting that the language used in the policy statement and accreditation standards is "provocative if not contradictory" and that social work educators tend to deem unreasonable the expectation that they prepare undergraduate and graduate students to achieve the same level of mastery of research content.

In the personal conversation cited earlier, Nancy Randolph, CSWE's accreditation director, acknowledged that the Accreditation Commission, after finding that its new standards governing research were difficult to interpret, reworded in 1985 the language of the standards to make it less "grandiose." In this connection, Smith, DeWeaver, and Kilpatrick (1986) pointed out the omission from the "guides" section of the accreditation handbook of the phrase that expects BSW programs to prepare students to "contribute to the generation of knowledge for practice." But Smith et al. also argue "that if students are effectively evaluating their own practice and programs, *then they are generating knowledge*" (p. 66; their italics). Smith et al. therefore recommended more dialogue between CSWE leaders and program faculty to clarify what is meant.

Questioning whether it is unrealistic to expect undergraduate programs to prepare practitioners who are capable of evaluating their own practice is not the same as questioning whether content on practice evaluation should be taught at all. If practitioners at other levels will be evaluating their own practice (which at this point remains a big "if"), it is important for BSW level practitioners to understand the logic and value of their work, and perhaps utilize it, in the same way that they understand and utilize more traditional research methods associated with nomothetic designs. In other words, one could think that the current expectations go too far, but still believe that practice evaluation ought to be a major content area in the required research course.

Since a substantial minority of BSW graduates will go on to MSW programs, we should consider the above issues not just in terms of what BSW level practitioners will do, but also in terms of how we might best link the BSW and MSW curricula and minimize redundancy between the two levels. As noted earlier, most BSW programs require only one research course, and most of the others require one research course plus one statistics course. Is that enough research course work to adequately prepare students to be able to evaluate their own practice and to introduce them to such basic research content areas as problem formulation and conceptualization, measurement and observation issues, sampling, strengths and weaknesses of alternative data collection strategies, causal inference and group designs, internal and external validity, interpreting descriptive and inferential statistics and tables, and so on? If not, where do they become prepared to evaluate their own practice?

### Increase the Number of Research Courses?

One possible proposal might be to increase the number of required research courses. Perhaps all BSW programs could require two research methods courses: an introductory one on traditional topics and a second one on practice evaluation. A third required course in the research sequence might cover statistics, an area in which social work students currently tend to be particularly weak — perhaps too weak to be able to adequately critique research studies or contribute meaningfully to them (Glisson and Fischer, 1987). That would add up to three required research courses, more than most MSW programs require. A nice idea perhaps, but has its time come?

## Do Not Use Research Courses to Teach Practice Evaluation?

Another possibility would be to assign the prime responsibility for preparing practitioner-researchers to the practice and field curriculum. If we do that, what content do we sacrifice to make room for the comprehensive evaluation content? Are our BSW graduates currently so well prepared in practice methods that we can afford to trade off a big chunk of the existing practice and field curriculum in order to make room for much more practice evaluation content? And can we find or develop practice and field instructors capable of and willing to focus intensively on the evaluation content?

As noted earlier, the study of MSW practice courses by LeCroy and Goodwin (1988) found that although CSWE currently requires that recent research be taught in practice courses, very few practice courses include published research in their readings. Until practice and field instructors develop much greater expertise and commitment regarding practice evaluation, relying primarily on practice and field sequences to prepare BSW students with the research material they need to learn how to evaluate their practice appears to be a risky strategy from the standpoint of ensuring proper and enthusiastic compliance with and implementation of the curriculum policy. Of course, we could recommend research/practice team teaching throughout the curriculum as one way to deal with this problem. But the feasibility of that approach is also dubious.

## Abandon Traditional Research Methods Content?

Alternatively, some might advocate abandoning traditional research methods content and focusing the research courses on practice evaluation exclusively. That would mean abandoning the objective of preparing intelligent consumers of research in order to produce practitioners who can implement practice evaluation procedures without much understanding of other forms of research or their value. And what would happen when these practitioners encounter the severe barriers in agencies to conducting practice evaluation?

### Linkage Between the BSW and MSW Research Curricula

If we focus on preparing practitioners who can evaluate their own practice in BSW programs, what are MSW programs to do in their research curricula? Does the similarity of purpose for the BSW and MSW levels in the current curriculum policy really foster linkage? Or does it merely foster redundancy? Perhaps it makes more sense from a linkage standpoint to have different purposes for the two levels, preparing BSW students to understand and consume the gamut of research methods of value to social work, including an introduction to practice evaluation and its role vis-à-vis other research methods and models, and enabling them to move immediately into a more advanced concentration on practice evaluation in their MSW education.

## RECOMMENDATIONS

Although the foregoing analysis has posed more questions than it has answered, several tentative recommendations can be derived from it. One pertains to the CSWE accreditation policy governing research in BSW programs. That policy needs to be more clearly explicated regarding the roles and level of autonomy or competence in practice evaluation expected of BSW graduates and how the expectations for the BSW and MSW levels differ. Perhaps we ought to expect BSWs to be able to apply practice evaluation methods on a beginning level that does not involve the degree of scientific rigor that would warrant disseminating their work for the purpose of generating knowledge for practice. If so, toward what ultimate end? To be prepared for more advanced study of practice evaluation in graduate school? To guide their own practice with findings that are not worth disseminating to others? These issues need to be addressed and clarified.

Another recommendation pertains to obstacles to conducting meaningful practice evaluation in agency settings. Social work educators committed to preparing practitioners who will evaluate their practice will probably experience little success until agency disinterest and hostility to practice evaluation are significantly alleviated. We could, of course, cling to the hope that our educational efforts alone will ultimately be sufficient in alleviating these obstacles and that we just need additional time as the more recent graduates who have been trained in practice evaluation gradually replace those who resist it. Perhaps ten years or so is insufficient time to attain the changes we seek. While that may be true, relying exclusively on our education of students seems risky. Those who do might be overestimating our long-term impact on students and underestimating the ability of the agency environment to make much of what we teach seem irrelevant or impractical. A more comprehensive strategy therefore would be to focus much of our efforts on current agency administrators and practitioners in order to improve their support of practice evaluation.

Until that support improves dramatically, we ought to have modest expectations of BSW programs (and perhaps even MSW programs) in connection to practice evaluation. In his book, *Historic Themes and Landmarks in Social Welfare Research* (1977), Sidney Zimbalist noted

> an excessive tendency for social work to 'go overboard' with the latest wave of research — when one succeeds in catching on in this generally research-resistant profession. (p. 406)

> \* \* \*

> Perhaps the periodic overenthusiasm is fed by the relative neglect of research at other times, so that the one extreme is a reaction to the other. In any case, there has been an obvious readiness to embrace a promising research approach as a potential panacea and ready solution to highly intractable and deep-seated ills. We saw this long ago in the research on the causes of poverty, in the social survey movement, in the drive for social work measurement, and more recently in the study of the multiproblem family. . . . What is clearly needed is a more evenly balanced and steady commitment to research and to research criticism throughout the profession over the long haul. (pp. 406-407)

If, despite all the above problems, we decide that the current expectation that BSW programs prepare their graduates to evaluate their own practice is not another example of "going overboard with the latest wave of research," then we need to communicate to undergraduate social work educators a more persuasive rationale for the policy and why it is realistic. But if we decide that the policy does go too far in the extent to which it expects BSW programs to prepare students to evaluate their own practice, then we might recommend a more balanced approach in which practice evaluation and single-case designs take their place alongside other important research methods. Thus, as suggested above, we might prepare BSW students to understand and consume the gamut of research methods of value to social work, including an introduction to practice evaluation and its role vis-à-vis other research methods and models, and enable them to move immediately into a more advanced concentration on practice evaluation in their MSW education. In other words, practice evaluation and single-case designs would constitute one of several important content areas in the required research course (as well as being covered in practice courses).

Finally, regardless of how the foregoing practice evaluation issues are resolved, we ought to take a very hard look at the circumstances under which accreditation is and should be granted to undergraduate programs whose required research courses are taught by non-social work faculty. More than one-third of the BSW faculty members in the United States have earned their doctorates (Rubin, 1986). Although the research training in doctoral programs is uneven (Rubin and Davis, 1981), it seems reasonable to suppose that most faculty members with doctoral degrees ought to have the capacity to teach an undergraduate *introductory* social work research course. If this supposition is reasonable, then we should be skeptical when BSW programs with at least one doctoral level faculty member claim to lack the resources needed to teach the required research course within the social work department.

Consequently, a study should be conducted to assess whether accredited BSW programs that farm out their required research course really lack the resources to teach research within the social work department and whether their arrangements with the external department teaching the required research course really result in an acceptable degree of integration with social work. Although we do not want to be insensitive to the resource limitations some BSW programs have, particularly those programs that have no doctoral level faculty members, the results of such a study would help us decide whether we should continue to grant accreditation to programs that farm out the required research course on grounds of having good communication or an adequate relationship with the external department. Denying accreditation may seem harsh, but would we accredit schools that farm out their required *practice* courses on the grounds that they communicate well with the external department teaching practice and that they lack faculty with sufficient practice expertise? What are we telling our students about research and its utilization in social work practice when we send them outside of social work to learn it? And is it reasonable to expect non-social work faculty, even those having frequent communication with social work faculty, to be able to teach research methods courses in a manner that integrates practice and research adequately — especially when social work majors are mixed with other majors? To reiterate, my point here would be pertinent even without our current curriculum policy — even if all we sought to do was prepare research consumers.

As noted above, this chapter has raised many questions and answered few. Its recommendations have been posed tentatively and primarily for the purpose of stimulating discussion. Although many problems have been noted and many issues remain unresolved, research and its integration with practice has become a much greater priority in social work education during this decade. Let us hope we make as much progress in the next decade.

## REFERENCES

Attinson, Zita and Glassberg, Eudice, "After Graduation, What? Employment and Educational Experiences of Graduates of BSW Programs," *Journal of Education for Social Work*, Winter 1983, 19, 1, pp. 5-13.

Barth, Richard P., "Professional Self-Change Projects: Bridging the Clinical-Research and Classroom-Agency Gaps," *Journal of Education for Social Work*, Fall 1984, 20, 4, pp. 13-19.

Bogal, Rosemarie B. and Singer, Mark J., "Research Coursework in the Baccalaureate Social Work Curriculum: A Study," *Journal of Education for Social Work*, Spring 1981, 17, 2, pp. 45-50.

Briar, Scott, Weissman, Harold, and Rubin, Allen (Eds.), *Research Utilization in Social Work Education* (New York: Council on Social Work Education, 1981).

Dea, Kay L., "Project Recommendations," in Briar, Scott, Weissman, Harold, and Rubin, Allen (Eds.), *Research Utilization in Social Work Education* (New York: Council on Social Work Education, 1981), pp. 66-73.

Dean, Ruth G. and Reinherz, Helen, "Psychodynamic Practice and Single System Design: The Odd Couple," *Journal of Social Work Education*, Spring/Summer 1986, 2, pp. 71- 81.

Fanshel, David, *The Future of Social Work Research* (Washington, DC: National Association of Social Workers, 1980).

Faver, Catherine, Fox, Mary, Hunter, Mary, and Shannon, Coleen, "Research and Practice: Orientations of Social Work Educators," *Social Work*, July-August 1986, 31, pp. 282-286.

Fortune, Anne E., "Teaching Students to Integrate Research Concepts and Field Performance Standards," *Journal of Education for Social Work*, Winter 1982, 18, 1, pp. 5-13.

Gingerich, Wallace J., "The Evaluation of Clinical Practice: A Graduate Level Course," *Journal of Social Welfare*, Winter 1977, 4, pp. 109-118.

Gingerich, Wallace J., "Generalizing Single-Case Evaluation from Classroom to Practice Setting," *Journal of Education for Social Work*, Winter 1984, 20, 1, pp. 74-82.

Glisson, Charles and Fischer, Joel, "Statistical Training for Social Workers," *Journal of Social Work Education*, Fall 1987, 3, pp. 50-58.

Griffin, Jerry and Eure, Gerald, "Defining the Professional Foundation in Social Work Education," *Journal of Social Work Education*, Fall 1985, 1, pp. 77-91.

Hardcastle, David A., *The Social Work Labor Force* (Austin, TX: Social Work Education Monograph Series, 7, 1987).

Kirk, Stuart A., "Understanding Research Utilization in Social Work," in Allen Rubin and Aaron Rosenblatt (Eds.), *Sourcebook on Research Utilization* (New York: Council on Social Work Education, 1979), pp. 3-15.

Kraybill, Donald B., Iacono-Harris, David A. and Basom, Richard E. Jr., "Teaching Social Work Research: A Consumer's Approach," *Journal of Education for Social Work*, Fall 1982, pp. 18, 4, 55-61.

Lawson, T. R., and Berleman, W. C., "Research in the Undergraduate Curriculum: A Survey." *Journal of Education for Social Work,* 18, 1, Winter, 1982, pp. 86-93.

LeCroy, Craig W. and Goodwin, Cynthia C., "New Directions in Teaching Social Work Methods: A Content Analysis of Course Outlines," Journal of Social Work Education, Winter 1988, 4, pp. 43-49.

Lukton, Rosemary C., "Barriers and Pathways to Integrating Research and Practice in Social Work: Suggestions for Innovation in the MSW Curriculum," *Journal of Education for Social Work*, Spring 1988, 24, 2, pp. 20-25.

Meyer, Carol H., *Curriculum Policy Statements in Social Work Education*, Social Work Education Monograph Series, School of Social Work, University of Texas at Austin, Fall 1986.

Nelson, Kristine, "Differences in Graduate and Undergraduate Performance in a

Core Research Course," *Journal of Education for Social Work*, Spring 1983, 19, 2, pp. 77-84.

Poulin, John, "Practice Evaluation in Undergraduate Social Work Education: Assessments and Obstacles," *Proceedings of the 5th Annual Association of Baccalaureate Program Directors Conference*, Kansas City, Fall 1987.

Rabin, Claire, "Matching the Research Seminar to Meet Practice Needs: A Method for Integrating Research and Practice," *Journal of Social Work Education*, Winter 1985, 1, pp. 5-12.

Reid, William and Hanrahan, P., "Recent Evaluations of Social Work: Grounds for Optimism," *Social Work*, 27, 1982, pp. 328-340.

Reinherz, Helen, Regan, Joseph M., and Anastas, Jeane W., "A Research Curriculum for Future Clinicians: A Multimodel Strategy," *Journal of Education for Social Work*, Spring 1983, 19, 2, pp. 35-41.

Richey, Cheryl A., Blythe, Betty J., and Berlin, Sharon B., "Do Social Workers Evaluate Their Practice?" *Social Work Research & Abstracts*, Summer 1987, pp. 14-20.

Robinson, Elizabeth A. R., Bronson, Denise E., and Blythe, Betty J., "An Analysis of the Implementation of Single-Case Evaluation by Practitioners," *Social Service Review*, June 1988, pp. 285-299.

Rubin, Allen, "Practice Effectiveness: More Grounds for Optimism," *Social Work*, 30, 1985, pp. 469-476.

Rubin, Allen, *Statistics on Social Work Education in the United States: 1985* (New York: Council on Social Work Education, 1986).

Rubin, Allen and Davis, Robbie J., "The Elusive Doctoral Curriculum: A Dilemma for the Social Work Profession," *ARETE*, Spring 1981, pp. 1-10.

Rubin, Allen and Zimbalist, Sidney E., "Issues in the MSW Research Curriculum: 1968-1979," in Briar, Scott, Weissman, Harold, and Rubin, Allen (Eds.), *Research Utilization in Social Work Education* (New York: Council on Social Work Education, 1981), pp. 6-16.

Siegel, Deborah H., "Can Research and Practice be Integrated in Social Work Education?" *Journal of Education for Social Work*, Fall 1983, 19, 4, pp. 12-19.

Simons, Ronald, "The Impact of Training for Empirically Based Practice," *Journal of Social Work Education*, Winter 1987, 1, pp. 24- 30.

Smith, Michael Lane, DeWeaver, Kevin L., and Kilpatrick, Allie C., "Research Curricula and Accreditation: The Challenge for Leadership," *Journal of Social Work Education*, Spring/Summer 1986, 2, pp. 61-70.

Tropman, J.E. and Dluhy, M., "Politics and the Implementation of Policy," In Tropman, J.E. et al. (Eds.) *Strategic Perspectives on Social Policy* (New York: Pergamon Press, 1976), pp. 146-155.

Welch, G.J., "Will Graduates Use Single-Subject Designs to Evaluate Their Casework Practice?" *Journal of Education for Social Work*, 1983, 19, pp. 42-47.

Zimbalist, Sidney E., *Historic Themes and Landmarks in Social Welfare Research* (New York: Harper and Row, 1977).

# Research Utilization in an Agency-University Research Model: The Center for the Study of Social Work Practice

Shirley Jenkins

The bottom line for research utilization in social work is that the research findings must have utility for practice. Elegance of design, sophistication of statistics, and soundness of theory are all beside the point if the problem which is addressed has little relevance to client needs or service delivery. This does not mean that research with a theoretical base is not essential for knowledge development, but rather that theoretical studies are often couched in terms too abstract for application, or executed in highly selective, ungeneralizable sites. An interim step of application is often needed before findings can be operationalized. The complaint of researchers that practitioners are research shy is too often answered by practitioners who say, "Show me a finding relevant to my practice, and I will use it."

There are several structural factors in social work which interfere with the desired continuum from problem formulation to research utilization. Some of the difficulties relate to the duality in the profession itself, with one foot firmly planted in service and the other with a toe in knowledge building; to another duality in training, with the student doubly committed to academic study on the one hand and agency placement on the other; and to the competing demands of social action and program accountability. Another impor-

---

The Center for the Study of Social Work Practice is a joint enterprise of the Columbia University School of Social Work and the Jewish Board of Family and Children's Services.

tant factor is the late development of a corps of trained social work researchers who appeared on the scene decades after the profession was operational, and professional attitudes were already established. This sequencing can be contrasted with developments in other fields, where research findings preceded and laid the base for the profession, as well as for peer respect for research endeavors. The scientific model is to start with hypotheses, test them with research, build to theory, and then proceed to application. This difference in sequencing is often overlooked when issues of research utilization in social work are discussed. In social work research is too often considered to be an add-on feature for the field. Social work is typically problem and service driven.

In spite of all the difficulties encountered, it is nonetheless true that a substantial literature on social work research has been published, and that both universities and agencies have had a part in that development. Although this paper will speak to a particular model of university-agency collaboration, this is by no means suggested to be the only model. There are many examples of useful findings which have grown from a variety of other forms of collaborative or independent effort by both agencies and/or universities. There appear to be differences, however, in the level of research utilization which occurs, depending on research site and sponsorship.

## SIX STUDIES: UTILIZATION REVIEW

It may be self-serving to review one's own experiences, and they are certainly not generalizable. But experience provides insights which can lead to testable hypotheses and has face validity at the least. In this connection I reviewed six studies I have done in terms of whether the sponsorship was agency- or university-based, and what the outcome was in each study with regard to research utilization. What I came to realize was that the three of the six studies which were agency-based each had very specific research utilization of findings. The three which were university-based added to professional knowledge and may have influenced practice, but none had a specific utilization component.

Let me be more specific and briefly report on research utilization in four foster care studies, two agency-based and two university-based, and on two studies in the field of ethnicity, one agency-based and one university-based. The first study, an experimental design which tested the impact of intensive therapy on disturbed children in foster care was agency-based and executed, and had direct consequences for agency practice (DeFries, Jenkins, and Williams, 1964). A second study, also agency-based, described the course of entry into foster placement in a large city welfare department, and the findings included recommendations for changes in service patterns (Jenkins and Sauber, 1966). A research utilization follow-up to this study inaugurated a social worker hot line and homemaker weekend care which resulted in a substantially reduced child shelter population.

The third study, a university-based research project, was part of a larger program of longitudinal studies on children in foster care. The study involved three repeat interviews of a large sample of biological parents of children in foster care. Although the data base derived from cases of over 70 cooperating agencies, the research design, development, management, and analysis were university-based. Two books resulted from this work, *Filial Deprivation and Foster Care*, and *Beyond Placement: Mothers View Foster Care* (both Jenkins and Norman, 1972, 1975). In these studies, important ideas were developed on the roles and treatment needs of biological parents, and the new concept of filial deprivation was introduced. These ideas found their way into the professional literature, into concepts of practice in foster care, and even into state and federal legislation, but the specifics of research utilization, as narrowly defined, cannot be illustrated. At renewal time the question of how the findings were being used was actually asked by the granting agency. Our reply was, "I think we changed some peoples' minds." The response from Washington was, "That doesn't count."

The last university-based foster care study involved no direct contact with agencies, but was a secondary analysis of two national data sets, a stratified sample of census data on a county base, and national foster care placement data, by ethnicity, as collected by the Office of Civil Rights (Jenkins and Diamond, 1985). The analysis tested a series of hypotheses on ethnicity, foster placement, and poverty, and the published findings brought a wide response from the professional community. The major discernible research utilization, however, seems to be that other researchers are using or adapting the methodology in subsequent studies.

The two ethnic studies which I undertook show a direct contrast in utilization. The first was university-based and government-funded, and it explored ethnic factors in service delivery (Jenkins, 1981). Both national and international material was used. The book from the study was well received, and became part of a growing literature in ethnicity and service delivery. The second ethnic study was agency-based and foundation-funded, and dealt with ethnic associations both locally and internationally (Jenkins, ed., 1988). A subsequent foundation grant for local research utilization was used by the sponsoring agency to bring together ethnic leaders in an "Ethnic Network" and to develop goals and programs of mutual concern.

There are two conclusions from this highly selective sample of six. The first is that where the research was agency-based, the findings were implemented and research was directly utilized. Where the studies were university-based, the major outcomes were contributions to the professional literature. A second thought, however, is that the entire concept of research utilization typically tends to be narrowly defined in programmatic terms, and that "changing people's minds" may indeed be an important part of research utilization. Ideally, of course, research that affects both thought and behavior, and adds to knowledge as well as improving services, should be the desired goal.

## CHANGES IN AGENCY-BASED RESEARCH

The relative roles of university and agency in social work research have shifted over the years. As recently as 20 years ago, in New York City there were four voluntary agencies with significant research departments as well as other programs. The four were the Institute of Welfare Research at the Community Service Society, and research departments at the Child Welfare League, the Community Council of Greater New York, and the Family Service Association of America.

For one reason or another none of these agency research enterprises is functioning in New York today as a knowledge building enterprise for social work practice. The Family Service Association of America and the Child Welfare League have relocated to other cities, where they are now restating interest in research endeavors. FSA has a new vice-president for Research and Information Systems, and the Child Welfare League has a new Institute for the Advancement of Child Welfare Practice. The Community Council of Greater New York is dissolved; what was the Institute of Welfare Research, with its solid achievements in the movement scale and long- versus short-term treatment, is now a Department for Research, Policy, and Program Development, with a strong orientation to such areas as demography, income maintenance, and service delivery. This is useful work, but there is a void in the area of practice theory and research.

In the late 1960s the research pendulum began to swing to the universities; the enriched funding opportunities at the federal level with a premium on sophisticated methodology, the call for program evaluation as a component of program development, the growth industry of the lucrative private market for research consultants, the burgeoning of doctoral programs in social work with graduates trained in research methods, and the expansion of computer technology were all factors which had a negative impact on agency-based research. There was only one problem—the Willie Sutton factor. (When Sutton was asked why he robbed banks he said, "Because that's where the money is.") For practice research, the agency is where the clients are. Efforts at practice research outside the agency setting present real problems in access, relevance, and utilization.

At the same time that social work research was shifting from an agency to a university base, the expansion of federal funding for community-based programs gave a strong impetus to evaluation research. Scoring criteria for funding of federal grant applications contained a designated number of points for an evaluation methodology. Requests for program development were most likely to succeed if there was a strong and independent evaluation component, and the evaluators were frequently university-based researchers. Obvious problems surfaced: external evaluators faced defensive, often uncooperative program people; agency personnel knew their turf and clients, and sensed that university researchers had only a partial view of the totality of their problems. The literature on evaluation research expanded in the decade of the 1970s, and from the early shotgun marriage of program innovators and external evaluators there emerged some solid thinking on how to manage the process. An implicit, if not explicit goal was usually that of research utilization.

## GUIDELINES FOR WORKING WITH AGENCIES

Recognizing the importance of agency-based research for applied social work and the lack of criteria for investigators in this area, a group of intervention researchers have pulled together some guidelines to help researchers work in agency-based research (Schilling et al., 1988). Their proposals focus on four areas: developing research questions, client issues, costs, and recognition of service organizations.

A major client issue affecting researchers' access to agencies is whether or not there is a service component to the research, from which clients perceive that a tangible benefit will result. Reductions in funding have limited service delivery through regular channels, and clients and workers are often prepared to tolerate the added time and effort needed to comply with research protocols in order to secure otherwise unobtainable services. One anathema of research for agencies is the concept of the control group, and the need for clients to take pre-tests and post-tests in situations where no interventions are offered. The Schilling article suggests that the use of alternative treatments, rather than the "no treatment" option, would be a more acceptable design for agency-based studies, and that such a design can also have research validity.

Another relevant need is an even-handed approach to costs. Researchers are adept at creating line budgets which cover their own operations, but they often overlook costs to agencies of participation. For example, researchers place much importance on reliability involving independent judgments, and may not realize that when three workers evaluate a case, worker costs are tripled. Another sore point is client time to participate in research interviews. Compensation is rarely provided for clients, sometimes on the questionable grounds that money would corrupt client responses. But the message that comes across is that research interviewers are paid, their time is valuable; research respondents are not paid, their time is free.

A final grievance of agencies with the research process is that researchers tend to take the data and run, or at least publish, and they often forget to acknowledge the time and effort of agencies in the research enterprise. To whom do the findings belong: the researchers who conceptualized the problem and articulated the results, or the agencies, workers, and clients who gave the substance and content to the study? Or to both? Unless there is appropriate recognition of the agency contribution, the prospects for research utilization are limited.

## CENTER MODEL

Given the problems inherent in internal or agency-based research, and in external or university-based research, it becomes apparent that the need is to invent a new structure with a more viable base for both research and utilization. One model which has emerged, and is reported on here, is a research center jointly sponsored by a university, Columbia, and a major social agency, the Jewish Board of Family and Children's Services. Called the Center for the Study of Social Work Practice, it was formally established in 1988 as a joint enterprise — a partnership between a major research university and an agency which serves 45,000 clients a year. Partnerships between agencies and schools of social work in the area of training, and in the form of supervised field placements are inherent to social work education, and are accepted as mutually beneficial. The concept of partnership in research, however, is not generally recognized. Although it is not a problem-free model, it has much to recommend it.

Our Center for the Study of Social Work Practice is simple in conception, but complex in operation. The purpose is to add to knowledge, the means is by grounding research in practice. To this end we seek collaboration of research scholars with strong methods and computer competence, practitioners with practice wisdom and experience, and clients who have unsolved problems. We need each other as the medical school, the hospital, and the patient population need each other to make a collaborative effort. We have had a good start — at present six professors and four doctoral students from Columbia are involved in the Research Center, together with eight agency administrative and clinical staff.

The Center formally operates under a contract between Columbia University and the Jewish Board of Family and Children's Services, an agreement which specifies broad policies but allows flexibility in procedures. There is a Center administrative Core, comprising the Director on a part-time basis and an administrative assistant. The annual budget comes from the income from a $2 1/2 million endowment, raised by the Agency. Most of this is in place, in gifts and pledges, although all the funds will not be available for a few years. The funds come from private donors who want to encourage development of a strong research arm for the agency. They remain with the agency in an earmarked fashion, generating income which supports Core salaries, administrative expenses, and seed money for development of research projects. The advantage of the endowment is that it insures continuity and stability. The Director, who must have a University appointment, is responsible for research development, overall administration, and maintaining academic standards. There is a Professional Advisory Committee of four, composed of senior persons from both the School and the Agency, and a Development Council which includes prominent persons recommended by both institutions. The Center is located at the School of Social Work; committee meetings alternate between the School and the Agency.

In addition to the Core, the Center operates through separate research projects approved by the Professional Advisory Committee, each of which has its own director and separate funding. This allows for an accordion-like structure, with an endowed, modest, central administrative core not subject to the vagaries of annual shifts in funding, and a series of time-limited projects with different funding sources. Thus the overall activities can expand or contract, depending on project activity, without threatening the core budget.

In its initial organizational year, 1987-88, the Center completed the contractual arrangements between the University and the Agency, had its inaugural reception, received a Foundation grant, and saw a successful funding campaign of pledges and gifts to ensure the basic endowment.

The academic year 1988-89 was a year of research development; the major goal was to establish a sound substantive base of research activities. In May 1989 there were seven ongoing projects, in addition to discussions about future efforts. The range of subjects is wide, reflecting the varied interests and service areas of the agency. In terms of method, the research includes descriptive and analytical projects, follow-up and intervention studies, and hypothesis testing proposals. All studies draw data from Agency clients and workers, and all except one preexisting project jointly involve professional staff from both the School and the Agency. Common to all the projects is that each is related to a social work area, and each has implications for practice.

The seven ongoing projects vary in content, method, funding, and history. One which fits the projected model most closely is the "Bereavement" study. An Agency psychiatrist, Dr. Nina Koh, was concerned about the numbers of young children, primarily minority, who lost a parent through homicide, drugs, or other traumatic events. She wanted to develop group treatment for these youngsters, and to introduce an intervention method that would focus directly on their loss. Also concerned was Dr. Robert Abramovitz, Chief Psychiatrist at the Agency. Through the Center structure a research professor at the School, Dr. Rob Schilling, was involved in developing a design and method for this project, which had three co-investigators and Foundation support was secured. Beginning in one Agency office, the project now involves intervention groups in four different agency settings. The clinical interventions are undertaken by the Agency psychiatrist and specially trained social work therapists; the pre-test and post-test data on children and families are analyzed by the School's research team. Presentation of preliminary data was done at the March 1989 meeting of the American Orthopsychiatric Association, and findings will be reported in professional journals. Following the testing period, the methods used are likely to find their way into agency practice.

A second project has a similar history. A senior social worker at the Agency, Dr. Jonathan Rabinowitz, was concerned about decisionmaking in "Short versus Long Term Treatment." He collaborated with a research professor, Dr. Irving Lukoff, in the development of a design to study both worker and client characteristics and their impact on the decision process. With full administrative support, there was excellent worker response to the study instruments, which incorporate different versions of case vignettes. The data have been collected and are being analyzed.

There are three Center research projects arising from Agency programs. The Agency conducts a Cult Clinic, counseling former cult members as well as families with children in cults. A Foundation and a private donor support a research study, "Bridge to Adulthood: Personal History and Family Patterns among Former Cult-involved and Non-cult-involved Persons," to test certain hypotheses about conditions relevant to cult involvement and to compare family patterns of cult and non-cult persons. Co-investigators are Dr. Bruce Grellong, Chief Psychologist of the Agency, and Dr. Carol Marcus. Groups studied were former cult members, non-cult-involved persons currently receiving mental health services, and non-cult-involved persons not currently receiving such services. The questionnaires were concerned with patterns of family interaction and measured individual dynamics, personalities, and attitudes.

A program to serve the homeless is the site for two research enterprises. One is a six-month follow-up study on the "Outcome of Services to the Homeless," which explores the effectiveness of the Agency program. The second research is an exploratory study of the "Doubled-up Homeless." This research examines a substantial but little-studied group who live with relatives and friends, but lack a domicile of their own. Both studies were conducted by Dr. Ruth Fangmeier, with the latter study being her doctoral dissertation.

The Child Development Center of the Agency runs a Therapeutic Nursery School, which has had extensive experience in working with youngsters in need of special help. The "Child Development Study" involves following up 180 graduates of the Therapeutic Nursery School. The research design includes use of case records obtained when children were in the School, and extensive parent interviews on current functioning. School and community data will also be gathered. A major hypothesis is concerned with how problems of early language development relate to later functioning. The study is directed by Dr. Alice Frankel, C.D.C. Director, and the staff includes Rick Greenberg, research assistant, who is a doctoral student at the School.

The alliance between University and Agency pushed the issue of computerization of client data. A Task Force on Computerization was set up by the Center, including both School and Agency personnel, and a group of doctoral students undertook some exploratory studies on available data. The researchers' interest in computerization of clinical data was compatible with the agency executives' interest in documentation of their clients' problems. This concern was related both to treatment and to the need to secure an appropriate level of reimbursement for services. From this joining of interests, a new project, "The Patient Profile," was developed. Co-investigators include Drs. Abramovitz and Grellong, and Mark Mattaini, doctoral student at the School. A major study of approximately 1,000 current clients is underway, using agency workers as respondents. Computer technologies are being applied to organize, analyze, and report on a broad range of clinical issues and situations. This project is an initial step in developing a comprehensive information system for agency utilization.

In addition to program studies and computerization work, the Center is developing some more basic research with broader theoretical implications. The focus is in the area of social work assessment. A review of the literature in this field was undertaken by a doctoral student, and an article analyzing recent developments, co-authored by Mr. Mattaini and Professor Stuart Kirk, was presented at the meetings of the Council on Social Work Education, and publication is anticipated in a forthcoming issue of *Social Work*. A Task Force on Assessment, led by senior researcher Stuart Kirk and including both School and Agency staff, met over a period of several months to explore the possibility of developing a major research proposal in the area of social work assessment. One purpose will be the construction of instruments that go beyond diagnosis and are relevant to social work intervention.

Seven ongoing projects have been briefly described. There are discussions under way for new projects in the areas of family violence and battered spouses, and intervention with adolescents in residential and day treatment.

The Center structure maximizes the potential for research utilization of findings from agency-based research. But since all solutions create problems, the limitations also need to be noted. Although Center research is not confined to agency clients or programs, there is an implicit understanding that studies should be in areas congruent with the Agency agenda. The Center has viability because the Agency, the largest in the country, has a large and diverse clientele, and operates a broad range of programs. The readiness and capability of the Agency to assume responsibility for raising the basic endowment is a critical factor in the joint enterprise. The School, for its part, must have confidence in the Agency operations, and respect for the concerns of practitioners. Furthermore the Center as a model is only one of many research enterprises in the School of Social Work, where a large research faculty with diverse interests is involved in a variety of projects and programs.

On the positive side, the Agency, which has a reputation for professional practice and training, is now developing a research stance which is permeating program activity and planning. The School faculty, which has long bemoaned the lack of opportunities for practice research, now has easy access to a range of treatment programs and to thousands of clients, with due consideration for consent procedures. The Center has the security of endowment support, ensuring stability and continuity. Beyond the separate benefits to the School and the Agency, practitioner-research collaboration can lead to new approaches to problem solution.

In the effort to establish a more scientific base for practice, there is room for all types of research—from theoretical laboratory experiments to program evaluations in the field. Where research utilization is a primary goal, however, and if the integrity of the research method is preserved, the greater the collaboration of researchers and practitioners, the greater the chance that findings will have relevance and utility. The Center which has been described has a full agenda—and the next five years should give us time to test our model.

# REFERENCES

DeFries, Z., S. Jenkins, and E. C. Williams. "Treatment of Disturbed Children in Foster Care," *American Journal of Orthopsychiatry*, 34(4), July 1964, pp. 615-624.

Jenkins, S., ed. *Ethnic Associations and the Welfare State: Services to Immigrants in Five Countries*, Columbia University Press, New York, 1988.

Jenkins, S. *The Ethnic Dilemma in Social Services*, Free Press, New York, 1981.

Jenkins, S. and B. Diamond. "Ethnicity and Foster Care: Census Data as Predictors of Placement Variables," *American Journal of Orthopsychiatry*, 44(2), April 1985, pp. 267-276.

Jenkins, S. and E. Norman. *Beyond Placement: Mothers View Foster Care*, Columbia University Press, New York, 1975.

Jenkins, S. and E. Norman. *Filial Deprivation and Foster* Care, Columbia University Press, New York, 1972.

Jenkins, S. and M. Sauber. *Paths to Child Placement: Family Situations Prior to Foster Care*, Community Council of Greater New York, New York, 1966.

Schilling, R. F., P. Schinke, M. Kirkham, J. Meltzer, and K. L. Norelius. "Social Work Research in Social Service Agencies: Issues and Guidelines," *Journal of Social Service Research*, 11(4), 1988, pp. 75-87.

# Research Utilization and MSW Education: A Decade of Progress?

Stuart A. Kirk
Cindy E. Penka

Social work has confronted many challenges in the last 20 years. It has attempted to respond to new social needs and disadvantaged populations; it has defended itself from conservative federal administrations that have expected the profession to do more with less; it has watched nonprofessionals and other professions encroach on its traditional domain; and it has tried to be responsive to calls for accountability, both those stemming from reasonable concerns about its effectiveness and those that were barely disguised political attacks.

Schools of social work have felt these and other pressures. For example, applications to MSW programs—the life blood for all schools—have increased, dramatically declined, and are again rising for reasons few understand. Government funding for social work education has declined dramatically in two decades. Increased competition for students, funding, and jobs has been introduced by new schools of social work and emerging professions, such as family and marriage counseling. In addition, schools have experienced steady pressure from universities to increase the academic productivity of their faculties.

Schools have responded to these pressures in various ways. Curricula are now much less dominated by single theoretical and methodological approaches; a renewed emphasis on social reform made a noisy appearance in the late 1960s and early 1970s and then retreated; Master's curricula developed specializations by practice methods and/or field of practice to better prepare students for specialized practice; schools devised a variety of alternative, "nontraditional" programs to improve access, including part-time, work-study, advanced standing, and off-site arrangements; and in response to challenges to its scientific foundation and intervention effectiveness, schools gave increasing attention to the role of research in the profession.

This latter concern emerged, in part, from early studies of social workers' use of research that were interpreted to suggest that social workers were not particularly invested in supporting, using or doing research (for an alternative interpretation, see Kirk, 1990). Unfortunately, at the very same time, the Council on Social Work Education appeared to weaken the research standards for the accreditation of MSW programs (Rubin and Zimbalist, 1981). The National Association of Social Workers began accepting those with only bachelor's degrees into full membership and the Council on Social Work Education started accrediting BSW programs. Educational institutions responded to these changes by producing a stampede of new undergraduate programs, possibly draining resources from more research-oriented master's and doctoral programs.

Nevertheless, graduate social work programs have attempted to increase research and its use in several ways. One approach focuses on the research content in the curriculum and might be called the spinach strategy. Its premise is that scientific findings and methods are good for students, will make them stronger and better practitioners, but, like children and spinach, they will not partake of the stuff willingly. The curriculum tactic is to mix scientific findings and methods into their favorites so they won't taste so bad; in fact, they may hardly be able to detect what was consumed. Nevertheless, they and the profession will be strengthened.

In the parlance of social work, this is the strategy known as "integration." Instead of requiring more or beefier research and statistics courses—considered undigestible for MSW students—the research content is merged with other content in the curriculum (usually with practice and human behavior), where it is thought to be more palatable and perhaps even more relevant to the practice world that these students will inhabit.

A second approach uses the "proper tool" strategy. If you want practitioners to evaluate their clients' progress in an objective, research-based, and rigorous way, they will need the appropriate tools. We know that few clinicians in their everyday practice will have such flagrant disregard for practicality or zealous commitment

to experimental science to want to mount a pretest-posttest intervention with clients randomly assigned to treatment or control groups.
Recognizing this limitation has led clinical researchers (Jayaratne
and Levy, 1979; Bloom and Fischer, 1982; Barlow et al., 1984) to
design tools to fit practice.

This strategy is embodied in a collection of measurement techniques, research design innovations, and data analytic schemes that
had not been readily available previously. Rapid assessment instruments, single-case designs and time series analysis were packaged
together as the proper tool kit to allow and encourage every practitioner to evaluate their practice. The image of a practitioner-re-
searcher emerged to symbolize this new research craftsperson who
would contribute systematically to knowledge development.

These developments were captured in publications that came out
of a National Association of Social Workers' conference (Fanshel,
1980) and projects and conferences sponsored by the Council on
Social Work Education (Rubin and Rosenblatt, 1979; Weinbach
and Rubin, 1980; Briar, Weissman, and Rubin, 1981) in the late
1970s and ushered in a period of ferment, experimentation, and
optimism in schools of social work. The response of MSW programs was not uniform (Weinbach, 1981). In addressing the research curriculum, programs varied in their educational objectives,
required courses, and teaching methods. Some tried forms of curriculum integration, some emphasized educating practitioners as
consumers of research, a few encouraged students to be doers of
traditional research, and others promoted the emerging single-case
evaluation methods. Even the Council on Social Work Education,
reversing field, adopted in 1984 a new curriculum policy statement
and accreditation standards encouraging programs to train students
to evaluate their own practice.

Has this ferment, curricular experimentation, and optimism made
a difference? Prior to 1980 there was a rising tide of concern about
practitioners' research orientation and use, and about the apparently
weakened research curriculum (Rubin and Zimbalist, 1981). The
research curriculum was the subject of considerable attention during
the 1970s and throughout the 1980s. Are recent graduates more
involved in research than earlier ones? Has exposure to single-case
methodologies taken place in MSW programs? And if so, has it

made any difference in the practice of those graduates? Do recent graduates, more than earlier ones, have the skills needed to conduct single-subject clinical evaluations? In other words, what can we learn about MSW education by looking at graduates? These are the questions we sought to address in this study.

## METHODOLOGY

In the spring of 1988, a five page questionnaire and self-addressed, stamped return envelope were sent to a random sample of 500 *direct practice* social workers drawn from the National Association of Social Workers' current membership list. A month later, a follow-up letter and another copy of the questionnaire were sent to all those who had not responded to the first mailing.

The questionnaire borrowed and modified content used in other surveys.[1] There were sections containing items about the respondent's clinical world view and attitudes toward the usefulness of research. These data are discussed in another paper (Penka and Kirk, 1989). Other sections asked respondents about their level of skill and usage of various evaluation components, reasons why they use or do not use clinical evaluation methods, their exposure to single-subject evaluation content in their MSW program, their current involvement in research, and several items about their characteristics and practice.

### Variables

The questions pursued revolve around whether aspects of MSW education make a noticeable difference in the practice of social workers. There are five related MSW educational variables, the *independent variables*:

---

1. For example, we borrowed shamelessly, but with permission, from questionnaires used by Richey et al. (1987), Gingerich (1984), and Kirk et al. (1976) in their studies of social workers. In addition, items from a similar questionnaire used with clinical psychologists (Morrow-Bradley and Elliot, 1986) were reviewed. We also developed new items. Copies of the final questionnaire can be obtained from the senior author.

- the number of research and statistics courses completed;
- the number of research courses completed that focused primarily on single-subject design;
- whether respondents were encouraged to use single-subject design methods in field work;
- whether they conducted any single-subject design studies while in school; and
- the year they received the MSW degree.

There are six dependent variables, each measuring some aspect of social workers' involvement in research, either as a consumer or doer. These *dependent variables* include:

- the number of single-subject design studies conducted since graduating;
- the number of formal research projects of any kind conducted in the last two years;
- the number of clinical research articles using single-subject designs they read in an average month;
- the number of journal articles read in an average month;
- how skilled respondents thought they were in using each of 13 tasks that are major components of clinical evaluation; and
- the percentage of their clients with which they used each of the 13 clinical evaluation components.

These variables do not necessarily measure the most important educational experiences (e.g., role models) or the most valid outcome indicators. Nevertheless, they are the kinds of questions that have been asked in past surveys of practitioners and they are the sort of indicators faculty often mention when discussing intended outcomes of the research curriculum. These variables enjoy some obvious face validity.

## FINDINGS

### Description of Sample

The response to the initial and follow-up mailing was slightly higher than other similar surveys of social workers which have reported 40 to 50% response rates (Kirk et al., 1976; Kutchins and Kirk, 1988). From the 500 questionnaires mailed, six were returned as undeliverable and three were returned uncompleted because the respondent thought they were unable to respond for some explainable reasons (e.g., retired). That left 491 potential respondents from which we received 276 questionnaires, a 56% response rate.

The characteristics of the sample provide few surprises. The respondents are largely white (93%), female (80%), and employed full-time (71%). They have a median age of 41 with nine years of practice experience. A quarter of them received their MSW degrees prior to 1970 and 58% prior to 1980. The majority (65%) work primarily with individuals and groups, but an additional 28% have some involvement in multiple methods such as supervision, administration, and so forth. Respondents work in a variety of practice settings: social service agencies (16%), private practice (20%), hospitals (13%), out-patient facilities (16%), and in various combinations (14%). Theoretically, they spread across psychoanalytic/ego psychology (24%), eclectic (23%), behavioral/cognitive/task-centered (20%), and family systems (13%). Although there are no known parameters for direct practice NASW members, what is known from other surveys suggests that this sample is not remarkably dissimilar from others.

### Educational Exposure to Research

Almost all respondents had taken at least one research course in the MSW program. Only 3% had taken none; 30% one, 42% two, and 25% had taken three or more. Exposure to single-subject content was much less common. Sixty-six percent had no course that focused primarily on this content; 73% had not been encouraged to use such methods in field work; and 66% had never conducted a single-subject study while in graduate school. On the other hand, about a third of the respondents had single-subject courses, were encouraged in field placement to use them, and had conducted such a study while in school. Since roughly a third of all respondents had graduated before single-subject material had begun to appear in the social work literature (around 1973), the finding that a third of all respondents had some exposure to this content suggests relatively rapid dissemination among MSW programs during the last 15 years.

Table 1 presents the relationships among the five measures of educational exposure to research and clinical evaluation. Five of the ten relationships are statistically significant and in the expected direction. Those who have taken courses in single-subject design are significantly more likely to have been encouraged to use those procedures in field work and to have conducted such evaluations while in graduate school. These three variables "hang together" with moderately strong correlation coefficients (Pearson $r = .45; p < .01$). As might be expected, since they are not independent observations, the number of single-subject design courses completed is related to the total number of research and statistics courses taken ($r = .16; p < .01$). The year of MSW graduation, however, is not significantly related to either the number of research and statistics courses completed, the number of courses devoted primarily to single-subject design, or to the use of such procedures in field work. There is a weak but significant relationship between year of graduation and having conducted single-subject evaluations while in graduate school.

In general, these data suggest that those exposed to single-subject content in the MSW curriculum tend to be exposed to a collection of experiences involving classroom learning, encouragement in field placement, and experience doing such evaluation. These experiences appear not to be in addition to other research courses or, surprisingly, not to be strongly related to year of graduation. One could speculate from these data that total exposure to research content has not increased over the last decade, although some students, perhaps within certain schools, have been presented with somewhat different research experiences involving clinical evaluation.

### Consuming and Doing Research

Following graduation, do students read research content and do they engage in any research or single-subject evaluations? The vast majority read some journal articles each month (median = 3); few (8%) read none. A 1973 survey had reported median articles read as four per month (Kirk et al., 1976). Forty-three percent read on the

TABLE 1. Relationship Among Educational Variables (Pearson Correlation Coefficients)

|  | 1 | 2 | 3 | 4 | 5 |
|---|---|---|---|---|---|
| 1. Year of MSW graduation | — | .07 | .07 | .00 | .17* |
| 2. Number of research courses completed as MSW student | | — | .16* | .01 | .03 |
| 3. Number of single-subject design courses | | | — | .45* | .61* |
| 4. Encouraged to use single-subject methods in Field Work? (0 = no; 1 = yes) | | | | — | .59* |
| 5. Conducted single-subject studies in school? (0 = no; 1 = yes) | | | | | — |

Ns vary from 235 to 265.

* probability .01

average one to three articles; 24% four to five; and 25% read six or more. Fewer are regularly exposed to any articles reporting single-subject studies. Sixty-two percent report generally not reading such articles in a typical month; 24% read one and 14% read two or more.

As has been found in other surveys (e.g., Kirk et al., 1976), few social workers are actively engaged in any formal research. Eighty-one percent had not done any formal research during the last two years; 10% had done one project and 9% had done two or more. Involvement in doing single-subject design studies was also modest; 88% had conducted no such study since graduation, 6% had done one, and 6% had done two or more.

Those who read more journal articles (see Table 2) tend to read more articles on single-subject evaluations ( r = .39; $p$ < .01) and to have completed more research of some kind during the last two years (r = .18; $p$ < .01). Conducting single-subject design studies following graduation, however, is not related to these other activities.

TABLE 2. Relationship Among Outcome Variables (Pearson Correlation Coefficients)

|  | 1 | 2 | 3 | 4 |
|---|---|---|---|---|
| 1. Number of SSD studies conducted since graduation | ___ | .07 | .10 | .05 |
| 2. Number of SSD articles read each month |  | ___ | .39* | .18* |
| 3. Number of journal articles read each month |  |  | ___ | .20* |
| 4. Number of formal research projects conducted 2 years |  |  |  | ___ |

Ns vary from 234 to 255.

*probability .01

## Evaluation Skills and Usage

Doing clinical evaluation requires more than simple exposure to course content. It may depend on whether the practitioner feels competent in using certain procedures. Borrowing from the work of others (Richey, Blythe, and Berlin, 1987), we asked respondents how skilled they considered themselves to be with each of 13 components of clinical case studies. These 13 components included:

- operationalize or specify target problems;
- specify treatment goals;
- involve client in setting short-term and long-term goals;
- describe goals in measurable terms;
- write one or more treatment goals in the case notes;
- operationalize or specify intervention components;
- describe intervention techniques in case notes with enough specificity to allow another social worker to duplicate them;
- monitor client change over time;
- have clients self-monitor progress toward a goal;
- develop a questionnaire or rating form to measure a particular client's change;
- use a standardized questionnaire or rating form (e.g., the Beck Depression Inventory);

• use graphs to evaluate client change; and
• use statistical techniques to evaluate client change.

In general, there is a high degree of self-perceived skill on the first nine of the 13 questions. From 83 to 96% of the respondents thought that they had considerable or some skill in these areas. However, on the last four items, which are most specifically related to research operations (i.e., measurement and analysis), the proportion rating themselves as skilled dropped dramatically to between 29 and 50%.

Clinicians can feel skilled but not actually use those skills in practice. To study this, respondents were asked to estimate for each of the 13 skill areas the proportion of their clients for which they actually engaged in such activity. For the first nine items respondents claimed that they engaged in these evaluative activities with 75 to 98% (median) of their clients. Again, their responses to the final four items were strikingly different. On the last items the median percents were zero, indicating that few engaged in these procedures with their clients.

The relative lack of variability of the responses to these skill and usage items raises issues of validity. Are these data suggesting that almost all practitioners engage in what are considered activities involved in the systematic evaluation of clinical practice? Or, are these items too broadly stated and fail to measure clinical evaluative behaviors, but instead tap beliefs about good practice? A prior survey (Richey, Blythe, and Berlin, 1987), also found relatively high scores on many evaluative components, but low scores on the more research-oriented items.

### Relationship of Education to Outcomes

The primary concern of this paper is whether students' differential exposure to research experiences in the MSW program is related to their involvement in research in their later careers. Secondarily, has the last decade of curriculum innovation and methodological developments had a detectable impact on practice? Let us look at the second question first.

Surprisingly, there is no relationship between year of graduation and the subsequent practice of single-subject or other research. Similarly, the number of single-subject or general journal articles read was not related to year of graduation (Table 3). This finding held when using both Pearson r correlations and when recoding and collapsing the data into contingency tables and using Chi-square probabilities. In short, there is no linear relationship between graduation year and involvement in research in general or in single-subject evaluation in particular.

Similarly, the number of research and statistics courses taken while an MSW student does not appear to exert a significant influence on the graduates' involvement in research in subsequent years, contradicting one earlier survey (Kirk et al., 1976) which reported a significant relationship ( $r = 30; p < .01$).

By contrast, exposure to single-subject design content in graduate school appears to be significantly related to research involvement after graduation (see Table 3). Of the 12 relationships examined between the three single-subject educational experience variables and the four research involvement measures, eight are statistically significant and in the expected direction: more exposure to single-subject content was related to greater reading of single-subject articles and conducting research, both single-subject and other kinds. The relationships were of only modest strength, but noteworthy. Re-

TABLE 3. Relationship of Educational Experiences to Outcome Variables (Kendall's Tau B or C)

|  | POST GRADUATION | | | |
|---|---|---|---|---|
| IN SCHOOL | SSD STUDIES (3) | SSD ARTICLE (2) | ARTICLE READ (3) | RES. PROJ. (3) |
| 1. MSW Year (3)[a] | .07 | .04 | -.05 | .08 |
| 2. Number of Research Courses (3) | .00 | .08 | .07 | .00 |
| 3. Number of SSD Courses (2) | .16** | .20** | -.03 | .15** |
| 4. Encouraged in Field (2) | .18** | .13 | -.05 | .12* |
| 5. Conducted SSD in School (2) | .17** | .23** | .02 | .14* |

Ns vary from 225 to 259.

*probability  .05 using chi-square
**probability  .01 using chi-square

[a] Number of ordinal categories in the recoded variable are in parentheses.

search exposure was not related to the reading of general journal articles.

Earlier it was seen that the three indicators of exposure to single-subject content were significantly related to each other. And now each of these three variables tend to be related to the outcome variables. In order to further test these relationships, a simple exposure index was developed in which the scores on each of the three variables were combined. The Exposure Index, measuring exposure to single-subject experiences in MSW programs, had a range of possible scores from 0 to 4, with 4 representing someone who had at least two single-subject courses, was encouraged to use the content in field placement, and had conducted a single-case evaluation while in school. A score of 0 represented someone who had none of these experiences. Table 4 shows the relationship of the Exposure Index to the four outcome variables. As expected, there is a positive relationship between exposure and involvement in research after graduation. Those with more exposure to research content and experiences were more likely to have done at least one single-subject study, read at least one single-subject article per month, and to have done at least one formal research project in the last two years.

Few of the self-ratings on evaluative skills were related to educational exposure. Of the 65 relationships between the five educational exposure measures and the 13 skill areas, only nine were statistically significant, a number not much better than chance. Moreover, they occurred in no apparent pattern or cluster. Similarly, the use of these skills with clients was not related systematically to educational experiences. Among these 65 relationships, only four were significant and they did not fall in any pattern and are not more than would be expected by chance. Since there was little variation in the distribution of responses to the skill and usage items, perhaps it was to be expected that they would not be significantly related to educational experiences.

This study, of course, has its limitations. Has the response rate introduced some sampling bias? Are self-report instruments valid or reliable? Can one reasonably expect to detect any impact of curriculum change when it has been so unevenly implemented among schools? Do graduates of some programs become more involved in research than graduates of other programs? If so, is it because of their exposure to a research-oriented curriculum or because of self-

TABLE 4. Relationship of Educational Exposure to Outcome Variables (Percent)

| Number of SSD Studies Conducted Since Graduation | Exposure Index | | | | | Kendall's Tau C | P |
|---|---|---|---|---|---|---|---|
| | Low 0 | 1 | 2 | 3 | High 4 | | |
| None | 96 | 92 | 82 | 70 | 57 | .18 | .01 |
| 1 | 2 | 4 | 4 | 24 | 14 | | |
| 2+ | 2 | 4 | 14 | 6 | 29 | | |
| | 100 | 100 | 100 | 100 | 100 | | |
| **Number of SSD Articles Read 1 Month** | | | | | | | |
| None | 70 | 77 | 36 | 53 | 33 | .24 | .01 |
| 1+ | 30 | 23 | 64 | 48 | 68 | | |
| | 100 | 100 | 100 | 101 | 101 | | |
| **Number of Journal Articles Read 1 Month** | | | | | | | |
| 0-2 | 36 | 48 | 28 | 44 | 47 | -.01 | NS |
| 3-6 | 47 | 32 | 41 | 44 | 20 | | |
| 7+ | 17 | 20 | 31 | 12 | 33 | | |
| | 100 | 100 | 100 | 100 | 100 | | |
| **Number of Formal Research Projects 2 Years** | | | | | | | |
| None | 85 | 88 | 77 | 62 | 53 | .15 | .01 |
| 1-2 | 14 | 8 | 17 | 38 | 27 | | |
| 3+ | 1 | 4 | 7 | 0 | 20 | | |
| | 100 | 100 | 101 | 100 | 100 | | |

Ns vary from 219 to 231.

selection in deciding to enroll in certain schools? These and other pertinent questions are unanswered.

## DISCUSSION

There are data from this survey to fortify both optimists and pessimists. Those with sanguine predispositions can point to many encouraging developments. A clear majority of graduates have taken two or more research courses as MSW students. Already, despite the recency of single-case technology, about a third of practicing social workers have had some systematic exposure to these methods in class or field work. Almost all practitioners do some professional journal reading each month, although not many about clinical research. A small proportion of practitioners (about 10%) seem to be engaged in some formal research, a figure perhaps not too different from other practicing professions. But involvement in formal research is not a common major objective of MSW education; sensitivity to the need to evaluate clinical intervention systematically is a more appropriate goal. And in this regard there is considerable evidence of success. Almost all respondents indicated that they feel reasonably skilled in and use with most of their clients evaluative procedures that constitute the core components of single-subject design methods. Moreover, exposure to single-subject content in school is significantly related to involvement in reading and doing research following graduation. Not bad at all, say the optimists.

But, respond the pessimists, those observations do not necessarily indicate that any progress has been made. It is apparent that students are taking no more research courses than they were two decades ago. About a third of practitioners may have had some exposure to single-subject content, but this exposure is no greater for recent graduates than for graduates of many years ago. There is no evidence of a trend in which graduates are increasingly being exposed to such content or using it after graduation. Dissemination of single-subject methods, hailed in the 1970s as the way to wed practice to research, has been uneven, affected only a minority of graduates, and has had, at best, a relatively weak effect. The majority of practitioners who claim that they are using evaluation components are only providing socially desirable responses that social workers of 40 years ago would have given, long before the advent of single-case methodology. Social workers continue to read little and avoid research involvement. There is little evidence that things have changed much in recent years. Things are not good, say the pessimists.

Has there been a decade of progress or pretense for MSW education? Would we even know by surveying practitioners? Are we asking the right questions or asking them of the right people? Is there any consensus on what the right questions are? Is there any agreement on what could constitute good progress? Since this is being written to serve as a springboard for a conference discussion, it would be unwise to resolve these matters without the benefit of that thoughtful and vigorous exchange.

## REFERENCES

Barlow, David H., Steven C. Hayes, and Rosemary O. Nelson, *The Scientist Practitioner* (New York: Pergamon, 1984).

Bloom, Martin and Joel Fischer, *Evaluating Practice* (Englewood Cliffs: Prentice-Hall, 1982).

Briar, Scott, Harold Weissman, and Allen Rubin (Eds.), *Research Utilization in Social Work Education* (New York: Council on Social Work Education, 1981).

Fanshel, David (Ed.), *Future of Social Work Research* (Washington, DC: National Association of Social Workers, 1980).

Gingerich, Wallace J., "Generalizing Single-Case Evaluation from Classroom to Practice Setting," *Journal of Education for Social Work* 20(1), Winter 1984, pp. 74-82.

Jayaratne, Srinika and Rona L. Levy, *Empirical Clinical Practice* (New York: Columbia, 1979).

Kirk, Stuart A., Michael J. Osmalov, and Joel Fischer, "Social Workers' Involvement in Research," *Social Work* 21(2), March 1976, pp. 121-124.

Kirk, Stuart A., "The Substructure of Belief," *Advances in Clinical Social Work Research*, 1990, pp. 233-250.

Kutchins, Herb and Stuart A. Kirk, "The Business of Diagnosis: DSM-III and Clinical Social Work," *Social Work*, 33(3) May-June 1988, pp. 215-220.

Morrow-Bradley, Cheryl and Robert Elliot, "Utilization of Psychotherapy Research by Practicing Psychotherapists," *American Psychologist*, 41(2), February 1986, pp. 188-197.

Penka, Cindy E. and Stuart A. Kirk, "Clinical Mind-Set and Involvement in Research," paper presented at the annual meeting of the National Association of Social Workers, San Francisco, October 1989.

Richey, Cheryl A., Betty J. Blythe, and Sharon B. Berlin, "Do Social Workers Evaluate Their Practice?" *Social Work Research & Abstracts* 23(2), Summer 1987, pp. 14-20.

Rubin, A. and A. Rosenblatt (Eds.), *Sourcebook on Research Utilization* (New York: Council on Social Work Education, 1979).

Rubin, A. and S. Zimbalist, "Issues in the MSW Research Curriculum, 1968-1979," in Scott Briar et al. (Eds.), *Research Utilization in Social Work Education* (New York: Council on Social Work Education, 1981), pp. 6-16.

Weinbach, Robert W. and Allen Rubin (Eds.), *Teaching Social Work Research: Alternative Programs and Strategies* (New York: Council on Social Work Education, 1980).

Weinbach, Robert W., "Variations in Social Work Research Education" in Scott Briar, Harold Weissman, and Allen Rubin (Eds.), *Research Utilization in Social Work Education* (New York: Council on Social Work Education, 1981), pp. 40-47.

# How to Avoid Producing "A Faculty of Very Efficient Pedants and Dullards": Evaluating Doctoral Education in Social Work

Aaron Rosenblatt

Knowing the score and knowing how to score are American obsessions. We are a nation of counters, tracing descent from a nation of shopkeepers. In all sectors of our national life we measure perfomance by counting. Business corporations, sports clubs, movie stars, universities, even love and charity: for each of these the public relies on some simple count. Every year, for example, a magazine lists the members of the Fortune 500. With this information we keep track of those remaining at the top, those slipping back, and those forging ahead.

Every day newspapers publish the won-and-lost averages of sports clubs and the individual records of athletes in baseball or football, basketball or hockey. Scores tell us who won the World Series, the Super Bowl, the finals at Flushing Meadow and the final game of the Final Four. The highest number of ballots determines the winner of the annual Oscar awards for artistic merit in film. Every year the count of ballots elects mayors, judges, sheriffs, and every four years the count of electoral votes elects a president.

Counts of money, games won, yards gained, baskets and ballots, offer a ready-made way of reaffirming under many different masks an underlying commitment to knowing the score, to accepting standard methods of evaluating performance and determining ranks. Generally, variant standards proposed by experts receive little attention. The public relies on simple measures to determine who is number one.

In this chapter we look critically at the goals of doctoral education in social work and the methods that researchers use to measure the performance of graduate students and their professors. Specifically, we raise questions about accepting measures that one can count quickly, and the slighting of goals not easily counted such as creativity, originality, and thoughtfulness.

Many social workers take pride in being out of step with American society. We object to the low level of support granted to needy families, to the foot-dragging of federal officials when cleaning up our earth and air, our lakes and streams. We subscribe to the social values of a democratic society in which poor kids count as much as rich kids.

Remaining true to these values is no easy task. The dominant society has developed highly effective means for diffusing acquisitive, Social-Darwinian values to all levels of society. A threat, ever present, is that we will lose our way and become unwitting supporters of values to which we take exception, succumbing to the seduction of a pervasive culture, accepting false values without knowing it.

We researchers are especially partial to counts, to assigning ranks and making judgments. Therefore, we may be the most vulnerable members of the social work profession. Knowing that validity is more important than reliability, we must always ask ourselves these questions: Are we counting the right things? What have we decided not to count?

The goals of doctoral education for social workers vary from program to program. No national authority has the power to proclaim certain goals as legitimate and to deny legitimacy to others. (The Council on Social Work Education does not accredit doctoral programs. Neither does the Group for the Advancement of Doctoral Education.) Before conducting an evaluation one must first decide on the goals of each doctoral program and then decide on suitable measures. These decisions are critical. The answers will reveal the goals and measures that become the pivot of the research evaluation.

As a guide for identifying goals, we draw from the work of a philosopher, a master teacher who influenced education in England and the United States. During his academic career Alfred North Whitehead was an active partisan supporting the intellectual side of education. Internationally known as a mathematician, the collaborator with Bertrand Russell on the monumental *Principia Mathematica*, Whitehead taught for many years at Harvard after leaving the Imperial College of Science in London.

Sixty years ago he gathered together a collection of addresses and essays that were published under the title, *The Aims of Education* (1929). The main idea stated in the preface and running through all of the chapters is that, "students are alive, and the purpose of education is to stimulate and guide their self-development. It follows as a corollary from this premise that the teachers should also be alive with living thoughts. The whole book is a protest against dead knowledge . . ." (Whitehead, 1949, n.p.).

Whitehead's ideas are challenging. It would be contrary to his openness and searching mind if, in recalling his words, we presented them as carved in stone, to be accepted without question. Whitehead was no authoritarian, no antiquarian classicist. "Knowledge," he warns, "does not keep any better than fish" (Whitehead, 1949, p. 102). His warnings ring true. His thoughts still sound fresh, as if newly drawn from the sea although some were first put down on paper over 75 years ago.

Professor Whitehead's aims of education are broad, even when considering the purpose of a technical education such as that being offered at the then newly founded School of Business at Harvard. I quote him at length with little or no gloss. The following selection on the justification of university education is taken from the opening paragraphs of the second section in Chapter Seven, entitled "Universities and Their Function":

> The universities are schools of education, and schools of research. But the primary reason for their existence is not to be found either in the mere knowledge conveyed to the students or in the mere opportunities for research afforded to the members of the faculty.
>
> Both these functions could be performed at a cheaper rate, apart from these very expensive institutions. Books are cheap,

and the system of apprenticeship is well understood. So far as the mere imparting of information is concerned, no university has had any justification for existence since the popularisation of printing in the fifteenth century. Yet the chief impetus to the foundation of universities came after that date, and in more recent times has even increased.

The justification for a university is that it preserves the connection between knowledge and the zest of life by uniting the young and the old in the imaginative consideration of learning. The university imparts information, but it imparts it imaginatively. At least, this is the function which it should perform for society. A university which fails in this respect has no reason for existence. This atmosphere of excitement, arising from imaginative consideration, transforms knowledge. A fact is no longer a bare fact; it is invested with all its possibilities. It is no longer a burden on the memory: it is energising as the poet of our dreams, and as the architect of our purpose.

. . . The tragedy of the world is that those who are imaginative [youth] have but slight experience, and those who are experienced have feeble imaginations. Fools act on imagination without knowledge; pedants act on knowledge without imagination. The task of a university is to weld together imagination and experience. (Whitehead, 1949, pp. 97-98)

One way, then, to evaluate doctoral education is to determine if "it preserves the connection between knowledge and the zest of life" through uniting students and teachers in the imaginative consideration of knowledge. Professors must impart information imaginatively. This is an essential function that they perform for society. The position taken by Professor Whitehead suggests that a basic service of the university is not only teaching, but *imaginative* teaching.

If I read him correctly, Professor Whitehead would want to learn the ways in which teachers go about the task of welding together their experience and the imagination of students. This is no easy task, but information of this kind can be gathered in different ways. A panel of judges can examine a teacher's syllabus and course curriculum, next observe the teacher's performance in the classroom, and then measure the impact of these on the imagination of students.

Another way of obtaining information on teaching, oftentimes viewed with disfavor by faculty members, is to ask students to rate their performance. The State University of New York requires students to rate their professors every semester. The unit of analysis is the individual professor. The ratings are not combined for the purpose of evaluating teaching at the university or any of its departments, schools, or colleges. Such a task would be difficult to carry out since each unit devises its own unique evaluation form.

There is no need here to review all of the different methods used in evaluating inputs into doctoral education. The point being made is that serious evaluators must present an adequate discussion justifying the goals of doctoral education along with adequate discussion justifying the selection and rejection of various criterion measures. What are they planning to count? What are they excluding? Adequate discussion of goals and measures is essential. Without it, readers find themselves forced into the uncomfortable position of guessing about the reasons for avoiding this task. Unfortunately, the goals of education and measures of input and output receive little attention in an otherwise careful study bearing the title, "Evaluating Doctoral Programs in Social Work: A Case Study" (Rosen, 1979).

Professor Whitehead offers a clear, forceful argument against using a count of scientific books and papers as the primary measure of output for a university:

> It must not be supposed that the output of a university in the form of original ideas is soley to be measured by printed papers and books labeled with the names of their authors. Mankind is as individual in its mode of output as in the substance of its thoughts. For some of the most fertile minds composition in writing or in a form reducible to writing seems to be an impossibility. In every faculty you will find that some of the more brilliant teachers are not among those who publish. Their originality requires for its expression direct intercourse with their pupils in the form of lectures or of personal discussion. Some men [sic] exercise an immense influence; and yet, after

the generation of their pupils has passed away, they sleep among the innumerable unthanked benefactors of humanity. Fortunately, one of them is immortal — Socrates.

Thus it would be the greatest mistake to estimate the value of each member of a faculty by the printed work signed with his [sic] name. There is at the present day some tendency to fall into this error; and an emphatic protest is necessary against an attitude on the part of authorities which is damaging to efficiency and unjust to unselfish zeal.

But, when all such allowances have been made, one good test for the general efficiency of a faculty is that as a whole it shall be producing in published form its quota of contributions of thought. Such a quota is to estimated in weight of thought, and not in number of words . . .

The sole question is, What sort of conditions will produce the type of faculty which will run a successful university? The danger is that it is quite easy to produce a faculty entirely unfit — a faculty of very efficient pedants and dullards. The general public will only detect the difference after the university has stunted the promise of youth for scores of years. (Whitehead, 1949, pp. 103-104)

How refreshing to find this distinquished scholar warning university officials against producing a "faculty of very efficient pedants and dullards" by relying on a count of published work as a suitable measure of output. Professors make many worthwhile contributions to universities and their chosen professions, only one of which is conducting research studies and writing up the results. Those who elevate the manufacture of knowledge above all other objectives deny full legitimacy to equally worthwhile endeavors such as teaching, administration, and consultation. When socialized to accept research productivity above all other values, doctoral students seek to lead professional lives remote from clinical practice. Asked to state the ideal distribution of time to be spent on professional activities, graduates of one doctoral program said they preferred to devote almost 45% of their time to research and writing and only 2% to practice (Rosen, 1979).

Programs that promote the production of books, articles, and papers as the goal of doctoral education slight the importance of originality and substance, perhaps because these qualities are not easily measurable, or worse, because they are of secondary importance. With or without conscious intent, faculty adhering to such narrow goals encourage students to concentrate their efforts on the more conventional problems arising from what Thomas Kuhn has termed normal science.

"Under normal conditions," according to Kuhn (1977, p. 234), "the research scientist is not an innovator but a solver of puzzles, and the puzzles upon which he [sic] concentrates are just those which he [sic] believes can both be stated and solved within the existing scientific tradition." Deans and other academic officers tacitly lend support to such career choices when they select productivity as the major criterion determining promotion and retention at a university. These officers never say that they are opposed to creativity, originality, or thoughtfulness. They believe in their importance. Since these qualities are difficult to measure, they may think it prudent to encourage students to produce those things that can be counted — papers, articles, books.

In the early stages of their careers doctoral students seek to identify norms that can provide a measure of certainty as they make significant career choices while taking courses and thinking about selecting a dissertation topic. Faculty members who encourage doctoral students to work on problems within an accepted style cast a silent vote for traditional, safe, conservative approaches to research.

Students soon learn the score and what they should do. Trained to be acute observers and analysts, they quickly identify the standards affecting the promotion of their professors and the cohorts of students in advance of them. They soon learn the rules of the game. First, conduct research that raises no challenge to the standards currently dominant within a discipline or profession. Second, write articles and submit them to refereed journals (Gleick, 1987).

This message is by no means restricted to social work education. A rationale for the acceptance of productivity norms is set forth in a study two sociologists conducted in 1969 which purported to measure quality in graduate education. The "objective index of academic quality," which they accept without any serious reservation, "is the departmental publication record." Here is the argument in full:

> While such a measure has some obvious limitations, publication of articles and books would seem to represent the primary avenue by which any department attains national visibility and recognition.
>
> There is no widely acknowledged standard by which to measure the significance of any specific publication. Consequently, the number of articles and books is usually defined as an acceptable indicator of a scholarly contribution. However, it must be recognized that publication of an article or the review of a book — particularly in the most prominent journals in the discipline — does provide some positive professional evaluation of quality because of the judgment exercised by editors and reviewers prior to the decision to publish the article or to review the book. Thus, publications in leading journals are in some degree a measure of both productivity and quality, two of the factors upon which the status of any department depends. (Knudsen and Vaughan, 1969, p. 12)

This argument looks only at the advantages of using productivity as an index of quality. It ignores the qualifications of the referees and the need to fill the pages of serial publications on schedule, regardless of quality. It makes no reference to the rejection rates of different journals or to the fact, in my experience, that persistence pays off: sending out articles rejected at one journal almost always results in finding a home for them at another journal. Also, it is well known that many directors of professional associations that sponsor annual meetings intentionally select a large number of papers for presentation at the sessions in order to insure high attendance at the conference.

James Gleick, a historian tracing the development of the emerging science of chaos, notes certain hazards to innovation stemming from the acceptance of productivity norms. Faculty advisors encourage doctoral students to shy away from dissertation proposals that may not readily be turned into publishable articles. Dennis Gabor, a Nobel laureate in physics for his work on holography, makes a similar point in recalling why he did not invent the laser:

> I have been asked more than once why I did not invent the laser. In fact, I have thought of it. In 1950, thinking of the desirability of a strong source of coherent light, I remembered in 1921, as a young student in Berlin, I had heard from Einstein's own lips his wonderful derivation of Planck's law which postulated the existence of stimulated emission. I then had the idea of the pulsed laser: Take a suitable crystal, make a resonator of it by means of a highly reflecting coating, fill up the upper level by illuminating it through a small hole, and discharge it explosively by a ray of its own light. I offered the idea as a Ph.D. problem to my best student, but he declined it as too risky, and I could not gainsay it, as I could not be sure that we would find a suitable crystal. (Gabor, 1972, p. 313)

In this example both dissertation advisor and doctoral student walk away from the chance to make an important discovery because it is too risky in promoting a scientific career.

Science is not supposed to work this way. Its standards are universalistic, the flow of knowledge open (Merton, 1982). Recognizing the ongoing nature of discovery, it seeks to encourage creativity and originality. Physics has one of the fastest turn-around times from the submission of an article to its publication, but it took two years before the editors of the best academic journals stopped rejecting articles written by Mitchell J. Feigenbaum, a brilliant, creative physicist who eschewed *obvious* problems to work on the *not obvious*, those that would not give way without long looks into the "universe's bowels" (Gleick, 1987, p. 3). He and other scientists worked alone, feeling their way toward discovering the foundations of a new science. In this uncertain state they are "unable to explain where they are heading, afraid even to tell their colleagues what they are doing—that romantic image lies at the heart of Kuhn's scheme and it has occurred in real life time and time again in the exploration of choas" (Gleick, 1987, p. 37).

Is it inevitable that those breaking with firmly established traditions within a profession or science must meet with discouragement, at times even hostility, from colleagues and university officers? Tolstoy thought so. As a wealthy aristocrat he could afford to challenge traditional views without economic hardship, but he felt the sting of rejection from his contemporaries. In his opinion "most men [sic] . . . can seldom accept even the simplest and most obvious truth if it be such as would oblige them to admit the falsity of conclusions which they have delighted in explaining to colleagues, which they have proudly taught to others, and which they have woven, thread by thread, into the fabric of their lives" (Tolstoy, 1987, p. 39).

Social work education, like all social institutions, has its imperfections. Although divorced from expectations of perfectability, we are still wedded to the possibility of improving institutions. Rather than accept defective standards as inevitable, we meet together at conferences such as this one trying to bring about improvements, yet knowing full well that any changes may make matters worse.

We hope that others will agree that productivity is an unsatisfactory standard for evaluating doctoral education. The sociologists' justification mentioned earlier fails to convince. No hocus-pocus can turn quantity into quality. Neither is quantity to be preferred to imagination, creativity, or a substantive contribution. It seems dead wrong in my judgment to choose productivity as the goal by which to evaluate doctoral programs in social work.

Professor Whitehead draws attention to the contributions of teachers who publish few articles, of those using their talent to pursue other worthwhile goals. Not every graduate or faculty member can be as inventive as Mitchell Feigenbaum or as pioneering as Paul Lazarsfeld. Doctoral programs cannot be expected to produce clones of grand masters. A practice profession needs many different kinds of knowledge and skill. A profession is like a splendid mansion with many different rooms. An architect would be foolish to pick out one room as most important and then design all the other rooms from this model. Such a house would not be filled with kitchens or bathrooms, nurseries or libraries, attics or antechambers, ballrooms or bedrooms. No one would want to live in such a house.

Everyone can recognize the value of conducting research studies and writing up the results, or of looking at patterns of research productivity among the holders of social work doctorates (Abbott, 1985). But it is a giant step from observing patterns of productivity to touting them as the goals of education, and then making decisions about the granting of appointment, promotion, and tenure primarily on that basis. A number of adventitious changes follow from accepting this narrow measurement of educational goals.

The importance of teaching declines. So does the importance of students. So does service to the profession and service to the university. Civility among colleagues and students also declines. A faculty hard-driven to meet productivity norms becomes too busy to spend time shmoozing with colleagues and students. Have others here had the experience of chatting with colleagues, feeling that they were anxious to end the conversation in order to get back to really important matters? Others also must have observed colleagues reading professional articles and grading student papers during faculty meetings.

In these final paragraphs I draw on my own experience to illustrate the effect of adopting the publish-or-perish standard. I was a doctoral student at a large research university, and I served as a faculty member on promotion and tenure committees at the department and university level in two professional schools. Also, I witnessed the transformation of a university striving to throw off the traditions of a teachers college and become a research center able to attract extramural support.

I played the game at all of these universities. I knew what counted, and I knew how to score. I wrote to publish, secondarily to inform. Grinding out article after article, I was as wedded to production as a sorcerer's sausage machine. And I was rewarded. My career blossomed. I was appointed professor at three universities, granted tenure, invited to serve on a national committee reviewing proposals for the support of social work education. I prospered from playing the game.

When this game is played, students, I suspect, are the major losers. They know that their chance to learn conflicts with the desire of their teachers to publish. They experience firsthand the willingness of university officials to downgrade teaching. In courses that I teach on research methods, I have a chance to talk to students about the evaluation forms that the university asks them to complete every year.

Many are bitter at having to sit through lectures delivered by teachers primarily interested in scholarly publication. For professors hell-bent to gain a national reputation and win promotion, time spent advising students is time stolen from writing. Graduate assistants are a resource to be used for advancing a professor's career. Students know the score. They do not enjoy this kind of education, but they put up with it in order to get on with their careers.

Professor Whitehead's aim of education — to stimulate and guide the self-development of students — needs to be reaffirmed, not abandoned. Research and writing must take their place along side of, instead of ahead of, other legitimate goals of doctoral education.

As a postscript let me add this final paragraph. Having identified certain problems in evaluating doctoral programs and standards for the promotion of faculty, I cannot begin a serious discussion of meaningful solutions unless, at this point, I were to take on the additional task of writing another paper. These problems are complex and defy easy solutions. Furthermore, even if I were to write another paper, it is not false modesty to anticipate the effort might result in laboring mightily and bringing forth a mouse. I make no claim to being a prophet or a wise man. The limited role of critic or gadfly fits me better than that of evangelist, proselytizer, or problem solver. Therefore, I end with this plea to readers: Discount the polemical tone in this paper. Then ask yourself if the problems identified are real. If the answer is "yes" or "yes and no," talk to your colleagues and students, to deans and vice-presidents at your university about the kinds of change needed to improve social work education.

## REFERENCES

Gabor, D. "Holography, 1948-1971." *Science* 177 (1972): 299-313.

Gleick, J. *Choas: Making a New Science.* New York: Viking, 1987.

Knudsen, D.D. & Vaughan, T.R. "Quality in graduate education: A re-evaluation of the rankings of sociology departments in the Cartter Report." *The American Sociologist*, Feb. 1969, 12-19.

Kuhn, T. *The Essential Tension: Selected Studies in Scientific Tradition and Change.* Chicago: University of Chicago, 1977.

Merton, R.K. *Social Research and the Practicing Professions*, A. Rosenblatt & T.F. Gieryn, ed. Cambridge: Abt Books, 1982.

Rosen, A. "Evaluating doctoral programs in social work: A case study." *Social Work Research and Abstracts*, 1979, 19-27.

Tolstoy, L., as quoted by Gleick, J. *Chaos: Making a New Science*. New York: Viking, 1987.

Whitehead, A.N. *The Aims of Education*. New York: The New American Library, 1949.

# Conclusion –
# Information Utilization:
# A Decade of Practice

Anthony J. Grasso

The conference that generated this collection was innovative in several ways. First, the conference itself was the result of an unprecedented effort on the part of a social service agency, Boysville of Michigan, and a school of social work, Wayne State University, to bring together innovators in the field of research utilization in social work to discuss their work. In addition, many of the papers presented at the conference offered innovative suggestions and described new strategies to enhance practitioner use of research in agency settings. Finally, the conference raised new research and information utilization questions that merit future consideration in their own right.

Why did Boysville of Michigan initiate such a conference? To answer this question the reader needs some background information on Boysville and its unique approach to management information, program evaluation, and applied research.

## BOYSVILLE OF MICHIGAN

Boysville of Michigan is the state's largest private agency serving troubled adolescents. Since its founding in 1948 with 15 boys, the agency has grown to where it now serves 550 boys and girls with treatment centers located at its main campus in Clinton, a smaller campus in Saginaw, and group homes in Detroit, Ecorse, Mt. Clemens, Redford, Saginaw, Mt. Morris, Alpena, and Monroe, Michigan, and in Toledo, Ohio.

Historically, Boysville's treatment technology was based on a modified version of positive peer culture in which the natural influences of the adolescent peer group were enlisted to bring about change in client behavior and attitude. Over the last few years, however, Boysville has expanded its intervention repertoire to include an intensive family therapy program on the main campus for all youth in placement, specialized foster care for youth unable to return to their natural families, and a metro area emergency placement program.

While a growing number of Boysville youth are neglected/abused, most are adjudicated delinquents with serious behavioral, social, and educational problems. Most come from the tri-county Detroit area. Recently, in response to needs expressed by both the public and private sectors, Boysville expanded its mission to include services to girls.

## BOYSVILLE'S INTEGRATED MANAGEMENT, INFORMATION, PRACTICE DECISION MAKING, PROGRAM EVALUATION AND APPLIED SYSTEM (BOMIS)

As with many social work organizations, Boysville began as a small agency adopting a "human relations" administrative approach (Etzioni, 1964) and a participatory management style. However, as the organization grew in size, structural complexity, and intervention repertoire, its nonhierarchical human relations ethos became increasingly problematic.

Although the mission and goals of Boysville were clearly articulated, prior to the implementation of BOMIS, efforts to fulfill this mission were often undermined by different professional staff working on different aspects of program without a clear understanding of what their overall goals and objectives were. This led to specialties within the organization such as education, treatment, dorm living, family services, etc., working toward conflicting individual client objectives, thereby subverting efforts at achievement of desired overall goals (Katz and Kahn, 1978). This problem was intensified by a lack of clear specification of desired client outcome in the organization. Thus, different treatment specialties frequently tended to work toward achievement of client goals and objectives specific to their own expertise without any effort at treatment or programmatic integration (Perrow, 1974; Etzioni, 1960).

Because of conflicting definitions of goals and objectives, operations directors were faced daily with the necessity of making immediate and reactive decisions which often had a negative impact on the overall effectiveness of the organization. They did so without comprehending the organizational significance of these decisions. Nevertheless, the human relations model fit comfortably with the religious orientation of the Holy Cross Brothers employed by the Michigan Diocese to administer the agency. This fit manifested itself in administrative staff's genuine concern for the well being of "co-workers" and in the continuing effort to promote the idea of a "work community" at Boysville. Human relations motivational theory functioned as an ideological underpinning to all organizational decision-making.

However, the human relations ideology and its associated management style caused a great deal of uncertainty and ambiguity with regard to the decision-making at Boysville. It offered no clear delineation of roles or responsibilities at different levels of the organization. As a result, most conflicts in the organization were viewed as personality conflicts rather than as structural problems that might be resolved by a rational, analytic, organizational process (Katz and Kahn, 1966).

As the organization grew it became more decentralized, with subunits of varying size located throughout the state. A conflict inevitably emerged between a need for uniformity across programs and a need for responsiveness to local differences. Those at the executive level of the organization concerned with finances, control, and personnel issues tended to favor standardization and centralization (Handy, 1976). Resistance to this pressure came from the regional directors who favored decentralization and organizational diversity. Despite pressures toward centralization from some individuals on the executive staff, the prevailing ideological commitment to a human relations model persisted for some time.

As Boysville became more technologically complex, staff size increased, as did professional skill and diversity. With this increase in skill, specialization, and diversity came demands for higher quality and more specialized information that would facilitate practice decision making of various kinds at different levels in the organization by different kinds of practitioners. These specialized needs for practice-based information coincided with an increased need of central administration for quantitative program information for internal administrative decision making as well as for external accountability purposes and for program expansion. As Katz and Kahn predicted (1966), the greater the distance between the higher and the lower levels in an organization, the greater the dependence on quantitative versus qualitative information in decision making. This greater dependence on quantitative information for decision making was also consistent with the need felt by some at the executive level for greater uniformity and standardization within the organization.

Because of changes mentioned above, the treatment system at Boysville gradually became fragmented, uncoordinated, and unintegrated with specialties independently pursuing their own institutional priorities and goals. This meant, for example, that family workers tended to be exclusively interested in family process and saw their specialty as the central intervention approach of the agency. The same was true of group workers, treatment specialists, teachers, and so on. In addition, the work at different Boysville sites varied markedly because of the unique history and staffing patterns at these sites.

Officially, the coordinating body for each treatment unit was the treatment team. A treatment team was made up of one core teacher, two treatment specialists, a group leader, and one family worker for every 12 children in care. The teams met weekly and reviewed treatment plans and process, and developed an interdisciplinary treatment plan for each client that was to be monitored and updated on an ongoing basis while the child was in care. The treatment director (group therapist) in the program had traditionally been given informal authority to coordinate the efforts of the different treatment specialties on the team, but formally, they were seen as co-equal with all other team members. This structural contradiction, explained by the prevailing human relations orientation of the agency, subverted the coordination function of the treatment directors. In other words, they were given the responsibility for coordinating treatment at the team level, but they did not possess the formal authority to implement treatment decisions across different treatment specialties.

Higher level decision making was equally fragmented and contradictory. Despite the participatory ideology, the Executive Office generally made major agency decisions unilaterally. This might have been appropriate in a small, undifferentiated, centralized setting, but at Boysville it meant uncoordinated decision making throughout the agency. Thus, in 1982 Boysville had no long-range strategic plan in place. Most decisions were therefore made on an *ad hoc* basis. And, because of an informal structure which allowed lower-level managers easy access to the Executive Office, there was a great deal of pressure for immediate responses to problems as opposed to planful, coordinated problem resolution.

This is not unique to Boysville. Katz and Kahn (1966), for example, remark:

> Immediate pressure often seems so overriding to executives that they will accept some hasty solutions and bypass a thorough analysis of the problem and the careful weighing of the likely major consequences of their action. The objective circumstances may be of such an emergency nature, that decisive actions must be embarked upon immediately. Often, however, specific organizational pressure and personality considerations are responsible for decision being reached without an adequate analysis of the problem, or an intelligent assessment of the consequences. (p. 275)

From its external environment, Boysville was at this time experiencing pressure to change as well. In 1983 the Michigan Department of Social Services (MDSS) was developing purchase of services contracts requiring performance objectives related to number of program successes at time of program completion, placement status of the client after program completion, and client length of stay in agency programs. In addition, Boysville was being asked by MDSS to serve a more difficult client which required greater staff skills. Agency leadership recognized that to function effectively and efficiently under these changing conditions required a new approach to management decision making.

These organizational changes and problems suggested the need for a new management information, practice decision making, and program evaluation system at Boysville (BOMIS). Pressures from external accountability, funding, and accrediting systems reinforced this need.

## BOMIS: THEORY AND PRACTICE

Elsewhere, Grasso and Epstein (1988) had theorized that if properly conceptualized, packaged, and fedback, information from a management information system has multiple uses and can contribute to effective decision making at all levels of an organization. Based on this premise, they conceived of four organizational ranks of potential information users: Line Service Workers, Supervisors, Program Managers, and Executives. They also pointed out that conflicts between information needs at different organizational levels often lead to falsified and underutilized information systems. Finally, they suggested that information systems are often inadequate because their designers fail to attend to these conflicts. Or, because in responding to these conflicts, designers compromise the information needs of the direct service practitioner. Thus, they conclude, most MIS professionals and the systems they design tend to favor the accountability-oriented information needs of program managers and administrators.

There are many causes of this fundamental design error. One is that academic researchers who often have been responsible for designing information systems have inadequate knowledge of or interest in treatment technologies (Reid, 1980). Another is the understandable emphasis that program managers and administrators who contract with MIS designers place on accountability needs (Grasso and Epstein, 1987).

In some organizations, the result of this overemphasis on accountability information is goal-displacement (Conrad, 1985; Hasenfeld, 1983). In these organizations, direct service staff are burdened with data collection responsibilities but benefit little from the information collected (Hoshino, 1982). As a result, the quality and accuracy of this information is likely to be questionable (Walker, 1972).

In response to this dilemma, some strategies have been suggested for ensuring that information systems provide clinically useful information to treatment staff in return for their data collection efforts. One approach is to create systems designs and to choose interactive computer hardware and software that maximize the likelihood of integrating administrative and clinical information (Mutschler and Hasenfeld, 1986). Another, emphasizing single-subject methodology, suggests a more active role for direct service practitioners in designing their own single case evaluation systems (Blythe and Briar, 1985).

Typically, however, discussions of information systems design for the human services have presented unintegrated and undifferentiated models for "total" systems (Bronson, Pelz, and Trzcinski, 1988) or highly specific information systems that serve the decisional needs of one specific group of organizational actors while ignoring the others (Caputo, 1988).

By contrast, Boysville's approach (Grasso and Epstein, 1987) to system design can best be described as a *utilization-driven design that integrates clinical, supervisory, and administrative information, but begins with the information needs of the direct service practitioner.* This approach rests on the following design principles:

1. Effective integration of the service technology and the accountability of the agency requires that attention be given to actual as well as measured performance.
2. Effective integration of the service technology and the accountability system requires valid and reliable information from line staff.
3. Line staff will provide this information to the degree that they receive in return information feedback that is timely and readily applicable to their practice (Grasso and Epstein, 1989).

These design principles flow directly from the basic assumption that if management information systems are to be fully utilized, they must provide information to all levels of the organization. In so saying, it is essential that the system give priority to the information needs of the direct service practitioners who must gather the information in the first place. Finally, this clinically-relevant information must be further specified by the stage of client career in a program (Epstein and Grasso, 1987).

## CONFLICTS ASSOCIATED WITH DIFFERENT MODELS OF RESEARCH AND UTILIZATION

Boysville's effort to successfully integrate information and research utilization in practice is unique (Epstein and Grasso, 1989). Its uniqueness is underscored by the many discussions in the social work literature of the failure to incorporate research utilization into social work practice and administration. These discussions range from those placing blame on the conflicting attitudes of practitioners and researchers to those faulting the institutional commitments of academically oriented researchers. So, for example, Briar (1980) has explained the lack of integration of practice and research in the light of the practitioner's inability to formulate or resistance to formulating practice interventions and treatment objectives in measurable terms. As he puts it:

> It appears to be general principle in social work never to use a specifically descriptive term if a more abstract one is available. The nearer terms get to operational or behavioral specificity, the more social workers turn away from them. (p. 33)

In a more even-handed discussion of practitioner and researcher attitudes, Rothman (1974) locates the problem of nonutilization in the interaction between practitioner and researcher. He comments:

> Different styles and modes of thinking divide the two types (practitioner/researcher) which makes communication difficult and utilization of each other's contributions and products problematic. There exists formidable social distance characterized by mistrust, differing outlooks and ostensibly contrasting goals which, in the past, has inhibited fuller articulation between social scientists and social practitioners. (p. 545)

Rather than stressing the antiresearch attitudes, Gordon (1984) posits blame on practitioners' lack of skill in deriving practice applications from studies as one of the central points in the conflict.

Lewis (1980), on the other hand, is critical of the conceptual and methodological paradigms that researchers bring to the study of practice. Thus, he suggests:

> It is in the design of research including its implementation and the form in which its findings are developed that one must locate the principle impediments to utilization. (p. 26)

Similarly, in stressing formative rather than summative evaluative designs, Epstein and Tripodi (1977) have sought to develop conceptual frameworks that link research to program development and to clinical decision making (Tripodi and Epstein, 1980). Still other authors have located the problem or integration of research and practice with the products of research efforts themselves. Weiss (1972), for example, has noted that research findings are frequently not applicable to practice. Rothman (1974) suggests that findings, when applicable, still require too much translation for the practitioner to deem them as useful. Seidl (1980) has commented on the failure of researchers to produce their findings in a timely and usable form for practitioners.

A final set of explanations has to do with the structural and physical location of the researcher and the practitioner. Thus, Bushnell and O'Brien (1979) have discussed several reasons why university-based research is not likely to find itself applied in practice. Arguing instead for the location of research at the agency, Seidl (1980) notes that:

> If research is to be timely and space specific, and to deal in practitioner's language with relevant and able variables, it must be conducted where direct practice is carried out. (p. 60)

Even when research is agency-based, its applicability to practice can vary depending on the model of research employed. Thus, Kirk (1979) has discussed the utilization pros and cons of three models of agency-based research articulated by Havelock (1969):

The R&D models emphasized the role of the research and development and the rational planning of diffusion efforts but it pays little attention to the role of the consumer of knowledge. The social interaction model perspective carefully documents the importance of social networks and understanding the flow of knowledge and utilization through a user system, however, it fails to articulate the linkage between the producer and users of knowledge. The problem solver model directs attention to the psychological conditions under which a new knowledge may be sought out and used by consumers but it over-emphasizes the extent to which consumers are capable of generating their own solution to problems. (p. 7)

Placing emphasis on the service consumer rather than on the consumer, Weissman (1977) proposed an agency-based evaluation system based on client perception and satisfaction. However, he points out that such a system will only succeed to the extent that service providers are committed to it and it provides timely and useful information.

What remains clear is that the literature concerning research utilization suggests that there is no single correct explanation for the failure to incorporate research data into our models of social work. Nevertheless, programs designed to promote and assess utilization of research must address staff attitudes toward research, staff skills in utilizing research, the timeliness and applicability of the research products themselves, the location and orientation of the researchers, and the model of research employed.

In an effort to assess the effectiveness of the Boysville information system (BOMIS) in achieving this, Grasso, Epstein, and Tripodi (1988) explored the impact of the implementation of BOMIS on worker utilization of information in practice decision making. That study presents descriptive findings that indicate that in 1987 there was a moderately high reported utilization of the products of the system, less than totally positive perception of agency efforts to facilitate utilization, but increasingly positive attitudes toward research since the system was introduced. Multivariate analysis suggested that positive perceptions of structural facilitators are the most important predictors of utilization, but that pro-research attitudes make a contribution of their own. These attitudes are enhanced by agency-based training and, in turn, contribute to positive perceptions of utilization facilitators. Extramural education contributes to positive pro-research attitudes but to a lesser degree than does agency-based training. Finally, agency-based training, timeliness of reports, and usefulness of reports have an effect on staff willingness to use information to assess their own performance and effectiveness and to use BOMIS information in supervision.

More generally these authors' findings suggest that computerization of social agencies brings with it a positive potential for research and information utilization. However, to realize this potential agency-based research and evaluation units must attend to structural factors that facilitate this process, and must provide sufficient practice-oriented training to sustain and enhance pro-research attitudes and utilization behaviors. In this context, they found that academic education is necessary but insufficient.

In studying research and information utilization, the basic problems are fundamentally the same irrespective of whether they are conceptualized as management problems, research utilization problems or program evaluation problems. The manager needs to measure and document program functioning, the evaluator needs to measure and document program effect, and the researcher needs to measure and document the relationship between program functioning and effect. Hence, all share the problem of research measurement, documentation, and utilization for agency decision making. However, by viewing these as separate institutional problems we fail to benefit from recent gains made in each of these areas. In other words, by identifying problems as research utilization, information processing, or information products usage we do not take the most efficient route to their resolution. Instead what remains are unintegrated efforts to implement organizational solutions which are not adequate to the task.

The contributors to this book have suggested a number of strategies for solving the foregoing problems of research utilization. Nonetheless, the problem of research integration with practice requires bold solutions (Reid/Fortune). As direct service practitioners point out, the current models of research are often bivariate in nature and do not address issues of mutual causality which are reflective of the practice experience. Additionally, treatment models which are robust enough to address issues of generalizability also suffer from internal inconsistencies which summative research models expose. If, however, the internal inconsistencies are addressed, the models of practice are often too idiosyncratic to a particular setting to generalize to other settings. This narrowly focused explanation of the failure of research utilization creates a dilemma that by its nature limits the ability to achieve effective integration into direct practice (Tripodi).

If, for example, one wishes to promote the idea of a scientific practitioner (Briar), one must create organizational structures that support more scientific practice. If one wishes to create a D&D/R&D approach (Thomas, Rothman), one needs a new model of administration (Hasenfeld/Patti) that fosters the ability for the organization to learn from its practice. If one hopes to promote a practitioner that is constantly engaged in learning, one must create agencies that have a capacity to learn.

The greatest difference between the writings presented in this collection and the writings of the previous decade is that the present work emphasizes the need to reconcile utilization issues, with organizational issues, with larger system issues (Fanshel/Marsters/Finch/Grundy, Mizrahi), and with direct service delivery issues (McCubbin/McCubbin, Rose, Lewis, Raider/Moxley). The introduction of the personal computer made this new conception of research/information utilization and integration possible (Mutschler, Blythe, Schuerman). It is assumed that the practitioner who makes use of this evolving paradigm of research and service delivery will serve clients more effectively. Education for the requisite roles in practice-utilization is the primary task of social work schools (Rubin, Kirk, Rosenblatt). New models may derive as well from closer agency/university relationships (Jenkins, Rehr).

The Boysville model of integrating information, research, and practice decision making is a case of what is possible given the advances in computer technology and research utilization models developed over the past decade.

Instead of waiting for other disciplines to bridge the research/practice gap, social work researchers must be in the forefront of the research and information utilization "movement." To further this movement let this conference be the final conference devoted to research utilization per se, and the first on information-driven, practice decision making. A decade from now a new conference can determine whether this new conception results in more effective applications of research and information technology to social work practice.

# REFERENCES

Briar, S. Toward the integration of practice and research. *Future of Social Work Research*, D. Fanshel, ed. NASW, Washington, DC, 1980: 31-37.

Blythe, B. and Briar, S. Developing empirically based models of practice. *Social Work*, Vol. 30, No. 6, 1985, 483-488.

Bronson, D. Pelz, D., and Trzcinski, E. *Computerizing Your Agency's Information System*. Sage Human Services Guide, Vol. 54, first printing 1988.

Bushnell, J. L. and O'Brien, G. M. Strategies and tactics for increasing research production and utilization in social work education. *Sourcebook on Research Utilization*. A. Rubin and A. Rosenblatt, eds. Council on Social Work Education, NY, 1979: 169-188.

Caputo, R. *Management and Information Systems in Human Services — Implications for the Distribution of Authority and Decision Making*. The Haworth Press, Binghamton, NY, 1988.

Conrad, K. Promoting quality of care: the role of the compliance director. *Child Welfare*, November-December 1985: 639-649.

Epstein, I. and Grasso, A. Integrating management information and program evaluation: the Boysville experience, in *Preventing Low Birthweight and Infant Mortality: Programmatic Issues for Public Health Social Workers*. J. Morton, M. Balassone, and S. Guendelman, eds. University of California, Berkeley, 1987: 141-152.

Epstein, I. and Grasso, A. Using agency based available information to further practice innovation, in *Serious Play: Creativity and Innovation in Social Work*, H. Weissman, ed. NASW Press, New York, 1989.

Epstein, I. and Tripodi, T. *Research techniques for program planning, monitoring and evaluation*. Columbia University Press, New York, 1977.

Etzioni, A. *Modern organizations*. Prentice-Hall, Englewood Cliffs, NJ, 1964.

Etzioni, A. Two approaches to organization analysis: a critique and a suggestion. *Administrative Quarterly*, 1960, 5: 257-278.

Gordon, J. E. Creating research based practice principles: a model. *Social Work Research and Abstracts*, Spring 1984: 3-6.

Grasso, A. and Epstein, I. Management by measurement: organizational dilemmas and opportunities. *Administration in Social Work*, Vol. 2 No. 3, 1987, 89-100.

Grasso, A., and Epstein, I. Agency based research utilization in a residential child care setting, *Administration in Social Work* Vol. 12, No. 4, 1988, 61-80.

Grasso, A. and Epstein, I. The Boysville experience: integrating practice decision-making, program evaluation, and management information. *Computers in Human Services*, Vol. No. 4, 1&2, 1989: 85-95.

Handy, C. *Understanding organizations*. Penguin, New York, 1976.

Hasenfeld, Y. *Human service organizations*. Prentice-Hall, Englewood Cliffs, NJ: 1983.

Havelock, R. G. *Planning for innovations: through dissemination and utilization of knowledge*. Institute for Social Research, Ann Arbor, 1969.

Hoshino, G., Computer tools of management and social work practice. *Applying Computers in Social Service and Mental Health Agencies*. Simon Slavin, ed. The Haworth Press, Binghamton, NY, 1982: 5-10.

Katz, D. and Kahn, R. *The social psychology of organizations*. 2nd Ed. New York, Wiley, 1978.

Katz, D. and Kahn, R. The social psychology of organizations. Wiley, New York, 1966.

Kirk, S. Understanding research utilization in social work. *Sourcebook on Research Utilization*. A. Rubin and A. Rosenblatt, eds., Council on Social Work Education, NY 1979: 132-140.

Lewis, H. Toward a planned approach in social work research. *Future of Social Work Research*. D. Fanshel, ed. NASW 1980: 19-28.

Mutschler, E. and Hasenfeld, Y. Integrated information systems for social work practice. *Social Work*, Vol. 31, No. 5, September-October 1986: 345-349.

Perrow, C. *The analysis of goals in complex organizations in HSO*. Hasenfeld and English, eds. Ann Arbor, University of Michigan, 1974: 214-229.

Reid, W. J., Research strategies for improving individualized services. D. Fanshel, ed. *Future of Social Work Research*. NASW, Washington, DC, 1980: 38-52.

Rothman, J. *Planning and organizing for social change*. Columbia University Press, New York, 1974: 531-576.

Seidl, F. Making research relevant for practitioners. *Future of Social Work Research*, D. Fanshel, ed. NASW, Washington, DC, 1980: 53-62.

Tripodi, T. and Epstein, I. *Research Techniques for Clinical Social Work*. Columbia University Press, New York, 1980.

Walker, R. The ninth panacea: program evaluation. *Evaluation* 1, 1972: 45-53.

Weiss, C. *Evaluating Action Programs: Readings in Social Action and Education*. Allyn and Bacon, Boston, 1972: 10-11.

Weissman, E. Clients, staff, and researchers: their role in management information systems. *Administration in Social Work*, Spring 1977: 43-51.

# Index

In this index, page numbers followed by the letter "f" designate figures; those followed by "t" designate tables.